Cancer Risk by Social Class and Occupation

Contributions to Epidemiology and Biostatistics
Vol. 7

Series Editor   *Jürgen Wahrendorf,* Heidelberg

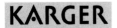

Basel · Freiburg · Paris · London · New York ·
New Delhi · Bangkok · Singapore · Tokyo · Sydney

Cancer Risk by Social Class and Occupation

A Survey of 109,000 Cancer Cases among Finns of Working Age

E. Pukkala
Finnish Cancer Registry, Helsinki, and
School of Public Health, University of Tampere,
Tampere, Finland

45 figures and 104 tables, 1995

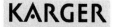

Basel · Freiburg · Paris · London · New York ·
New Delhi · Bangkok · Singapore · Tokyo · Sydney

Contributions to Epidemiology and Biostatistics

Founder and Editor from 1979 to 1984
M.A. Klingberg, Ness-Ziona/Tel Aviv

Library of Congress Cataloging-in-Publication Data
Pukkala, Eero I.
Cancer risk by social class and occupation: a survey of 109,000 cancer cases among Finns of working age / E. Pukkala.
(Contributions to epidemiology and biostatistics: vol. 7)
Includes bibliographical references and index.
1. Cancer – Finland – Epidemiology. 2. Occupational diseases – Finland. I. Title. II. Series.
[DNLM: 1. Neoplasms – epidemiology – Finland. 2. Neoplasms – etiology – Finland.
3. Social Class – Finland. 4. Occupations – Finland. 5. Risk Factors – Finland.
W1   CO778RC v. 7 1995 / QZ 200 P979c 1995]
RC279.F5P85 1995
614.5′999′094897-dc20
DNLM/DLC   95-1186
ISBN 3–8055–6152–0 (alk. paper)

Drug Dosage. The authors and the publisher have exerted every effort to ensure that drug selection and dosage set forth in this text are in accord with current recommendations and practice at the time of publication. However, in view of ongoing research, changes in government regulations, and the constant flow of information relating to drug therapy and drug reactions, the reader is urged to check the package insert for each drug for any change in indications and dosage and for added warnings and precautions. This is particularly important when the recommended agent is a new and/or infrequently employed drug.

All rights reserved. No part of this publication may be translated into other languages, reproduced or utilized in any form or by any means, electronic or mechanical, including photocopying, recording, microcopying, or by any information storage and retrieval system, without permission in writing from the publisher.

© Copyright 1995 by S. Karger AG, P.O. Box, CH–4009 Basel (Switzerland)
Printed in Finland on acid-free paper by Print PunaMusta, Helsinki
ISBN 3–8055–6152–0

Contents

Editors' preface	VIII
Acknowledgements	IX

I. Introduction	1
Aims of the study	2
Structure of the report	2

II. Background	3
Earlier occupational cancer surveillance systems	3
Carcinogenic agents	5
Health-related habits in Finland	7
Health care in Finland	11

III. Materials and Methods	12
Census 1970	12
Follow-up for death, person-years at risk	14
Finnish Cancer Registry	14
Record linkage	16
Cancer risk estimates	17
Output selections	18
Inclusions and exclusions	19

IV. Results	22
Cancers of the mouth and pharynx	22
Lip	22
Tongue and salivary glands	23
Oral cavity and pharynx	24
Cancer of the gastrointestinal tract	28
Oesophagus	28
Stomach	29
Small intestine	33
Colon	34
Rectum	39
Cancer of other digestive organs	39
Liver	39
Gallbladder and biliary ducts	42
Pancreas	44

Cancer of the respiratory organs	46
Nose and nasal sinuses	46
Larynx	48
Lung	51
Mesothelioma	57
Cancer of the breast	59
Cancer of the female genital organs	63
Cervix uteri	63
Corpus uteri	67
Ovary	68
Other female genitals	69
Cancer of male genital organs	73
Prostate	73
Testis	75
Other male genitals	76
Cancer of the urinary organs	76
Kidney and renal pelvis	76
Bladder, ureter and urethra	80
Cancer of the skin	82
Melanoma	82
Non-melanoma skin cancer	86
Basal cell carcinoma	90
Cancer of the eye and nervous system	90
Eye	90
Nervous system	92
Cancer of the endocrine glands	96
Thyroid	96
Other endocrine glands	99
Cancer of the bone and connective tissue	99
Bone	99
Soft tissue	100
Cancer at unspecified sites	102
Haematological cancers	103
Non-Hodgkin's lymphoma	103
Hodgkin's disease	107
Multiple myeloma	108
Leukaemia	110
Cancer at all sites	112
V. Cancer profiles of selected occupations	117
Physicians	117
Teachers and labourers	117
Tobacco industry workers	118
Economically inactive persons	119

	VI. General discussion	123
	Quality of the data sources	123
	Population Census 1970	123
	Record linkage and follow-up for death	123
	Cancer Registry	124
	Comparison to other types of study	125
	Ecological vs. individual level	125
	Mortality vs. incidence	127
	Proportionate analyses	128
	General case-control vs. general cohort study	129
	Specific studies vs. general surveillance system	132
	Limits of present study	135
	Classification of social class and occupation	135
	Job exposure matrices	136
	Social class in controlling for confounding	138
	Multiple tests	139
	Age, period, latency	140
	Upper social classes as predictors of future cancer incidence	142
	Preventability	143
	Social class variation	143
	Occupational variation	147
	VII. Summary and Conclusions	150
	Method	150
	Findings	151
	VIII. References	153
	Appendix tables	161
A.	Average number of persons under follow-up, by occupation, social class and sex	163
B.	Numbers of cancer cases and standardised incidence ratios, by primary site, sex, social class and period	181
C.	Numbers of cancer cases, and crude and social class adjusted standardised incidence ratios for all occupational branches, and for specific occupations with at least five expected cases or with an SIR significantly different from 1.0, by primary site and sex	203

Editors' preface

This book presents the results of an epidemiologic cohort study which links the data of a population census with the data of a cancer registry. Eero Pukkala has taken the data of the population census which was conducted routinely in Finland in 1970 and followed up its participants individually in order to identify the cases of cancer which have occurred in the meantime. The Finnish Cancer Registry was the source from which he could accurately obtain the cancer diagnoses. The author was able to establish a cohort of enormous size with individually determined occupational and social class information of high quality. Though the study population was restricted to persons aged between 35 and 69 years at cancer diagnosis, the number of cancer cases was huge and amounted to about 109,000. Therefore, it was possible to include rare cancer sites into the evaluation as well as women whose occupational cancer risks are seldom quantified due to the small number of women exposed.

Although the survey does not formally match the criteria which are set for dedicated occupational cancer studies, i.e., the levels of particular types of occupational exposures or durations of exposures are not specified as they are in the best occupational follow-up studies, the results achieved by this approach very much resemble those of the more specific studies. The item social class (which, besides occupation, covers a broad range of lifestyle factors including use of medical care) is used for separating the roles of the general life-style factors from the real occupational ones. The social class differences in cancer incidence themselves given systematically for all main cancer sites reflect the patterns of established or suspected lifestyle dependent risk factors.

Overall, the book is valuable proof of the consistency and public health relevance of many findings of dedicated epidemiologic studies and constitutes a bridge between the observational level of those studies and a birds-eye-view of descriptive epidemiology on risk patterns in the total population.

Heidelberg, January 1995
N. Becker
J. Wahrendorf

Acknowledgements

This study was carried out at the Finnish Cancer Registry. Doctors Matti Hakama and Marja Jylhä from the School of Public Health of the University of Tampere, Elina Hemminki from the Finnish National Research and Development Centre for Welfare and Health and Nikolaus Becker from the German Cancer Research Center in Heidelberg carefully reviewed the manuscript and gave useful suggestions for clarifying the presentation. Several other persons in various institutes in Finland and other countries provided valuable information about their specialized fields.

The computer graphs were made by Mr. Bengt Söderman from the Finnish Cancer Registry, and the English language was revised by Mrs. Luanne Siliämaa, Harare, Zimbabwe.

This study was supported financially by the Cancer Society of Finland and by the Finnish Work Environment Fund.

I. Introduction

Factors associated with social class play an essential role in cancer causation. Doll and Peto estimated in 1981 that 30% of cancer deaths in the U.S.A. can be accounted for by smoking, 35% by diet, 7% by reproductive behaviour and 3% for alcohol drinking [1]. However, the estimated confidence intervals for many of these percentages were broad, e.g., for dietary factors from 10% to 70%. The burden of occupational cancer in industrialised countries is generally considered to be less than 6% of all cancer cases [1-5].

Routine statistics on the general mortality in different occupational categories have been published in England from the middle of the 19th century [6], and the decennial supplements of England and Wales have subsequently reported on cancer mortality rates systematically by occupation [7]. Since the late 1970s surveillance systems of occupational cancer risk have been created in several other countries, including all the Nordic countries.

Specific reports — case reports and publications of analytical studies — on the association between certain occupational exposures and cancer have been published in mass quantity since 1775 when Percival Pott observed that among chimney sweeps in London there were exceptionally many cases of cancer of the scrotum [8]. Some of the surveillance systems of cancer risk include tabulations, not only by occupation but also by social class or socioeconomic status. Occupation and social class variables are closely intercorrelated. Even in the studies not explicitly mentioning the concept of social class there is a background idea that the occupation represents the way of life more generally than just exposures in the working environment. Although occupational classifications can be brought somewhat closer to occupation-specific exposures, e.g., by dividing the occupational titles according to the type of industry, even the most exact classifications include such a burden of general life-style associated factors that the separation of real occupational hazards is problematic, if not impossible. It has been estimated from a set of British data that 88% of the occupational variation was due to social class, ethnicity and smoking, and only 12% due to directly occupational exposures [9].

Many studies have been conducted in which social class or some other factor describing the socioeconomic conditions has been taken as a determinant of morbidity or mortality. There are, however, very few, if any, really large studies in which both occupation and social status have been analysed simultaneously. The present epidemio-logical study attempts to distinguish between the general role of social class and the more specific role of occupation. The study cohort includes the entire population aged 25-64 residing in Finland in 1970, with data on occupation and social class as they were recorded in the 1970 Population Census. This cohort was followed up for cancer incidence through the nationwide population-based Finnish Cancer Registry.

Contrary to most earlier studies, women are also included in an equal way remembering that the number of economically active women is approaching that of men in many countries, and the occupation-related risks among women are becoming increasingly important issues of public health.

Aims of the study

The aims of the present study were

1. to describe systematically the social class and occupational variation in the incidence of all major cancer types among working-aged Finnish men and women,

2. to discuss the role of possible risk factors associated with the general lifestyle of various social classes, and

3. to demonstrate the residual occupational variation after adjustment for social class and search for clues for occupation-specific factors.

The occupation-specific factors are understood here to include not only factors such as chemicals and dusts in the working environment which workers cannot avoid in their work, but also factors associated with the typical behaviour among persons in certain occupations, e.g., the easy access to alcoholic beverages among waiting personnel. Going deep into specific occupational risk factors such as individual chemical agents is avoided.

The main focus is put on aim 3. Thus, the selection of social class variable criteria such as usefulness in social class adjustment and simplicity in understanding the order of the social classes in terms of living standards were preferred. If social aspects had been the main focus, a more sophisticated measure of socio-economic status would have been used.

Structure of the report

First in this report, in chapter II, earlier internationally known surveillance systems are briefly described, and a short summary of today's consensus of known and suspected carcinogenic agents is given. In the same chapter, some background information of the Finnish way of life and health care — with special reference to social class and occupational differences — is also given for the orientation of the readers.

Chapter III includes a description of the materials and method used for the present study. All major sites of cancer diagnosed in Finland in 1971-85, when necessary even by histological or otherwise defined subcategory, are analysed in a systematic way, and the social class differences in cancer incidence are shown. Cancer risks for more than 400 occupational categories are tabulated with and without adjustment for social class. In chapter IV, site-specific observations are presented. Similarities with earlier occupational results and potential new associations are picked up and shortly discussed. The result section is supported by extensive appendix tables showing social class and occupation-specific results by primary site in a systematic way. These tables may include much information of less general interest; they are mainly intended to offer the Finnish data available as references for other occupational cancer risk studies and for meta-analyses.

Examples of occupation-specific cancer profiles, i.e., risk patterns of various cancer forms in certain occupations, are picked up in chapter V. Examples about the weaknesses and strengths of record linkage-based cancer surveillance systems like the present one, including comparisons with other types of studies on cancer, social class and occupation, are given in chapter VI. A discussion about the attributable risks and magnitudes of realistic potential for prevention conclude the report.

II. Background

Earlier occupational cancer surveillance systems

In the decennial supplements of England and Wales, the numbers of cancer deaths by occupation were known from death certificates, and the sizes of the corresponding populations from the census data [7]. Similar tabulations on both mortality and incidence have been published since the late 1970s in the Nordic countries, which typically cover the whole populations and are based on record linkages between the death or disease register and the population census register (table 1). Representative samples of the total population have been used in Japan [35], Great Britain [28, 33], and Canada [27].

In proportional studies, the proportions of various types of cancer in a given occupation out of all cancers in that occupation is compared with the corresponding proportion in the reference population. Proportional analyses have been done in some states within the U.S. using cancer registry or death certificate data, including codes of occupation (e.g. [12-16, 36]). A proportional study has also been conducted in New Zealand [17] and in Denmark [18].

Table 1. Examples of surveillance systems of occupational cancer (modified from [10])

Study	Period	N[1]
Unlinked death certificate and census data		
Decennial Supplement for England and Wales [7]	1979-80, 1982-83	148,000
Cancer mortality in New Zealand [11]	1974-78	5,000
Death certificate data		
Washington State, U.S.A. [12]	1950-79	?
Rhode Island, U.S.A. [13]	1973-78	?
State of California, U.S.A. [14]	1959-61	199,000
Massachusetts, U.S.A. [15]	1971-73	17,000
Cancer registry mortality data		
Los Angeles County Cancer Surveillance Program, U.S.A. [16]	1972-74	60,000
New Zealand Cancer Registry [17]	1979-83	2,700[2]
Linked cancer registry incidence and pension scheme data		
Pension scheme data for cancer patients, Denmark [18]	1970-79	94,000
Interview incidence data		
Roswell Park Memorial Institute, U.S.A. [19]	1956-65	14,000
Third National Cancer Survey, U.S.A. [20]	1969-71	7,500
Case-referent study in Montreal, Canada [21]	1979-85	4,600
Linked death certificate and census data		
Occupational mortality, Norway [22]	1970-80	27,000
Occupational mortality, Sweden [23]	1961-70	120,000
Occupational mortality, Finland [24]	1971-80	20,000
Occupational mortality, Denmark [25]	1970-80	60,000
Occupational mortality, Nordic countries [26]	1971-80	141,100
Ten percent sample of labor force, Canada [27]	1965-73	4,200
Longitudinal mortality study, U.K. [28]	1971-75	?
Linked cancer registry incidence and census data		
Cancer incidence by occupation, Norway [29]	1961-84	163,000
Cancer environment register, Sweden [30]	1961-79	605,000
Cancer incidence by occupation, Finland [31]	1971-80	39,000
Occupational cancer study, Denmark [32]	1970-80	115,000
Longitudinal cancer study, U.K. [33]	1971-75	8,000
Linked hospital discharge registry incidence and census data		
Occupational hospital discharge, Denmark [34]	1981-84	?

[1] Number of cancer cases or deaths.
[2] Only leukemia and controls.

Large scale case-referent interview studies like those done in North America [20, 21] can also result in an occupational surveillance system comparable to those based on record linkages.

There is a large number of smaller cohort studies including one or a few occupations, and case-referent studies with one or a few cancer sites, where often very detailed occupational exposure histories have been available. A library search of cancer studies with the keyword "occupation" published between January 1992 and October 1993 in CANCER-CD [37] resulted in a list of 1089 papers.

One or two studies indicating a previously unknown association between certain occupational factor and cancer risk do not usually convince the scientific world of the real causal nature of the association, especially if the biological mechanism is not clear. Therefore — and also to restrict the abundance of details — reviews and meta-analyses of all published studies presenting the current status of agreement of each association are preferred as references in this book.

Carcinogenic agents

The International Agency for Research on Cancer (IARC) has in the first 60 volumes of its Monograph series evaluated the carcinogenicity of over 700 chemicals, groups of chemicals, complex mixtures, occupational exposures and cultured habits [38]. In the first 16 volumes of the Monograph series the assessments of evidence of carcinogenicity in humans and in animals were made separately, but in 1977 a scheme for the categorization of the degree of evidence based both on human and animal studies was developed using terms such as "sufficient", "limited", "inadequate", and later, "evidence suggesting lack of carcinogenicity". The assignment into a given group is a matter of scientific judgement, reflecting the strength of the evidence derived from studies in humans and in experimental animals and from other relevant data, including data on possible mechanisms of action. The categorization refers to the strength of the evidence that an agent is carcinogenic, and not to carcinogenic strength or potency.

The first 42 volumes of the Monograph series were updated in 1987 [39], and a periodical of the IARC [38] always gives the most recent lists of all evaluated agents with references to the complete documentation of the evaluation. In October 1994 there were 67 agents in group 1 (carcinogenic to humans; table 2), 51 in group 2A (probably carcinogenic to humans; table 3), 210 in group 2B (possibly carcinogenic to humans), 454 in group 3 (unclassifiable as to carcinogenicity to humans) and one agent — caprolactam — in group 4 (probably not carcinogenic to humans). In Finland, workers reported to the national registry on the manufacture and use of carcinogenic agents (as defined by the International Labor Office [40]) in 1987 accounted for 0.6% of the total work force [41]. However, not all persons exposed to carcinogenic or probably carcinogenic agents are included in that registry, and the true proportion of exposed persons is estimated to be between 60,000 and 80,000, i.e., 2-3% of the work force [41].

Table 2. Overall Evaluations of Carcinogenicity to Humans in IARC Monographs volumes 1-62: group 1 — *The agent (mixture) is carcinogenic to humans* [38]

Agents and groups of agents

Aflatoxins
4-Aminabiphenyl
Arsenic and arsenic compounds[1]
Asbestos
Azathioprine
Benzene
Benzidine
Beryllium and beryllium compounds[2]
N,N-Bis(2-chloroethyl)-2-naphthylamine (Chlornaphazine)
Bis(chloromethyl)ether and chloromethyl methyl ether (technical-grade)
1,4-Butanediol dimethanesulfonate (Myleran)
Cadmium and cadmium compounds[2]
Chlorambucil
1-(2-Chloroethyl)-3-(4-methylcyclohexyl)-1-nitrosourea (Methyl-CCNU)
Chromium[VI] compounds[2]
Ciclosporin
Cyclophosphamide
Diethylstilboestrol
Erionile
Ethylene oxide[3]
Heliobacter pylori (infection with)
Hepatitis B virus (chronic infection with)
Hepatitis C virus (chronic infection with)
Melphalan
8-Methoxypsoralen (Methoxsalen) plus ultraviolet A radiation
MOPP and other combined chemotherapy including alkylating agents
Mustard gas (Sulfur mustard)
2-Naphthylamine
Nickel compounds[2]
Oestrogen replacement therapy
Oestrogens, nonsteroidal[1]
Oestrogens, steroidal[1]
Opisthorchis viverrini (infection with)
Oral contraceptives, combined[4]
Oral contraceptives, sequential
Radon and its decay products
Schistosoma haematobium (infection with)
Solar radiation
Talc containing asbestiform fibres
Thiotepa
Treosulfan
Vinyl chloride

Mixtures

Alcoholic beverages
Analgesic mixtures containing phenacetin
Betel quid with tobacco
Coal-tar pitches
Coal-tars
Mineral oils, untreated and mildly-treated
Salted fish (Chinese-style)
Shale-oils
Soots
Tobacco products, smokeless
Tobacco smoke
Wood dust

Exposure circumstances

Aluminium production
Auramine, manufacture of
Boot and shoe manufacture and repair
Coal gasification
Coke production
Furniture and cabinet making
Haematite mining (underground) with exposure to radon
Iron and steel founding
Isopropanol manufacture (strong-acid process)
Magenta, manufacture of
Painter (occupational exposure as a)
Rubber industry
Strong-inorganic-acid mists containing sulfuric acid (occupational exposure to)

---

[1] This evaluation applies to the group of chemicals as a whole and not necessarily to all individual chemicals within the group.
[2] Evaluated as a group.
[3] Overall evaluation upgraded from 2A to 1 with supporting evidence from other relevant data
[4] There is also conclusive evidence that these agents have a protective effect against cancers of the ovary and endometrium.

Table 3. Overall Evaluations of Carcinogenicity to Humans in IARC Monographs volumes 1-62: group 2A — *The agent (mixture) is probably carcinogenic to humans* [38]

Agents and groups of agents

Acrylamide
Acrylonitrile
Adriamycin
Androgenic (anabolic) steroids
Azacitidine
Benz[*a*]anthracene
Benzidine-based dyes
Benzo[*a*] pyrene
Bischloroethyl nitrosourea (BCNU)
1,3-Butadiene
Captafol
Chloramphenicol
1-(2-Chloroethyl)-3-cyclohexyl-1-nitrosourea
para-Chloro-*ortho*-toluidine and its strong
 acid salts; evaluated as a group
Chlorozotocin
Cisplatin
Clonorchis sinensis (infection with)
Dibenz[*a,h*]anthracene
Diethyl sulfate
Dimethylcarbamoyl chloride
Dimethyl sulfate
Epichlorohydrin
Ethylene dibromide
N-Ethyl-*N*-nitrosourea
Formaldehyde
IQ (2-Amino-3-methylimidazo[4,5-*f*]quinoline)
5-Methoxypsoralen
4,4'-Methylene bis(2-chloroaniline) (MOCA)
N-Methyl-*N*'-nitro-N-nitrosoguanidine
N-Methyl-*N*-nitrosourea
Nitrogen mustard
N-Nitrosodiethylamine
N-Nitrosodimethylamine
Phenacetin
Procarbazine hydrochloride
Silica, crystalline
Styrene-7,8-oxide
Tris(2,3-dibromopropyl)phosphate
Ultraviolet radiation A
Ultraviolet radiation B
Ultraviolet radiation C
Vinyl bromide

Mixtures

Creosotes
Diesel engine exhaust
Hot mate
Non-arsenical insecticides (occupational
 exposures in spraying and application of)
Polychlorinated biphenyls

Exposure circumstances

Art glass, glass containers and pressed ware
 (manufacture of)
Hairdresser or barber (occupational exposure
 as a)
Petroleum refining (occupational exposures in)
Sunlamps and sunbeds (use of)

Health-related habits in Finland

Studies on health inequalities between population subgroups have a long history in Western Europe. The results have been consistent: persons in good social positions live longer and are, in general, healthier than the poor ones [42-45]. In the early 1970s differences in mortality between socioeconomic classes, education categories and main occupational categories in Finland were larger than those in the other Nordic countries, and the variation was increasing: e.g., the general mortality of male white-collar workers during the period 1971-85 decreased by 27%, but that of unskilled workers only by 13%. The largest fraction of this difference can be accounted for by cardiovascular diseases [46].

Table 4. Total expenditure and consumption per capita of some dietary components and tobacco in Finland during a one-year period (1966), by socioeconomic class [47]

	Socioeconomic class							
	Farmers	Other self-employed	Managerial	Clerical	Skilled workers	Unskilled workers	Inactive	Total population
Total consumption[1]	69	118	170	120	97	80	99	100
Flour, groats and bread (kg)	118	87	68	76	77	83	76	88
Fresh and prosessed meat (kg)	29	44	36	33	35	32	20	33
Fish (kg)	7.7	5.4	5.5	4.3	5.0	4.4	8.0	5.8
Butter and margarine (kg)	20	18	15	15	16	15	14	17
Milk (l)	301	235	214	185	206	201	184	228
Fruits and berries (kg)	25	42	54	45	34	27	35	35
Potatoes and other roots (kg)	137	87	67	63	80	93	67	92
Tomatoes and cucumber (kg)	2.7	3.9	5.9	5.9	4.7	3.1	3.9	4.2
Sugar (kg)	35	30	23	25	28	31	28	29
Salt (kg)	3.1	1.9	1.7	1.6	2.0	2.0	3.0	2.4
Coffee (kg)[2]	4.8	5.8	3.8	4.7	4.7	5.0	6.5	4.8
Tobacco (FIM)[2]	72	116	115	105	144	150	73	110

[1] Index; total population=100.
[2] Consumption per adult.

Even in Finland, known for its excellent statistics, there are relatively little systematically collected data about the prevalence of aetiological factors of cancer risk, especially from earlier decades which would be most relevant as background for the cancers of the 1970s and 1980s. The samples of, e.g., Finnish household studies including extensive data about consumption of various food items, alcohol, tobacco and other goods, are so small that occupation-specific tabulations are seldom meaningful. Some information is available on the level of socio-economic classes.
From the Household Study from 1966 [47] we know that men and women of the highest socio-economic classes used to eat more meat, vegetables and fruit, but less cereals, salt and sugar than those in the lower ones (table 4). Families of blue-collar workers bought more tobacco than the rich ones, but this difference was attributable to men only (fig. 1). Women of the low social classes smoked less than highly educated, urban women [48].

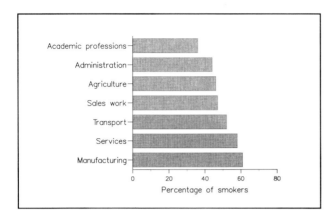

Fig. 1. Prevalence of smokers among adult Finnish men in 1968, by occupational branch (modified from [48]).

There are more data about lifestyle factors of various population subgroups from newer periods. Since 1978 the National Public Health Institute of Finland has regularly carried out a questionnaire survey on health related lifestyles, "Monitoring Health Behaviour among Adult Finns", based on annual samples of 3000-5000 Finns [49]. These data show, for instance, that the prevalence of an unhealthy lifestyle, measured by numerous single variables, varied greatly by social class. Upper white-collar male workers smoked less, exercised more and had a healthier diet, but drank more alcohol than men of the other groups (fig. 2). A nationwide randomised health survey in 1979-81 indicated that the better the level of education, or the higher the socioeconomic class, the greater the proportion of people whose diet was good and varied [50].

There was a change towards a healthier lifestyle during the period from the early 1970s to the late 1980s, and the occupational differences tended to diminish [49, 51]. However, the trends of these lifestyle factors can not necessarily be extrapolated backwards to the earlier decades. Even the order of the classes can change: for instance, smoking among women is now least common in the highest social class in which the prevalence of female smokers was by far still the highest in the 1960s [48, 52]. Similar changes have also occurred in animal fat consumption in both sexes [49]. In general, the differences among men tend to be larger and more stable over time than among women.

On the other hand, women have additional factors strongly affecting their cancer risk, namely reproductive factors. Women with higher education have their first birth later than average, and their fertility has been lower [53]. The age at menarche has strongly decreased in Finland during this century, but the differences between social classes have persisted, the higher social classes having the earliest menarche [54].

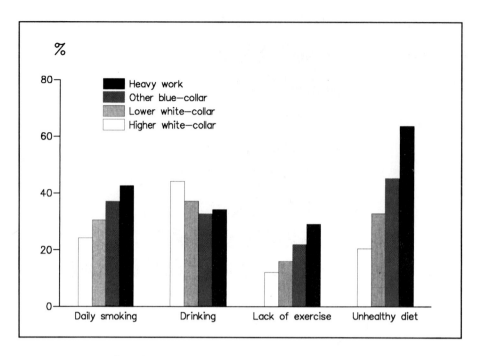

Fig. 2. Age-adjusted prevalence of some health related life styles among Finnish men aged 30-49 in 1978-90, by occupational class (modified from [49]). *Heavy work:* forestry, stevedoring, agriculture and construction industries. *Drinking:* more than 8 portions/week. *Lack of exercise:* free-time exercise only few times a year. *Unhealthy diet:* much fat and sugar, little vegetables.

Rather little has been published about the typical health behaviour of single occupational groups. In most cases the roles of possible non-occupational confounders among persons in certain occupations have to be evaluated from what is known about the social class to which they belong, or from "common knowledge" alone. However, the drinking habits of the main occupational branches have been documented precisely since the 1970s [55], and alcohol abuse in several occupational categories can be roughly estimated from the alcohol-related utilisation of health care resources by these categories in 1972 [56]. The highest indices for alcohol-related utilization of health care resources among men were obtained for labourers, followed by painters, seamen, construction workers, forestry workers, and artists and journalists. The indices were low for farmers, managers and car drivers. The alcohol-related utilization of health care resources among women was much smaller than among men, but the order of occupations was similar [56]. Social problems connected with drinking have been most frequently encountered in blue-collar occupations, even though average consumption has been higher in some other fields [55].

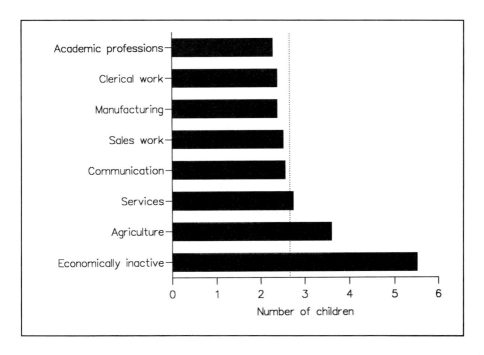

Fig. 3. Average number of children of 40-49 year-old women on 31 December 1985, by main occupational branches [57].

The average number of children and mean age at first birth in 1985 by occupation were estimated in a data series produced specifically for the needs of the present study by Statistics Finland [57]. The average number of children among women aged 40-49 in the main occupational branches ranged from 2.3 among women in academic professions to 3.6 among those in agriculture (fig. 3).

Health care in Finland

The health care system in Finland (population 5.0 million) is comparable with that in the other Nordic countries [58]. In 1975 there were 1.4 physicians and 5.0 qualified nurses per 1,000 inhabitants. The infant mortality was one of the lowest in the world; less than 1% of children died under one year of age. The expectation of life at birth in 1975 was 67 years for males and 76 years for females, and it increased to 71 and 79, respectively, around the year 1990 [59].

During the observation period of this study, 1971-85, Finland was divided into 21 central hospital districts. The diagnosis and treatment of cancer were only centralised to a certain extent. Cancer surgery was practised in all central hospitals and also in many smaller units. Facilities for radiotherapy were available in nine hospitals [60].

Since 1972, every Finnish person is entitled to consult a physician at a municipal health centre free of charge (or in recent years for a small charge), and the costs incurred in purchasing drugs or staying in hospital are also strongly subsidised. There were certain inequities in the provision and utilization of health care services in Finland before the 1970s, but after the implementation of the National Sickness Insurance Scheme in 1964 and the Primary Health Care Act in 1972, the regional and social class differences in the availability of medical care and diagnostic facilities can be regarded as small [61-63]. However, long distances and other geographical reasons still cause some regional variation in the utilisation of public health services, and the availability of specialised private sector medical care is better in the area of the capital than in remote areas of Finland [64], but the differences are not much attributable to education or socio-economic status [65].

III. Materials and Methods

Census 1970

An official census describing the Finnish population on the last day of 1970 was organised by Statistics Finland [66]. Everyone living in Finland on that day was expected to complete a questionnaire including questions on family structure, living conditions, work etc. The response rate was 98% [67]. The questionnaires were coded and entered into the computer at Statistics Finland.

Occupation was taken to mean the activity or work a person performed to get income, independent of branch, industrial status or education. In addition to this income criterion, a time criterion was used: a person was considered as economically active only if she/he had been working at least half of the normal working time of the branch. If a person carried out many trades during a year, she/he had to state the occupation to which she/he was devoting the most time. Temporally unemployed persons were classified according to their latest occupation. In other cases occupation referred to the circumstances on January 1, 1971. When a family member assisted another member of the household in his/her occupation for at least half of the normal working hours, she/he was considered economically active.

Employers who performed practical work, e.g., shopkeepers or owners of shoemaker shops, were classified as their employees. Vocationally trained apprentices were classified under the occupation for which they were practising.

The classification of occupations in the 1970 Population Census was based on the Nordic Classification of Occupations of 1963 and on the International Classification on Occupations, published by the International Labour Office in 1958 [66]. The first digit of the three-digit occupation code indicates the *main occupational branch* grouped as follows:

0   technical, physical science, social science, humanistic and artistic work,

1   administrative and clerical work,

2   sales work,

3   farming and forestry work, fishing and hunting,

4   mining and quarrying,

5   transport and telecommunication work,

6/7 manufacturing and construction work,

8   service work, and

9   other and unclassified work.

The two first digits of the occupation code indicate the *occupational branch* (e.g., 05 Teaching work), and all three digits together the *specific occupation* (052 Primary school teachers). There are altogether 70 occupational branches divided to 335 specific occupations. The hierarchy of the codes, with the average numbers of persons under follow-up in each category, is shown in appendix table A.

During the follow-up period 1971-85 there were three occupations with only female workers (midwives, beauticians and pedicurists) and eleven occupations with only male workers (forestry managers, ship pilots, chief engineers in ships, engine room crew, pilots and flight engineers, engine drivers, linemen, reinforced concreters and stonemasons, firemen, and officers), i.e., the actual number of specific occupations was 332 among men and 324 among women. Since there were no women working in occupational branches of pilots and flight engineers or engine drivers, the actual number of branches among women was only 68. Fifteen occupational branches in men and thirteen among women included only one specific occupation; in these cases the results are given for the branch only. Thus the actual numbers of reportable one, two and three-digit occupational categories were 9, 70 and 320 among men and 9, 68 and 311 among women, respectively. The group of economically inactive people (i.e., those not working at all or working less than half of normal working time of the occupation) was a separate category in the analyses.

In line with the aim of this study, with its main focus on occupational factors, a simple social class classification with four ordinary classes was chosen out of the various classifications describing *social class* in the 1970 Population Census. This classification was formed on the basis of occupation, education, industrial status and industry groupings by socio-economic status as used in the Census [66]. It was mainly based on the prestige of the occupation, taking into account the special features of social strata in Finnish society [68]. Financially dependent persons (e.g., housewives and students) were classified by the occupation of their supporter and economically active persons by their current or former occupation.

The four social classes were defined as follows:

I   managers and other higher administrative or clerical employees, farmers owning more than 50 hectares of land,

II lower administrative or clerical employees, small-scale entrepreneurs, farmers owning 15 to 49.9 hectares of land,

III skilled and specialised workers, farmers owning 5 to 14.9 hectares of land, and

IV labourers, farm and forestry workers, institutions inmates, farmers owning less than 5 hectares of land, pensioners whose former occupation is unknown.

Persons with unknown social class (1.5% of the total population or 1.0% of the economically active population; mainly farmers and fishermen) were included the social class III. The number of persons by social status is given in appendix table A which also indicates the relationships of occupation and social class.

Follow-up for death, person-years at risk

To be able to count the exact numbers of person-years under follow-up, the 1970 Population Census file was linked with the annual death files from the years 1971-85. The annual death files of Statistics Finland include death certificate information of all deaths in Finland. These data are used, e.g., for producing the official mortality statistics of Finland.

The numbers of person-years for each occupational category further divided into social classes were counted by five-year birth cohort (year of birth 1906-10, ..., 1941-45), separately for males and females. The follow-up period started on January 1, 1971 and came to an end at death or on the closing-date (December 31, 1985), whichever was earliest. The follow-up period was divided into three five-year parts (1971-75, 1976-80 and 1981-85).

Finnish Cancer Registry

The Finnish Cancer Registry — The Institute for Statistical and Epidemiological Cancer Research has collected data on all indicent cancer cases and all cancer deaths in Finland since 1953. All hospitals, medical practitioners, and institutions with hospital beds are obliged to notify the Finnish Cancer Registry about all cancer cases that come to their attention. Moreover, pathological laboratories send information on all tissue and cytological specimens with a diagnosis of cancer. Statistics Finland sends a report whenever cancer is mentioned on the death certificate. An average of five notifications per case are received during various phases of the disease. The unique personal identification number given to every resident of Finland used as a registration key helps to avoid double registrations.

Since 1961 the reporting of cancer cases has been compulsory, based on a letter of instruction from the Medical Board of Health (part of whose work is now continued by the National Research and Development Centre for Welfare and Health, NAWH). According to that letter, all malignant tumours and certain benign lesions must be reported to the cancer register which is run by the Finnish Cancer Registry on the premises of the Cancer Society of Finland.

The cancer notifications from hospitals, private physicians and laboratories to the Cancer Registry come either on manually completed cancer notification forms, or increasingly since 1986, automatically on floppy disks or magnetic tapes from informants' computerised registers. The contents of information in manual and computerised reporting are identical. Nowadays the data about all death certificates in which cancer is mentioned as the underlying or contributory cause of death are also transferred on magnetic tape from the files of Statistics Finland to the Finnish Cancer Registry. At the Cancer Registry all the data are manually entered or automatically transferred into the data base. If there are only laboratory notifications or death certificate information from a cancer case, the Cancer Registry sends a request for clinical data to the treating hospital(s).

Soon after the arrival of the first notification of the cancer, usually some months after the diagnosis of cancer, a summary record including essential data fields concerning, e.g., primary site, histology, stage and treatment, are coded at the Finnish Cancer Registry by making use of all information about that patient as stored in the data base. The coding is nowadays done by trained secretaries under the supervision of a pathologist. Earlier, up to the cancers diagnosed in 1982, all coding was done by a physician. According to internal quality control studies, the change in the coding practise did not affect the quality of coding. If new data for a patient (e.g. the death certificate) comes after the initial coding, the coding will be re-evaluated and, if necessary, changed. Recoding of old records may also be needed in the context of various quality control check-ups performed actively by the Registry.

The summary record alone is sufficient for most of the statistical uses and also detailed enough for many analytical studies as such. However, summary records are often used just as keys to the cases of interest, and the more detailed data are identified from the complete notifications of the Cancer Registry files, or even from the original hospital records or laboratory specimen.

In this study, the following data items of the summary record of the Cancer Registry were used:

- Personal identification number of the patient (including the date of birth and gender).

- Primary site: the code of the International Classification of Diseases from 1955, 7th revision (ICD-7), modified and extended by the Finnish Cancer Registry.

- Date of diagnosis, i.e, date when the cancer was verified by a physician.

- Malignancy of the cancer: true malignant tumours; borderline tumours; in situ cancers; lesions such as basal cell carcinoma of the skin, carcinoma in situ of the cervix, and papilloma of the bladder, which are notified to the Cancer Registry but not usually included in the official cancer statistics.

- Histology of the cancer: code of Manual of Tumor Nomenclature Coding [69].

- Stage of the disease at diagnosis: localised; non-localised, with metastasis only in regional lymph nodes; non-localised, with distant metastases; non-localised, extent not known; stage not known.

When coding the above data items, several other data, e.g., those indicating the means of confirmation of diagnosis, treatment, and date and cause of death have been utilised, i.e., these items also have an indirect effect on the accuracy of the data set for this study.

In the present study all primary site categories were analysed one by one. Cancers of the lung and thyroid were further divided into subcategories by histology, because the subtypes are considered to have different aetiologies. Tumours of the nervous system and leukaemias were also divided into more homogeneous subcategories, and skin tumours were studied by skin area. Extranodal lymphomas were not classified according to their target organs, but were analysed as a subcategory of non-Hodgkin's lymphomas. Tumours of the pleura and the peritoneum histologically defined as mesotheliomas were handled as a separate group. Carcinoma in situ of the cervix uteri and basal cell carcinoma of the skin were analysed as separate categories but not included in the sum category of total cancer.

Record linkage

Linking the 1970 Population Census file with both the annual death files and Cancer Registry file was performed automatically by making use of the unique personal identifier (PID) given to all persons having resided in Finland since January 1, 1967. The PID includes the date of birth, a three-digit running number given by the Population Register Center (odd for men, even for women), and a check digit (number or letter selected on the basis of modulo 31 of a number formed as a catenation of the date of birth and the running number). This PID is used as the identifier in all main personal registers in Finland.

Cancer risk estimates

The risk estimates in this study were calculated for strata defined by the following variables:

Gender: males, females,

Occupation: all 1, 2 and 3-digit occupation codes (399 categories for men and 388 for women), and the category of economically inactive persons,

Social class: four classes (I, II, III, IV),

Period: three 5-year periods (1971-75, 1976-80, 1981-85), and

Age: six five-year age groups (35-39, ..., 60-64 years) at the beginning of each calendar period.

Restricting the analysis to birth cohorts which were 35 to 64 years of age at the beginning of each observation period means that those under follow-up in the first period (1971-75) were born in 1906-35 and those in the last period (1981-85) in 1916-45 (fig. 4). Whenever age is mentioned in this report, it always means the age at the beginning of each follow-up period, although the persons at the end of each five-year follow-up period were, if alive, actually five years older.

For each stratum defined by sex, calendar period and age-group and by occupation or social class, three types of indicators of cancer frequency were calculated:

1. Observed number of cases.

2. Incidence rate: observed number of cases divided by the stratum-specific number of person-years, given per 100,000 person-years.

3. Standardised incidence ratio (SIR): ratio of the observed (Obs) and expected (Exp) number of cases. The expected number of cases was achieved by multiplying the stratum-specific number of person-years by sex, period and age-specific incidence rate of the reference population. In calculations of social class-specific SIRs and *crude* occupation-specific SIRs (marked with SIR_c), the expected numbers were based on the incidence of the total *economically active* Finnish population of the same sex. For occupational categories *social class adjusted* SIRs (SIR_a) were also calculated. In that case the expected number of cases (Exp_a) for each stratum defined by sex, calendar period and age for each occupation was calculated according to the formula

$$Exp_a = \sum_{j=1}^{4} P_j I_j,$$

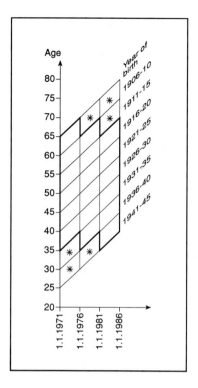

Fig. 4. Birth year cohorts under follow-up in 1971-75, 1976-80 and 1981-85. Birth cohort-period combinations excluded from the present study are marked with an asterix (*).

where P_j is the number of person-years in that occupation belonging to social class j, and I_j is the cancer incidence in social class j.

The total SIRs over ages, periods, etc. were calculated as ratios of the sums of the observed numbers of cases to the sums of expected numbers of cases in the respective strata. The 95% confidence intervals (95% CI) for each SIR were defined under the assumption that the observed number of cases followed a Poisson distribution. Incidence rates in the figures and text are always — if not otherwise stated — age-adjusted totals, i.e., weighted averages of the six age-group specific incidence rates. The weights are based on the age distribution of all person-years (males and females combined) in the study series.

Output selections

The number of strata for each cancer site and sex is some 28,000 (about 400 occupational categories, 4 social classes, 3 calendar periods and 6 age groups). Therefore, it is necessary to make a strong reduction in data before presenting them. Any reducing of the data covers some pertinent aspects, i.e., a compromise between various possible choices always has to be made. This choice strongly depends on the aims of the study.

In the present study, the following selection of results (or part of it) is shown for each site and gender:

- The age-adjusted incidence rates by social class and period. These data — mainly given as graphs — indicate the absolute incidence level, differences between social classes, and trends in incidence by social class over time. If social class patterns of many cancer-sex combinations are presented in the same picture, the SIRs are shown instead of incidence rates. All social class-specific SIRs together with 95% confidence intervals and absolute numbers of cases are given systematically by primary site in the appendix table B.

- The observed numbers of cases and standardised incidence ratios (both SIR_c and SIR_a) for all main (one-digit) occupational branches and for two and three-digit occupational categories with at least 5 expected cases (Exp_c or Exp_a) or with an SIR (SIR_c or SIR_a) differing statistically significantly ($p<0.05$) from 1.0 are given systematically for all sites with substantial numbers of cases in appendix tables C1-C42.

- Observed numbers of cases and standardised incidence ratios (both SIR_c and SIR_a) for occupational categories with known or suspected occupational aetiology, as well as occupations with high or low SIRs in the present series, are shown in text tables. The occupations are ordered by SIR_a, i.e., occupations with a cancer incidence differing most from the national average incidence of their socio-economic class are on the top and on the bottom of the list. Even significantly high SIRs without additional knowledge about possible aetiological mechanisms are usually ignored if they are based only on one or two observed cases.

Results by age or birth cohort are given only when there are obvious risk differences by these factors.

Inclusions and exclusions

Almost 40,000 cancers of persons born in 1906-45 diagnosed in 1971-85 were excluded because they were younger (6% of the excluded cases) or older (94%) than the age range selected for this study (i.e., 35-64 years at the beginning of each 5-year follow-up period). The total number of cancer cases included in the analyses was about 47,000 in each gender (table 5). The annual number of cases among men slightly decreased by calendar time. Among women there was a 9% increase between 1971-75 and 1981-85. Among persons born after 1925 there were more cancer cases in women than in men, whereas in the older birth cohorts men were dominating.

Table 5. Numbers of cancer cases (any site) included in the analyses, by birth cohort, observation period and sex (M = males, F = females)

Year of birth	Sex	Observation period			Total included
		1971-75	1976-80	1981-85	
1906-10	M	5,824	(6,757)[1]	(6,607)[1]	5,824
	F	4,179	(5,232)[1]	(5,899)[1]	4,179
1911-15	M	4,281	5,611	(6,508)[1]	9,892
	F	3,353	4,289	(5,382)[1]	7,642
1916-20	M	2,554	3,792	5,090	11,436
	F	2,549	3,484	4,369	10,402
1921-25	M	1,781	3,077	4,464	9,322
	F	2,293	3,057	3,860	9,210
1926-30	M	1,033	1,829	2,938	5,830
	F	1,617	2,356	2,938	6,911
1931-35	M	492	834	1,519	2,845
	F	924	1,457	2,225	4,606
1936-40	M	(316)[1]	529	865	1,394
	F	(544)[1]	1,017	1,693	2,710
1941-45	M	(268)[1]	(397)[1]	635	635
	F	(352)[1]	(714)[1]	1,193	1,193
Total included	M	15,965	15,672	15,541	47,178
	F	14,915	15,660	16,278	46,853

[1] Excluded from the analysis.

More than 2,200 eligible cancer cases (2.3%) had to be excluded because these patients were not found in the 1970 Population Census. The rate of undercoverage varied by primary site from 0.4% (vulva) to 4.8% (larynx). The numbers of included and excluded cases for the cancer categories used in this study are given in table 6. Adding the separately analysed in situ lesions of the cervix uteri and basal cell carcinomas of the skin to the amount of malignant cancers raises the sum of all cancer cases in this study to 109,000.

Table 6. Numbers of cancer cases included in the analyses (by sex), and the proportion of excluded cases because of missing 1970 Population Census data, by primary site

Primary site (ICD-7)	Included			Excluded	
	Men	Women	Total	Total	%
ALL SITES (140-204)	47,178	46,853	94,031	2,208	2.3
Lip (140)	1,046	86	1,132	21	1.9
Tongue (141)	188	131	319	4	1.3
Salivary glands (142)	143	135	278	9	3.2
Oral cavity (143-144)	189	129	318	6	1.9
Nasopharynx (146)	84	41	125	2	1.6
Other pharynx (145,147,148)	231	101	332	13	3.9
Oesophagus (150)	599	462	1,061	37	3.5
Stomach (151)	4,364	2,698	7,062	169	2.4
Small intestine (152)	166	143	309	5	1.6
Colon (153)	1,744	2,031	3,775	74	2.0
Rectum (154)	1,678	1,588	3,266	59	1.8
Liver (155.0)	658	375	1,033	32	3.1
Gallbladder and biliary tract (155.1)	341	752	1,093	29	2.7
Pancreas (157)	1,891	1,350	3,241	81	2.5
Nose (160)	149	84	233	4	1.7
Larynx (161)	1,269	104	1,373	66	4.8
Lung and trachea (162.0-1)	15,613	1,868	17,481	496	2.8
adenocarcinoma	1,687	565	2,252	62	2.8
small cell carcinoma	2,512	303	2,815	107	3.8
squamous cell carcinoma	5,373	346	5,719	141	2.5
Mesothelioma (pleura/peritoneum)	130	65	195	5	2.6
Breast (170)	47	13,782	13,829	294	2.1
Cervix uteri (171)	.	1,917	1,917	46	2.4
Corpus uteri (172)	.	3,842	3,842	56	1.5
Ovary (175)	.	3,366	3,366	58	1.7
Other female genitals (176)	.	418	418	4	1.0
vulva (176.0)	.	274	274	1	0.4
vagina (176.1)	.	106	106	3	2.8
Prostate (177)	3,270	.	3,270	32	1.0
Testis (178)	184	.	184	3	1.6
Other male genitals (179)	116	.	116	3	2.6
penis (179.0)	107	.	107	3	2.8
scrotum (179.1)	4	.	4	-	-
Kidney (180)	1,864	1,269	3,133	71	2.3
renal pelvis (180.1)	114	60	174	1	0.6
Bladder, ureter and urethra (181)	2,121	564	2,685	51	1.9
Skin melanoma (190)	1,148	1,234	2,382	58	2.4
head and neck (190.0-4)	130	151	281	5	1.8
trunk (190.5)	711	382	1,093	27	2.5
limbs (190.6-7)	252	659	911	23	2.5
Non-melanoma skin cancer (191)	745	548	1,293	27	2.1
head and neck (191.0-4)	430	331	761	15	2.0
trunk (191.5)	104	69	173	4	2.3
limbs (191.6-7)	164	122	286	5	1.7

Table 6 (continued)

Primary site (ICD-7)	Included			Excluded	
	Men	Women	Total	Total	%
Eye (192)	181	171	352	9	2.6
Brain and nervous system (193)	1,504	1,943	3,447	71	2.1
malignant brain tumours	928	840	1,768	34	1.9
glioma	709	606	1,315	27	2.1
benign brain tumours	427	903	1,330	30	2.3
meningeoma	334	844	1,178	26	2.2
Thyroid (194)	302	1,081	1,383	41	3.0
folliculary	74	256	330	5	1.5
localized	39	151	190	5	2.6
papillary	144	654	798	24	3.0
localized	82	443	525	14	2.7
Other endocrine glands (195)	111	75	186	5	2.7
Bone (196)	156	95	251	6	2.4
Soft tissue (197)	308	321	629	9	1.4
Unspecified cancer (199.1-9)	857	866	1,723	45	2.6
Non-Hodgkin lymphoma (200,202)	1,328	1,049	2,377	46	1.9
nodal	941	746	1,687	25	1.5
extranodal	387	303	690	21	3.0
Hodgkin's disease (201)	428	261	689	16	2.3
Multiple myeloma (203)	563	532	1,095	14	1.3
Leukaemia (204)	1,163	967	2,130	40	1.9
chronic lymphatic leukaemia (CLL)	413	253	666	9	1.4
acute myelocytic leukaemia (AML)	364	360	724	19	2.6
other	386	354	740	12	1.6
Not included above:					
Ca in situ of the cervix uteri	.	1,374	1,374	29	2.1
Basal cell carcinoma of the skin	6,263	7,218	13,481	259	1.9

IV. Results

Cancers of the mouth and pharynx

Lip

There were 1,046 lip cancer cases in men and 86 in women. The SIR among men in the lowest social class was almost five-fold that of the lowest one (fig. 5). This difference is one of the largest among all sites presented in this report. Fishermen had the highest SIR_a, followed by timber workers and agricultural workers (table 7, *appendix table C1*). Indoor occupations, some of them with rather high chemical or dust exposures, typically showed low SIRs.

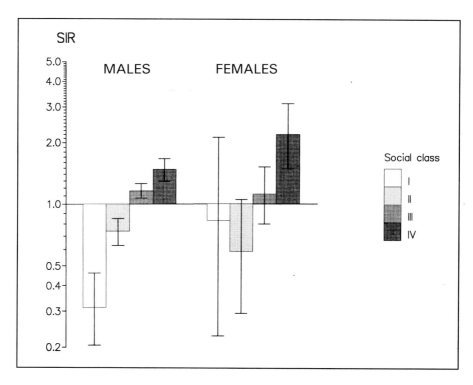

Fig. 5. Standardized incidence ratios (SIR), with 95% confidence intervals, for lip cancer among working-aged Finns in 1971-85, by sex and social class. Reference: economically active population.

Also in women the incidence of lip cancer was highest in social class IV (SIR 2.19, 95% CI 1.49-3.11; fig. 5). The small number of cases did not allow for proper detailed occupational comparison. However, in women nonsignificantly elevated risks were also obtained for farmers and farm workers (*appendix table C2*). The SIR_a for chefs and cooks was 5.19 (1.42-13.3).

Comment. The results for lip cancer completely fit the known aetiology of lip cancer, i.e., the joint effect of outdoor work and smoking [70]. The significantly elevated SIR for chefs and cooks may be a clue for new aetiological factors, e.g., cooks are likely to burn their lips when tasting the food they prepare.

Tongue and salivary glands

There was no variation in the risk by social class among the 319 cases of cancer of the tongue. The only significant occupation-specific risk based on more than one observed case was that of male motor-vehicle drivers (17 cases observed, SIR_a 1.77, 95% CI 1.03-2.83).

Table 7. Lip cancer, men: number of cancer cases (Obs.) and crude and social class adjusted standardized incidence ratios (SIR) with 95% confidence intervals (95% CI) for selected occupational categories in 1971-85

Occupation		Obs.	Crude		Adjusted	
			SIR	95% CI	SIR	95% CI
330	Fishermen	8	3.69	1.59-7.27	3.24	1.40-6.39 *
670	Round-timber workers	5	3.42	1.11-7.97	3.06	0.99-7.13 *
310	Agricultural workers	27	2.80	1.84-4.07	2.22	1.47-3.23 *
671	Timber workers	19	2.36	1.42-3.68	2.15	1.29-3.35 *
302	Forestry managers	11	1.50	0.75-2.68	2.11	1.05-3.77 *
300	Farmers, silviculturists	306	1.56	1.39-1.73	1.46	1.30-1.63 *
698	Roadbuilding hands	25	1.80	1.17-2.66	1.24	0.80-1.83 *
	- - -					
66	Electrical work	9	0.48	0.22-0.90	0.42	0.19-0.80 *
655	Welders and flame cutters	3	0.48	0.10-1.40	0.42	0.09-1.22
11	Corporate administration	3	0.12	0.02-0.35	0.36	0.07-1.05 *
654	Plumbers	3	0.37	0.08-1.07	0.33	0.07-0.97 *
650	Turners, machinists	4	0.29	0.08-0.74	0.26	0.07-0.67 *
013	Mechanical technicians	1	0.13	0.00-0.72	0.18	0.00-1.00 *
58	Postal services/couriers	1	0.19	0.00-1.05	0.17	0.00-0.94 *
22	Sales representatives	1	0.12	0.00-0.64	0.16	0.00-0.90 *
02	Chemical/physical/biological work	-	exp 5.2	0.00-0.71	exp 2.6	0.00-1.40 *
675	Bench carpenters	-	exp 3.7	0.00-0.99	exp 3.7	0.00-1.00 *
70	Printing	-	exp 4.2	0.00-0.87	exp 4.8	0.00-0.77 *

Age 35-64 years at the beginning of each 5-year follow-up period. Ordered by the social class adjusted SIR. Reference: economically active population. * Crude and/or social class adjusted SIR significant (p<0.05).

The 278 cases of cancer of the salivary glands did not reveal any major social class or occupation-specific risks.

Comment. There are a few earlier observations suggesting that drivers or persons repeatedly sucking machine oils have increased risk of cancer of the tongue [71]. The only significantly high SIR in the present data set was obtained among motor-vehicle drivers and might be associated with similar risk factors. The results for cancer of the salivary glands are in line with the view that there are almost no external risk factors for this cancer.

Oral cavity and pharynx

The incidence of cancer of the *oral cavity* among women clearly increased with increasing social status (fig. 6). The SIR for social class I was 1.62 (0.88-2.71) and that for social class IV 0.69 (0.39-1.12). In men there was an increase in high social class and a decrease in the lowest one. The incidence among the whole population

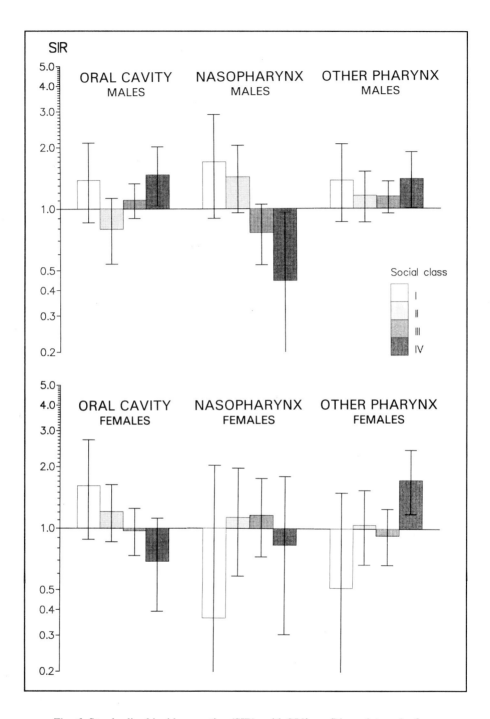

Fig. 6. Standardized incidence ratios (SIR), with 95% confidence intervals, for cancers of the oral cavity, nasopharynx, and other pharynx among working-aged Finns in 1971-85, by sex and social class. Reference: economically active population.

Table 8. Cancer of the oral cavity: number of cancer cases (Obs.) and crude and social class adjusted standardized incidence ratios (SIR) with 95% confidence intervals (95% CI) for selected occupational categories in 1971-85

	Occupation	Obs.	Crude		Adjusted	
			SIR	95% CI	SIR	95% CI
MEN						
9	Work not classified elsewhere	4	3.52	0.96-9.01	3.74	1.02-9.57 *
4	Mining and quarrying	3	3.41	0.70-9-96	3.38	0.70-9.89
660	Electricians (indoors)	6	3.07	1.13-6.69	3.02	1.11-6.58 *
34	Forestry work	9	1.72	0.79-3.27	1.51	0.69-2.86
- - -						
67	Woodwork	7	0.65	0.26-1.34	0.65	0.26-1.35
30	Agricultural/forestry management	18	0.55	0.33-0.88	0.58	0.35-0.92 *
69	Construction work NOS	5	0.57	0.19-1.33	0.51	0.17-1.20
11	Corporate administration	3	0.67	0.14-1.94	0.46	0.10-1.35
673	Construction carpenters	2	0.30	0.04-1.09	0.30	0.04-1.09
WOMEN						
562	Railway traffic supervisors	2	21.9	2.64-78.9	18.9	2.29-68.4 *
054	Vocational teachers	3	12.6	2.60-36.9	11.4	2.35-33.3 *
82	Waiters	5	3.18	1.03-7.42	2.86	0.93-6.67 *
- - -						
3	Farming, forestry and fishing	12	0.71	0.37-1.24	0.75	0.38-1.30

Age 35-64 years at the beginning of each 5-year follow-up period.   Ordered by the social class adjusted SIR.
Reference: economically active population.   * Crude and/or social class adjusted SIR significant (p<0.05).

increased in both sexes by some 40% in ten years. Male miners and electrical workers had an elevated risk of oral cancer (table 8). In women there was a tendency towards an increased incidence in service occupations. The lowest SIRs were obtained among agricultural and construction workers.

Cancer of the *nasopharynx* was studied separately from other pharynx cancers because of the difference in the aetiology. Although there were only 84 cases of nasopharyngeal cancer among men, a significant increasing social class trend was seen (fig. 6). The SIR in the highest social class was more than three-fold that of the lowest one. The SIR_a for male mechanical technicians was 5.20 (1.91-11.3) and for farmers 0.40 (0.15-0.88). In women there were only 41 cases of nasopharyngeal cancer in the study series. No associations with social class or occupation were seen.

The risk of cancer of the *pharynx other than nasopharynx* was significantly elevated among women in social class IV (SIR 1.73, 1.18-2.44) but otherwise there was no consistent trend in cancer incidence by social class (fig. 6).

Table 9. Cancer of the pharynx other than nasopharynx: number of cancer cases (Obs.) and crude and social class adjusted standardized incidence ratios (SIR) with 95% confidence intervals (95% CI) for selected occupational categories in 1971-85

Occupation		Obs.	Crude		Adjusted	
			SIR	95% CI	SIR	95% CI
MEN						
072	Lawyers	2	21.4	2.59-77.4	14.9	1.80-53.7 *
620	Shoemakers and cobblers	2	12.9	1.55-46.4	12.5	1.51-45.0 *
663	Electronics and telefitters	2	10.3	1.25-37.2	10.8	1.30-38.8 *
096	PR officers	3	8.21	1.69-24.0	7.25	1.49-21.2 *
780	Dockers	4	4.54	1.24-11.6	4.82	1.31-12.3 *
08	Artistic and literary professions	6	5.74	2.11-12.5	4.75	1.74-10.3 *
697	Building hands	9	2.24	1.02-4.25	1.96	0.90-3.72 *
2	Sales professions	13	1.61	0.86-2.76	1.61	0.86-2.76
- - -						
3	Farming, forestry and fishing	33	0.69	0.47-0.97	0.70	0.48-0.98 *
11	Corporate administration	4	0.82	0.22-2.09	0.68	0.19-1.74
65	Machine shop/steelworkers	6	0.50	0.18-1.08	0.53	0.19-1.15
01	Technical work	2	0.35	0.04-1.26	0.35	0.04-1.25
WOMEN						
620	Shoemakers and cobblers	1	94.3	2.39-526	87.6	2.22-488 *
77	Machinists	2	11.3	1.37-40.9	9.22	1.12-33.3 *
- - -						
31	Farming, animal husbandry	8	0.88	0.38-1.73	0.87	0.38-1.71
0	Technical, humanistic, etc. work	2	0.34	0.04-1.22	0.58	0.07-2.08

Age 35-64 years at the beginning of each 5-year follow-up period. Ordered by the social class adjusted SIR. Reference: economically active population. * Crude and/or social class adjusted SIR significant (p<0.05).

Among men with a total of 231 cases, the highest SIRs were found among lawyers, shoemakers, electrical workers, PR officers, dockers, building hands and sales professionals (especially commercial travellers), i.e., in occupations with very different socioeconomic backgrounds (table 9). The incidence was significantly below the Finnish average only among men in farming, forestry and fishing. Among women there were only 101 cases and the only significantly high risks (shoemakers, machinists) were based on 1-2 observed cases only (table 9).

Comment. The socioeconomic pattern of oral cancer roughly corresponds to the smoking pattern of Finns, i.e., the present results fit with the known smoking aetiology. The incidence pattern of nasopharyngeal cancer is dissimilar to the smoking pattern in Finland. This is in accordance with an earlier observation suggesting that there is no association between smoking and nasopharyngeal cancer [72]. The risk of cancer of other parts of pharynx does not follow the smoking pattern, either. Many of the high-risk occupations of pharyngeal cancer (e.g. shoemakers, commercial travellers and building hands) are traditionally thought or known [56] to include exceptionally high proportions of heavy drinkers. Alcohol abuse seems to be a clearly more important risk factor for pharyngeal cancer than smoking in Finland.

No excess risk of oral cancer was seen among asbestos, steel, metal or textile workers as suggested by some earlier studies [71, 73]. Leather production workers showed an increased risk of pharyngeal cancer in an earlier study [74], and in the present one there was a significantly high risk of pharyngeal cancer among both male and female shoemakers. A potential candidate for an occupational association to be tested in future studies is also the excess risk of both oral cancer and pharyngeal cancer among electrical workers, seen at least in one earlier study [75].

Cancer of the gastrointestinal tract

Oesophagus

The incidence of oesophageal cancer was highest in low socioeconomic classes (fig. 7). Among women the incidence in social class IV was 3.8-fold that of the social class I, and the relative difference increased with time. The risk pattern did not depend on age. Although oesophageal cancer is much more common among men than in women in most western countries [76], working-aged Finnish women of low social class experienced a higher incidence of oesophageal cancer than men of social classes I-II.

The occupation-specific SIR_as for male workers were highest for greasers, cabinetmakers, miners and indoor electricians (table 10, *appendix table C3*). Painters, building hands, labourers and machinists also had SIR_as above 1.5. Female furriers and building hands had elevated SIRs (table 10, *appendix table C4*), and the whole branch of industrial and construction workers had an SIR_a of 1.28 (95% CI 0.97-1.66).

Teachers had low SIR_es. Adjustment for social class raised the SIR for female teachers above 1.0, but for male teachers even the SIR_a was as low as 0.32. Some occupations in farming and domestic work also showed rather low SIRs.

Comment. The elevated SIRs of oesophageal cancers among male labourers, building hands of any gender, and among men with an unknown occupation may reflect a higher than average alcohol consumption [56] or a diet poor in fresh fruit and vegetables [49, 77]. However, other high-risk occupations suggest that dust and fibres from stone, metal, wood or even from fur and textiles may explain part of the elevated SIRs. This is in line with an earlier suggestion that exposure to metal dust and asbestos might increase the risk of oesophageal cancer [73].

The numbers of cases in the present study were not large enough to confirm or disprove earlier observations [78] of elevated risks of barmen (combined number of cases for males and females 3, SIR_a 1.31, 95% CI 0.27-3.83), commercial travellers

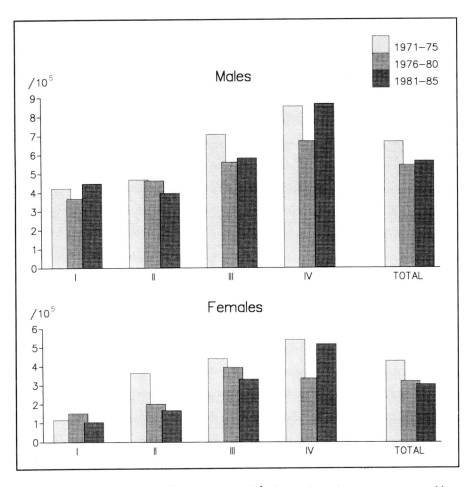

Fig. 7. Age-adjusted incidence rates per 10^5 of oesophageal cancer among working-aged Finns in 1971-85, by sex, social class and period.

(4 cases, SIR_a 1.12, 95% CI 0.31-2.87) or chimney sweeps (no cases observed, Exp_a 0.6).

Stomach

The incidence of stomach cancer decreased over the period 1971-75 to 1981-85 by 24% in males and by 20% in females. The incidence decreased with increasing welfare (fig. 8). In men the downward time trend in cancer incidence was larger the higher the social class was, and the social class difference thus increased with calendar time. In social class II-IV for women there was a change from a negative social class gradient (i.e., higher incidence in lower classes) to a positive one during

Table 10. Cancer of the oesophagus: number of cancer cases (Obs.) and crude and social class adjusted standardized incidence ratios (SIR) with 95% confidence intervals (95% CI) for selected occupational categories in 1971-85

Occupation		Obs.	Crude		Adjusted	
			SIR	95% CI	SIR	95% CI
MEN						
91	Occupation not specified	5	4.45	1.44-10.4	4.34	1.41-10.1 *
774	Greasers	4	4.37	1.19-11.2	4.27	1.16-10.9 *
676	Cabinetmakers etc.	5	4.11	1.34-9.60	4.11	1.33-9.59 *
4	Mining and quarrying	8	3.25	1.40-6.40	3.13	1.35-6.17 *
660	Electricians (indoors)	12	2.38	1.23-4.16	2.31	1.20-4.04 *
680	Painters	11	1.96	0.98-3.50	1.95	0.97-3.48
697	Building hands	21	1.99	1.23-3.04	1.54	0.95-2.35 *
79	Labourers not classified elsewhere	11	1.95	0.97-3.49	1.51	0.75-2.70
77	Machinists	17	1.44	0.84-2.30	1.40	0.82-2.24
34	Forestry work	19	1.34	0.81-2.09	1.04	0.63-1.62
- - -						
0	Technical, humanistic, etc. work	23	0.57	0.36-0.85	0.72	0.45-1.08 *
73	Chemical process/paper making	3	0.56	0.12-1.65	0.54	0.11-1.58
80	Watchmen, security guards	4	0.50	0.14-1.29	0.53	0.15-1.37
31	Farming, animal husbandry	4	0.63	0.17-1.61	0.52	0.14-1.34
05	Teaching	2	0.24	0.03-0.87	0.32	0.04-1.17 *
652	Machine and motor repairers	2	0.28	0.03-1.00	0.28	0.03-0.99 *
WOMEN						
612	Furriers	2	11.5	1.39-41.6	12.2	1.48-44.2 *
697	Building hands	6	3.93	1.44-8.56	2.85	1.05-6.21 *
60	Textiles	10	1.88	0.90-3.46	1.89	0.91-3.47
05	Teaching	4	0.50	0.13-1.27	1.05	0.29-2.69
- - -						
831	Cleaners	30	1.33	0.89-1.89	0.97	0.66-1.39
81	Housekeeping, domestic work, etc.	17	0.90	0.53-1.44	0.78	0.46-1.25
14/15	Clerical work NOS	10	0.60	0.29-1.11	0.77	0.37-1.41
30	Agricultural/forestry management	14	0.75	0.41-1.26	0.69	0.37-1.15

Age 35-64 years at the beginning of each 5-year follow-up period. Ordered by the social class adjusted SIR. Reference: economically active population. * Crude and/or social class adjusted SIR significant ($p < 0.05$).

the study period. The downward trend in the SIR for women of social class IV was mostly attributable to the youngest birth cohorts.

The only occupation with a significantly low SIR_a among women, i.e., book-keepers and accountants, showed a significantly increased SIR_a in men (tables 11-12, *appendix tables C5-6*). Otherwise the list of high and low risk occupations was also inconsistent between genders.

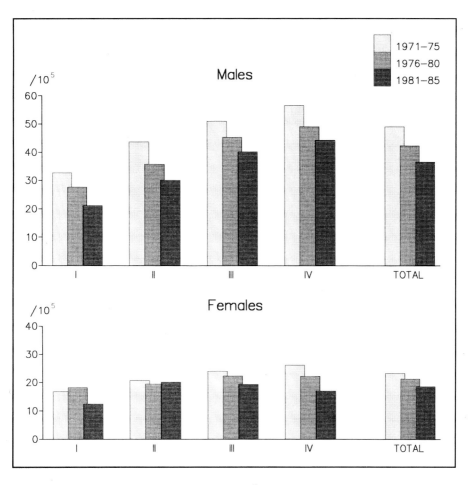

Fig. 8. Age-adjusted incidence rates per 10^5 of stomach cancer among working-aged Finns in 1971-85, by sex, social class and period.

Comment. Stomach cancer is not usually thought to have an occupational exposure aetiology [73, 79]. The observations of the present series confirm this view. Despite the large number of cases (4,364 in men and 2,698 in women) there were only nine occupational categories in males and four in females with an SIR_a significantly ($p<0.05$) different from 1.0. The elevated risk among male miners and blasters (SIR_a 1.80) could, however, be associated with the only suspected occupational risk factors, i.e., radiation and dusts [73].

Gardeners in both sexes had reduced SIRs which may reflect the known protective effect of fresh fruits and vegetables in the causation of stomach cancer. Although bakers also had low SIRs in both sexes, pastry products are not known to reduce the risk of stomach cancer.

Table 11. Cancer of the stomach, men: number of cancer cases (Obs.) and crude and social class adjusted standardized incidence ratios (SIR) with 95% confidence intervals (95% CI) for selected occupational categories in 1971-85

Occupation		Obs.	Crude		Adjusted	
			SIR	95% CI	SIR	95% CI
021	Physicists	2	5.88	0.71-21.3	9.55	1.16-34.5 *
088	Film and radio producers	3	3.61	0.74-10.6	5.91	1.22-17.3 *
120	Book-keepers, accountants	13	1.64	0.87-2.80	2.02	1.08-3.46 *
40	Mining and quarrying	24	1.90	1.22-2.83	1.80	1.15-2.68 *
312	Livestock workers	10	1.96	0.94-3.61	1.78	0.85-3.27
699	Construction workers NOS	15	1.68	0.94-2.77	1.63	0.91-2.69
695	Insulators	9	1.71	0.78-3.25	1.62	0.74-3.07
752	Plastics	9	1.68	0.77-3.19	1.58	0.72-3.00
670	Round-timber workers	10	1.63	0.78-3.00	1.54	0.74-2.82
672	Plywood makers	15	1.63	0.91-2.69	1.52	0.85-2.51
71	Glass and ceramic work	14	1.60	0.88-2.69	1.51	0.82-2.53
725	Butchers and sausage makers	12	1.61	0.83-2.81	1.50	0.78-2.63
655	Welders and flame cutters	38	1.47	1.04-2.02	1.37	0.97-1.88 *
634	Blacksmiths	13	1.31	0.70-2.24	1.30	0.69-2.23
580	Postmen	19	1.40	0.85-2.19	1.30	0.78-2.03
34	Forestry work	169	1.43	1.22-1.66	1.22	1.04-1.41 *
79	Labourers not classified elsewhere	62	1.33	1.02-1.70	1.13	0.87-1.45 *
05	Teaching	47	0.66	0.49-0.88	0.99	0.73-1.32 *
00	Technical professions	23	0.61	0.38-0.91	0.98	0.62-1.47 *
01	Technical work	101	0.82	0.67-0.99	0.94	0.76-1.13 *
112	Commercial managers	13	0.52	0.28-0.89	0.82	0.44-1.41 *
09	Humanistic and social work etc.	12	0.55	0.29-0.97	0.75	0.39-1.31 *
220	Commercial travellers, etc.	21	0.64	0.40-0.98	0.74	0.46-1.14 *
773	Operators of stationary engine	20	0.79	0.48-1.21	0.74	0.45-1.14
56	Traffic supervisors	11	0.57	0.28-1.02	0.70	0.35-1.26
10	Public administration	8	0.37	0.16-0.73	0.59	0.25-1.15 *
231	Shop personnel	27	0.58	0.39-0.85	0.54	0.36-0.79 *
311	Gardeners	4	0.61	0.16-1.55	0.52	0.14-1.33
030	Medical doctors	3	0.32	0.07-0.93	0.51	0.10-1.49 *
562	Railway traffic supervisors	4	0.42	0.11-1.07	0.50	0.14-1.29
53	Engine drivers	8	0.54	0.23-1.07	0.50	0.22-0.98 *
721	Bakers and pastry chiefs	2	0.30	0.04-1.08	0.29	0.04-1.05
701	Printers	1	0.19	0.00-1.04	0.17	0.00-0.97 *

Age 35-64 years at the beginning of each 5-year follow-up period. Ordered by the social class adjusted SIR.
Reference: economically active population.   * Crude and/or social class adjusted SIR significant (p<0.05).

Table 12. Cancer of the stomach, women: number of cancer cases (Obs.) and crude and social class adjusted standardized incidence ratios (SIR) with 95% confidence intervals (95% CI) for selected occupational categories in 1971-85

Occupation		Obs.	Crude		Adjusted	
			SIR	95% CI	SIR	95% CI
110	Corporate managers	7	3.59	1.44-7.40	4.46	1.79-9.18 *
69	Construction work NOS	19	1.80	1.09-2.82	1.75	1.05-2.73 *
035	Psychiatric nurses	9	1.66	0.76-3.16	1.75	0.80-3.32
123	Shop and restaurant cashiers	16	1.53	0.87-2.48	1.61	0.92-2.62
159	Clerical workers NOS	14	1.37	0.75-2.31	1.44	0.79-2.42
703	Bookbinders	7	1.47	0.59-3.03	1.41	0.57-2.91
019	Laboratory assistants	7	1.26	0.51-2.59	1.34	0.54-2.75
672	Plywood makers	14	1.38	0.75-2.31	1.31	0.72-2.20
040	Pharmacists	6	0.93	0.34-2.01	1.30	0.48-2.82
820	Waiters in restaurants	18	1.28	0.76-2.03	1.22	0.72-1.93
032	Nurses	25	1.12	0.72-1.65	1.21	0.78-1.79
811	Chefs, cooks etc.	33	1.24	0.86-1.75	1.21	0.83-1.69
76	Packing and labelling	30	1.26	0.85-1.79	1.19	0.80-1.70
- - -						
721	Bakers and pastry chiefs	11	0.77	0.38-1.37	0.74	0.37-1.33
570	Post/telecommunications officials	7	0.63	0.26-1.31	0.66	0.27-1.37
58	Postal services/couriers	10	0.67	0.32-1.24	0.65	0.31-1.19
311	Gardeners	6	0.65	0.24-1.42	0.62	0.23-1.35
810	Housekeepers	6	0.59	0.22-1.28	0.61	0.23-1.34
09	Humanistic and social work etc.	7	0.51	0.20-1.04	0.60	0.24-1.24
145	Bank clerks	7	0.54	0.22-1.11	0.58	0.23-1.20
051	Subject teachers	5	0.38	0.12-0.89	0.57	0.18-1.32 *
08	Artistic and literary professions	2	0.31	0.04-1.14	0.40	0.05-1.43
120	Book-keepers, accountants	7	0.36	0.15-0.74	0.38	0.15-0.78 *
092	Librarians, museum officials	-	exp 4.2	0.00-0.87	exp 3.5	0.00-1.04 *

Age 35-64 years at the beginning of each 5-year follow-up period. Ordered by the social class adjusted SIR.
Reference: economically active population. * Crude and/or social class adjusted SIR significant (p<0.05).

Small intestine

The incidence of cancer of the small intestine (excluding lymphomas which constitute one quarter of cancers in the small intestine) was significantly elevated among men of the highest social class (fig. 9). In women the incidence decreased towards the lower social classes in the 1970s, but this trend disappeared by 1981-85. The significantly elevated crude SIRs for male corporate managers and teachers decreased close to 1.0 after adjustment for social class (table 13).

Comment. The causes of this rare cancer form are by and large unknown [71, 80]. The social class pattern somehow fits with the observation of an association

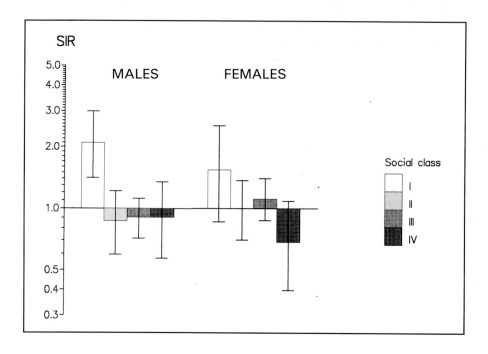

Fig. 9. Standardized incidence ratios (SIR), with 95% confidence intervals, for cancer of the small intestine among working-aged Finns in 1971-85, by sex and social class. Reference: economically active population.

between red meat consumption and cancer of the small intestine [81]. The whole of the occupations with elevated SIR_as in the present study give an impression that there might be an occupational (chemical?) component included in the aetiology of cancer of the small intestine. However, the observed numbers of cases were small; the total number of cases in the whole series was only 309.

Colon

In the early 1970s colon cancer was clearly a cancer of affluence in both sexes (fig. 10). Later on, the social class gradient disappeared among women and strongly diminished among men. In women of the highest social class, the incidence of colon cancer has even been decreasing since 1971-75. The social class difference greatly varied by birth cohort and was most prominent among the oldest men (fig. 11).

Among occupations with high SIRs there were many precision work technical professions (tables 14-15, *appendix tables C7-8*). All categories of managerial jobs (males only) experienced SIR_cs of 1.5-1.7 and SIR_as around 1.2. Men and women in agricultural and forestry work had relatively low risks of colon cancer, but there was a miscellaneous collection of occupations with even lower SIRs (tables 14-15).

Table 13. Cancer of the small intestine: number of cancer cases (Obs.) and crude and social class adjusted standardized incidence ratios (SIR) with 95% confidence intervals (95% CI) for selected occupational categories in 1971-85

Occupation		Obs.	Crude		Adjusted	
			SIR	95% CI	SIR	95% CI
MEN						
631	Hardeners, temperers, etc.	1	33.8	0.85-188	39.5	1.00-220 *
731	Cookers (chemical processes)	2	16.9	2.05-61.1	19.4	2.35-70.1 *
540	Motor-vehicle and tram drivers	12	1.34	0.69-2.35	1.54	0.80-2.69
11	Corporate administration	10	2.32	1.11-4.26	1.09	0.52-2.01 *
05	Teaching	6	1.97	0.72-4.28	1.04	0.38-2.26
- - -						
8	Services	4	0.68	0.19-1.74	0.77	0.21-1.98
69	Construction work NOS	6	0.70	0.26-1.52	0.76	0.28-1.66
2	Sales professions	5	0.69	0.22-1.60	0.75	0.24-1.74
WOMEN						
741	Cigar makers	1	88.3	2.23-492	76.6	1.94-427 *
084	Journalists	3	18.6	3.84-54.5	22.5	4.64-65.8 *
230	Buyers, office sales staff	2	13.2	1.60-47.6	14.1	1.71-50.9 *
831	Cleaners	5	0.76	0.25-1.78	1.29	0.42-3.01
03	Medical work and nursing	6	1.24	0.46-2.70	1.19	0.44-2.59

Age 35-64 years at the beginning of each 5-year follow-up period.   Ordered by the social class adjusted SIR.
Reference: economically active population.   * Crude and/or social class adjusted SIR significant (p<0.05).

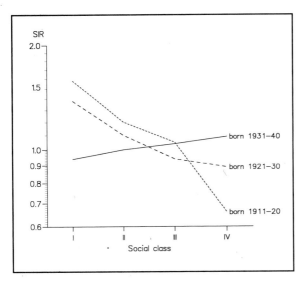

Fig. 11. Standardized incidence ratios (SIR) of colon cancer among Finnish men in 1971-85, by birth cohort and social class. Reference: economically active population.

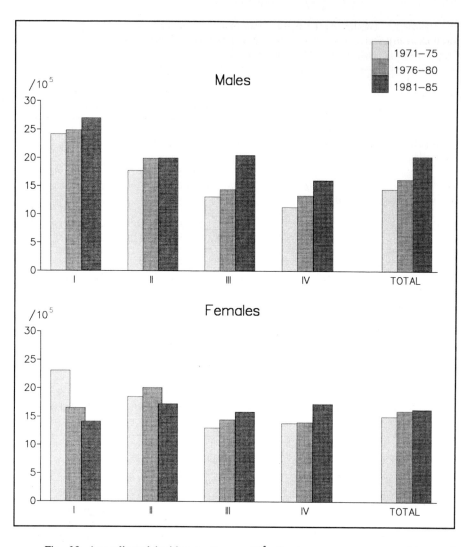

Fig. 10. Age-adjusted incidence rates per 10^5 of colon cancer among working-aged Finns in 1971-85, by sex, social class and period.

Comment. The typical incidence pattern of colon cancer of Western countries with the highest incidence rates in upper income classes was seen also in Finland, especially in the birth cohorts born before the 1930s. The socioeconomic variation in Finland can best be accounted for by differences in meat consumption, which until the 1970s was highest in upper social classes [47]. The correlation coefficient between meat consumption and colon cancer incidence in six main socioeconomic categories in 1971-75 was 0.98 [82]. During recent decades the lower social classes have

Table 14. Cancer of the colon, men: number of cancer cases (Obs.) and crude and social class adjusted standardized incidence ratios (SIR) with 95% confidence intervals (95% CI) for selected occupational categories in 1971-85

Occupation		Obs.	Crude		Adjusted		
			SIR	95% CI	SIR	95% CI	
644	Goldsmiths, silversmiths etc.	5	3.52	1.14-8.21	3.48	1.13-8.11	*
239	Sales staff NOS	5	3.16	1.03-7.38	3.24	1.05-7.56	*
007	Engineers NOS	4	4.00	1.09-10.2	2.93	0.80-7.50	*
70	Printing	16	2.09	1.19-3.39	2.17	1.24-3.53	*
660	Electricians (indoors)	32	1.76	1.20-2.48	1.83	1.25-2.58	*
734	Pulp mill workers	8	1.57	0.68-3.09	1.66	0.72-3.27	
61	Cutting/sewing etc.	8	1.61	0.69-3.17	1.59	0.68-3.12	
780	Dockers	11	1.42	0.71-2.53	1.53	0.77-2.74	
773	Operators of stationary engine	15	1.44	0.80-2.37	1.52	0.85-2.52	
231	Shop personnel	28	1.38	0.92-2.00	1.43	0.95-2.07	
664	Telephone installers and repairmen	7	1.36	0.55-2.81	1.43	0.57-2.94	
652	Machine and motor repairers	35	1.35	0.94-1.88	1.39	0.97-1.93	
550	Railway staff	19	1.37	0.82-2.14	1.38	0.83-2.16	
010	Civil engineering technicians	29	1.50	1.01-2.16	1.37	0.92-1.97	*
01	Technical work	76	1.44	1.13-1.80	1.32	1.04-1.65	*
08	Artistic and literary professions	16	1.68	0.96-2.73	1.30	0.74-2.11	
030	Medical doctors	7	1.75	0.70-3.60	1.29	0.52-2.65	
801	Policemen	15	1.34	0.75-2.22	1.24	0.69-2.04	
112	Commercial managers	18	1.67	0.99-2.64	1.24	0.73-1.95	
201	Retailers	27	1.37	0.90-1.99	1.22	0.80-1.78	
013	Mechanical technicians	18	1.30	0.77-2.05	1.20	0.71-1.90	
00	Technical professions	26	1.54	1.01-2.26	1.16	0.76-1.70	*
110	Corporate managers	33	1.64	1.13-2.30	1.14	0.78-1.60	*
- - -							
79	Labourers not classified elsewhere	13	0.71	0.38-1.21	0.92	0.49-1.57	
698	Roadbuilding hands	14	0.60	0.33-1.00	0.78	0.43-1.31	
300	Farmers, silviculturists	228	0.69	0.60-0.78	0.72	0.63-0.82	*
302	Forestry managers	10	0.78	0.38-1.44	0.71	0.34-1.30	
34	Forestry work	28	0.56	0.37-0.82	0.68	0.45-0.98	*
052	Primary school teachers	10	0.83	0.40-1.53	0.64	0.31-1.18	
651	Fitter-assemblers etc.	6	0.56	0.20-1.22	0.58	0.21-1.27	
693	Concrete/cement shutterers	3	0.40	0.08-1.17	0.42	0.09-1.23	
735	Paper and board mill workers	2	0.28	0.03-1.02	0.30	0.04-1.07	

Age 35-64 years at the beginning of each 5-year follow-up period. Ordered by the social class adjusted SIR.
Reference: economically active population. * Crude and/or social class adjusted SIR significant (p<0.05).

increased their meat consumption, and many persons in higher social classes turned over to a diet rich in vegetables. This change may be associated with the change in the social class pattern of the incidence of colon cancer after the mid-1970s.

Table 15. Cancer of the colon, women: number of cancer cases (Obs.) and crude and social class adjusted standardized incidence ratios (SIR) with 95% confidence intervals (95% CI) for selected occupational categories in 1971-85

Occupation		Obs.	Crude		Adjusted	
			SIR	95% CI	SIR	95% CI
001	Civil engineers	2	31.7	3.84-114	21.1	2.55-76.1 *
050	University teachers	4	5.56	1.52-14.2	4.57	1.24-11.7 *
540	Motor-vehicle and tram drivers	5	3.40	1.10-7.93	2.95	0.96-6.87 *
572	Switchboard operators	8	2.36	1.02-4.66	1.96	0.84-3.85 *
053	Teachers of practical subjects	11	1.89	0.94-3.39	1.60	0.80-2.87
73	Chemical process/paper making	10	1.40	0.67-2.58	1.55	0.74-2.86
821	Waiters in cafés etc.	21	1.52	0.94-2.32	1.49	0.92-2.28
570	Post/telecommunications officials	16	1.71	0.98-2.78	1.42	0.81-2.30
616	Garment workers	31	1.25	0.85-1.78	1.39	0.94-1.97
820	Waiters in restaurants	14	1.18	0.65-1.98	1.27	0.69-2.12
01	Technical work	11	1.49	0.75-2.67	1.26	0.63-2.26
035	Psychiatric nurses	7	1.52	0.61-3.13	1.26	0.51-2.60
145	Bank clerks	16	1.43	0.82-2.32	1.24	0.71-2.01
23	Sales work	110	1.12	0.92-1.34	1.19	0.98-1.43
052	Primary school teachers	27	1.26	0.83-1.83	1.14	0.75-1.66
032	Nurses	24	1.26	0.81-1.87	1.08	0.69-1.61
144	Office clerks	79	1.24	0.98-1.55	1.04	0.82-1.30
312	Livestock workers	151	0.85	0.72-0.99	0.88	0.75-1.03 *
60	Textiles	18	0.71	0.42-1.13	0.77	0.46-1.22
811	Chefs, cooks etc.	15	0.69	0.38-1.13	0.75	0.42-1.24
300	Farmers, silviculturists	48	0.67	0.49-0.88	0.71	0.52-0.94 *
813	Domestic servants	14	0.62	0.34-1.04	0.70	0.38-1.17
30	Agricultural/forestry management	48	0.65	0.48-0.86	0.69	0.51-0.91 *
120	Book-keepers, accountants	12	0.74	0.38-1.29	0.61	0.32-1.07
672	Plywood makers	4	0.47	0.13-1.20	0.52	0.14-1.34
311	Gardeners	3	0.40	0.08-1.16	0.45	0.09-1.31
611	Dressmakers	4	0.43	0.12-1.11	0.38	0.10-0.97 *

Age 35-64 years at the beginning of each 5-year follow-up period. Ordered by the social class adjusted SIR. Reference: economically active population. * Crude and/or social class adjusted SIR significant (p<0.05).

Occupational studies have not shown consistent patterns for colon cancer. Increases in some sedentary occupations have been reported [83, 84]. Some observations of the present study (e.g., elevated risks in presicion work professions) suggest that sedentary work may play a role in the aetiology of colon cancer, but there were also typical sedentary occupations among those with low SIRs. Work stress may cause irregularity in bowel function and may contribute to the causation of colon cancer.

The stress, increasing with increasing educational level [85] or responsibility [86], may explain part of the social class variation and also the elevated incidence in managerial occupations even in comparison with the average of their own social class.

The high SIR_a among indoor electricians (1.83) based on a large number of cases, and the elevated SIRs among printing workers and chemical process (especially pulp mill) workers in both sexes should be studied in more detail in order to reveal possible occupation-related risk factors.

Rectum

There was no variation in the incidence of rectal cancer between social classes and no change with time during 1971-85. Only one three-digit occupational category in males (forestry consultants) and one in females (livestock workers) showed an SIR_a significantly below 1.0 (table 16, *appendix tables C9-10*). Men in artistic and literary professions had an SIR_a of 2.33 (sculptors and painters even 5.45, 95% CI 2.00-11.9), and elevated SIRs were obtained also in many occupations in metal industry. Machine shop workers, waitresses in cafés and nurses were the only occupations with significantly increased SIRs among women.

Comment. There were many occupations with an elevated risk of both rectal cancer and colon cancer. These include printing, chemical and paper work, and smelting and foundry work where the presence of occupational carcinogens clearly could be suspected. If there are occupational factors behind some of these excesses, they seem to be similar for both cancers of the colon and rectum.

The lack of socioeconomic variation suggests that general lifestyle factors such as dietary ones may be less important in the causation of rectal cancer than in colon cancer. A high risk of rectal cancer among artists and some other occupations with likely higher than average beer consumption [56], is in line with earlier observations about the role of nitrosamines associated with excessive beer drinking as a cause of rectal cancer [87, 88].

Cancer of other digestive organs

Liver

The incidence of liver cancer among men of the lowest social class was slightly above and among women of the highest class slightly below the national sex-specific average (fig. 12). Men of social class I and women of social class IV showed the strongest increase in the incidence with time. The highest birth-cohort specific SIRswere obtained among men of social class IV born after 1920 (combined SIR for birth cohorts 1921-45 was 1.51, 95% CI 1.10-2.01).

Elevated SIRs were found among men and women in miscellaneous occupations in service, sales and industry (table 17). The few low-incidence occupations were in farming and forestry.

Table 16. Cancer of the rectum: number of cancer cases (Obs.) and crude and social class adjusted standardized incidence ratios (SIR) with 95% confidence intervals (95% CI) for selected occupational categories in 1971-85

Occupation		Obs.	Crude		Adjusted	
			SIR	95% CI	SIR	95% CI
MEN						
08	Artistic and literary professions	22	2.46	1.54-3.72	2.33	1.46-3.52 *
775	Industrial personnel, riggers	10	1.93	0.93-3.56	2.02	0.97-3.72
09	Humanistic and social work etc.	17	1.97	1.15-3.16	1.79	1.04-2.86 *
013	Mechanical technicians	23	1.79	1.14-2.69	1.58	1.00-2.37 *
64	Precision mechanical work	9	1.57	0.72-2.98	1.52	0.69-2.88
63	Smelting, metal and foundry work	21	1.42	0.88-2.17	1.46	0.90-2.22
801	Policemen	18	1.70	1.01-2.69	1.44	0.85-2.28 *
230	Buyers, office sales staff	9	1.62	0.74-3.07	1.43	0.65-2.71
10	Public administration	12	1.40	0.72-2.45	1.42	0.74-2.49
782	Warehousemen	24	1.24	0.79-1.84	1.37	0.88-2.04
21	Real estate, services, securities	8	1.55	0.67-3.06	1.36	0.59-2.67
650	Turners, machinists	30	1.31	0.88-1.86	1.35	0.91-1.93
540	Motor-vehicle and tram drivers	107	1.30	1.06-1.55	1.26	1.03-1.51 *
- - -						
31	Farming, animal husbandry	13	0.61	0.32-1.04	0.66	0.35-1.14
68	Painting and lacquering	13	0.65	0.34-1.11	0.66	0.35-1.12
772	Construction machinery operators	7	0.55	0.22-1.13	0.56	0.22-1.15
03	Medical work and nursing	4	0.59	0.16-1.51	0.55	0.15-1.42
052	Primary school teachers	6	0.55	0.20-1.19	0.49	0.18-1.07
735	Paper and board mill workers	3	0.45	0.09-1.32	0.48	0.10-1.39
144	Office clerks	3	0.54	0.11-1.58	0.47	0.10-1.37
028	Consultancy, forestry	-	exp 4.2	0.00-0.89	exp 4.4	0.00-0.85 *
WOMEN						
65	Machine shop/steelworkers	12	1.98	1.02-3.45	2.06	1.06-3.60 *
821	Waiters in cafés etc.	18	1.81	1.07-2.85	1.80	1.07-2.85 *
311	Gardeners	10	1.75	0.84-3.23	1.73	0.83-3.18
032	Nurses	22	1.67	1.05-2.53	1.60	1.01-2.43 *
75	Industrial work NOS	14	1.48	0.81-2.49	1.54	0.84-2.59
810	Housekeepers	9	1.44	0.66-2.73	1.39	0.64-2.64
672	Plywood makers	8	1.28	0.55-2.52	1.33	0.58-2.63
01	Technical work	7	1.36	0.55-2.81	1.33	0.54-2.75
611	Dressmakers	9	1.29	0.59-2.46	1.28	0.59-2.44
602	Weavers	8	1.24	0.54-2.45	1.28	0.55-2.53
120	Book-keepers, accountants	15	1.27	0.71-2.09	1.23	0.69-2.02
813	Domestic servants	21	1.23	0.76-1.88	1.20	0.74-1.84
831	Cleaners	91	1.18	0.95-1.45	1.15	0.93-1.41
- - -						
312	Livestock workers	92	0.70	0.56-0.85	0.71	0.57-0.87 *
201	Retailers	9	0.67	0.31-1.28	0.66	0.30-1.25
72	Food industry	11	0.58	0.29-1.04	0.61	0.30-1.08
051	Subject teachers	4	0.52	0.14-1.34	0.50	0.14-1.27
123	Shop and restaurant cashiers	3	0.48	0.10-1.39	0.46	0.10-1.36

Age 35-64 years at the beginning of each 5-year follow-up period.   Ordered by the social class adjusted SIR.
Reference: Economically active population.   * Crude and/or social class adjusted SIR significant ($p < 0.05$).

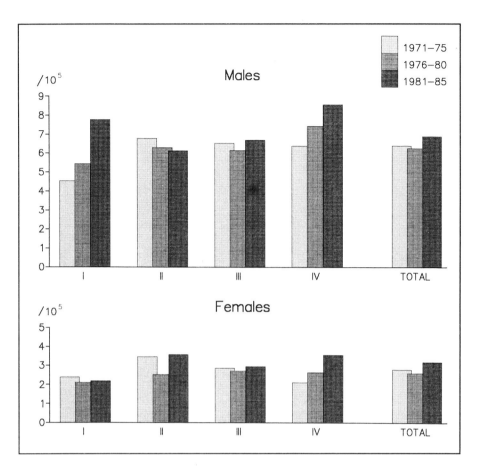

Fig. 12. Age-adjusted incidence rates per 10^5 of liver cancer among working-aged Finns in 1971-85, by sex, social class and period.

Comment. Most Western studies have shown an association between chronic alcohol abuse and hepatocellular carcinoma, which is by far the most common type of liver cancer [87, 89]. Very high occupation-specific risk ratios in occupations such as waiters, commercial travellers, civilian guards and warehousemen fit with the alcohol hypothesis [56]. The high incidence among young men of social class IV might also be associated with drinking.

Possible direct occupational factors may be hidden behind the strong effect of alcohol. The high risk among painters could in principle be attributable to solvents, but this is not likely since an elevated incidence has not been observed among painters in Sweden or Norway with roughly similar occupational exposures [90].

Table 17. Cancer of the liver: number of cancer cases (Obs.) and crude and social class adjusted standardized incidence ratios (SIR) with 95% confidence intervals (95% CI) for selected occupational categories in 1971-85

Occupation		Obs.	Crude		Adjusted	
			SIR	95% CI	SIR	95% CI
MEN						
820	Waiters in restaurants	2	12.6	1.53-45.6	12.6	1.52-45.3 *
750	Basket and brush makers	2	9.12	1.10-32.9	9.07	1.10-32.8 *
781	Freight handlers	7	4.33	1.74-8.91	3.93	1.58-8.11 *
804	Civilian guards	9	3.10	1.42-5.88	3.20	1.46-6.07 *
773	Operators of stationary engine	8	2.27	0.98-4.46	2.34	1.01-4.62 *
220	Commercial travellers, etc.	10	2.33	1.12-4.28	2.25	1.08-4.13 *
68	Painting and lacquering	15	2.17	1.21-3.58	2.23	1.25-3.68 *
80	Watchmen, security guards	17	1.85	1.08-2.96	1.90	1.11-3.04 *
698	Roadbuilding hands	16	1.91	1.09-3.10	1.80	1.03-2.93 *
782	Warehousemen	13	1.92	1.02-3.28	1.80	0.96-3.07 *
23	Sales work	16	1.59	0.91-2.58	1.62	0.93-2.63
652	Machine and motor repairers	12	1.47	0.76-2.57	1.53	0.79-2.67
150	Property managers, warehousemen	9	1.49	0.68-2.83	1.43	0.65-2.72
79	Labourers not classified elsewhere	9	1.38	0.63-2.63	1.30	0.60-2.48
- - -						
31	Farming, animal husbandry	5	0.69	0.22-1.62	0.66	0.21-1.54
34	Forestry work	10	0.62	0.30-1.14	0.56	0.27-1.03
300	Farmers, silviculturists	55	0.46	0.35-0.60	0.46	0.35-0.60 *
WOMEN						
759	Industrial workers NOS	3	6.25	1.29-18.3	6.30	1.30-18.4 *
150	Property managers, warehousemen	3	6.88	1.42-20.1	6.24	1.29-18.2 *
819	Housekeeping workers NOS	3	6.18	1.27-18.1	5.88	1.21-17.2 *
12	Clerical work	9	1.63	0.74-3.09	1.51	0.69-2.86
83	Caretakers and cleaners	26	1.34	0.88-1.96	1.39	0.91-2.03
14/15	Clerical work NOS	22	1.50	0.94-2.27	1.36	0.85-2.05
03	Medical work and nursing	13	1.28	0.68-2.19	1.28	0.68-2.19
- - -						
312	Livestock workers	21	0.71	0.44-1.08	0.69	0.43-1.06
300	Farmers, silviculturists	8	0.64	0.28-1.26	0.64	0.28-1.26
61	Cutting/sewing etc.	4	0.56	0.15-1.43	0.56	0.15-1.43

Age 35-64 years at the beginning of each 5-year follow-up period. Ordered by the social class adjusted SIR. Reference: economically active population. * Crude and/or social class adjusted SIR significant (p<0.05).

Gallbladder and biliary ducts

There was no consistent social class trend in the incidence of cancer of the gallbladder and biliary ducts (fig. 13). The male-female difference in the incidence was diminishing along with the increase of incidence among men of the lowest social classes.

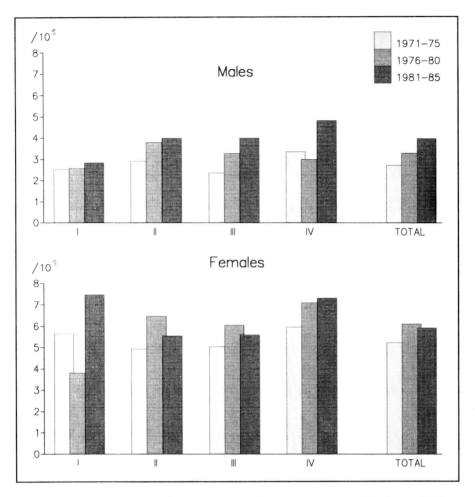

Fig. 13. Age-adjusted incidence rates per 10^5 of cancer of the gallbladder and biliary tract among working-aged Finns in 1971-85, by sex, social class and period.

There were very few occupations with SIRs significantly different from 1.0 (table 18). The only significantly reduced SIR_a (0.52, 95% CI 0.24-0.98) was observed among women in medical work and nursing. Women in housekeeping and domestic work also showed generally low SIRs.

Comment. It has been estimated that 50% of gallbladder cancers among whites are attributable to gallstones [91]. Whether women with a low cancer incidence working in hospitals, restaurants and home kitchens have lower risk of gallstones than other women, is not known. This study did not confirm earlier observations of elevated risks in rubber, textile or metal workers [71, 92].

Table 18. Cancer of the gallbladder and biliary tract: number of cancer cases (Obs.) and crude and social class adjusted standardized incidence ratios (SIR) with 95% confidence intervals (95% CI) for selected occupational categories in 1971-85

Occupation		Obs.	Crude		Adjusted	
			SIR	95% CI	SIR	95% CI
MEN						
66	Electrical work	9	1.44	0.66-2.73	1.48	0.68-2.81
697	Building hands	10	1.48	0.71-2.72	1.38	0.66-2.53
- - -						
78	Dock and warehouse work	3	0.49	0.10-1.42	0.46	0.09-1.34
WOMEN						
670	Round-timber workers	2	13.8	1.67-49.8	15.9	1.93-57.5 *
562	Railway traffic supervisors	3	5.99	1.23-17.5	5.74	1.18-16.8 *
201	Retailers	9	1.63	0.75-3.09	1.57	0.72-2.98
83	Caretakers and cleaners	48	1.35	0.99-1.79	1.13	0.83-1.49
- - -						
811	Chefs, cooks etc.	5	0.75	0.24-1.74	0.87	0.28-2.02
812	Kitchen assistants	7	0.98	0.39-2.02	0.79	0.32-1.64
82	Waiters	5	0.68	0.22-1.58	0.72	0.23-1.67
03	Medical work and nursing	9	0.49	0.22-0.93	0.52	0.24-0.98 *
310	Agricultural workers	3	0.47	0.10-1.37	0.48	0.10-1.41
813	Domestic servants	4	0.56	0.15-1.44	0.48	0.13-1.22

Age 35-64 years at the beginning of each 5-year follow-up period.   Ordered by the social class adjusted SIR.
Reference: economically active population.   * Crude and/or social class adjusted SIR significant (p<0.05).

Pancreas

The incidence of pancreatic cancer was stable during the follow-up period. There was almost no variation by social class, either. The highest occupation-specific SIR_as among men were observed among sauna attendants and hairdressers (table 19, *appendix table C11*). Female sauna attendants and hairdressers also had elevated SIR_as (table 20, *appendix table C12*). Various occupations with solvent and dust exposures, e.g., painters, plumbers and miners, were on the top of the list of the highest SIRs.

Comment. While numerous occupations, including those involving exposure to petroleum products and paint thinners, have been reported to be associated with a moderate increase in risk, no obvious common exposure has been detected [73]. In the present study, numerous high occupation-specific SIRs were found, obviously not only by chance. The high risk of pancreatic cancer among barbers and hairdressers (SIR_a among men 9.04 and among women 1.84) is similar to that obtained in a traditional cohort study of the female members of the Finnish Hairdressers Association [93]. Although the cohort and observation period of that study largely overlaps with those of the present study, the SIR for pancreatic cancer obtained in the Hairdresser

Table 19. Cancer of the pancreas, men: number of cancer cases (Obs.) and crude and social class adjusted standardized incidence ratios (SIR) with 95% confidence intervals (95% CI) for selected occupational categories in 1971-85

Occupation		Obs.	Crude		Adjusted	
			SIR	95% CI	SIR	95% CI
843	Sauna attendants etc.	2	11.2	1.36-40.6	12.1	1.46-43.6 *
840	Hairdressers and barbers	3	7.80	1.61-22.8	8.31	1.71-24.3 *
656	Plate/constructional steel workers	12	3.57	1.85-6.24	3.54	1.83-6.19 *
303	Horticultural managers	5	3.14	1.02-7.34	3.37	1.09-7.87 *
654	Plumbers	32	2.17	1.49-3.07	2.16	1.48-3.05 *
550	Railway staff	24	1.63	1.05-2.43	1.65	1.05-2.45 *
4	Mining and quarrying	14	1.56	0.86-2.62	1.56	0.85-2.61
655	Welders and flame cutters	17	1.51	0.88-2.42	1.49	0.87-2.39
68	Painting and lacquering	32	1.45	0.99-2.05	1.46	1.00-2.06
72	Food industry	18	1.45	0.86-2.29	1.45	0.86-2.29
781	Freight handlers	8	1.56	0.67-3.07	1.41	0.61-2.79
782	Warehousemen	32	1.51	1.03-2.13	1.38	0.95-1.95 *
010	Civil engineering technicians	26	1.29	0.84-1.89	1.38	0.90-2.02
735	Paper and board mill workers	10	1.38	0.66-2.54	1.36	0.65-2.51
651	Fitter-assemblers etc.	15	1.37	0.77-2.26	1.36	0.76-2.24
201	Retailers	27	1.26	0.83-1.84	1.34	0.88-1.95
80	Watchmen, security guards	37	1.30	0.91-1.79	1.33	0.93-1.83
110	Corporate managers	26	1.20	0.79-1.76	1.25	0.81-1.83
697	Building hands	51	1.34	0.99-1.76	1.21	0.90-1.59
54	Road transport	105	1.15	0.94-1.39	1.18	0.96-1.41
- - -						
300	Farmers, silviculturists	294	0.80	0.71-0.89	0.80	0.71-0.89 *
650	Turners, machinists	14	0.55	0.30-0.93	0.55	0.30-0.92 *
659	Machine shop/steelworkers NOS	5	0.47	0.15-1.10	0.47	0.15-1.10
693	Concrete/cement shutterers	3	0.38	0.08-1.11	0.38	0.08-1.11
052	Primary school teachers	4	0.33	0.09-0.86	0.36	0.10-0.92 *
775	Industrial personnel, riggers	1	0.18	0.00-0.98	0.17	0.00-0.97 *
06	Religious professions	-	exp 3.8	0.00-0.96	exp 3.6	0.00-1.02 *

Age 35-64 years at the beginning of each 5-year follow-up period. Ordered by the social class adjusted SIR.
Reference: economically active population. * Crude and/or social class adjusted SIR significant (p<0.05).

Association study was only 1.46 (95% CI 0.67-2.77), i.e., the barbers not being members of the Association seem to have higher risk of pancreatic cancer than the members, possibly due to worse working conditions.

There was a high risk among Finnish steambath sauna attendants. Although sauna attendants may also be exposed to various chemicals, their high risk may be a clue for studying the role of heat-related factors in cancer causation, e.g., the consequences of excessive use of liquids. Other examples of occupations with warm working conditions and a high risk of pancreatic cancer were flame cutters and cooks.

Table 20. Cancer of the pancreas, women: number of cancer cases (Obs.) and crude and social class adjusted standardized incidence ratios (SIR) with 95% confidence intervals (95% CI) for selected occupational categories in 1971-85

Occupation		Obs.	Crude		Adjusted	
			SIR	95% CI	SIR	95% CI
655	Welders and flame cutters	2	9.41	1.14-34.0	10.4	1.26-37.7 *
681	Lacquerers	3	7.32	1.51-21.4	7.93	1.64-23.2 *
050	University teachers	3	7.92	1.63-23.2	6.92	1.43-20.2 *
843	Sauna attendants etc.	4	3.68	1 00-9.42	3.65	1.00-9.35 *
73	Chemical process/paper making	9	2.07	0.95-3.94	2.30	1.05-4.37 *
570	Post/telecommunications officials	12	2.21	1.14-3.86	1.96	1.01-3.42 *
840	Hairdressers and barbers	11	2.00	1.00-3.58	1.84	0.92-3.29
123	Shop and restaurant cashiers	10	2.01	0.96-3.70	1.80	0.86-3.32
811	Chefs, cooks etc.	18	1.32	0.78-2.08	1.46	0.87-2.31
820	Waiters in restaurants	9	1.32	0.60-2.50	1.42	0.65-2.69
821	Waiters in cafés etc.	11	1.38	0.69-2.47	1.37	0.68-2.44
310	Agricultural workers	17	1.30	0.76-2.08	1.33	0.78-2.13
672	Plywood makers	6	1.18	0.43-2.58	1.31	0.48-2.85
72	Food industry	18	1.17	0.69-1.84	1.28	0.76-2.02
13	Stenographers and typists	10	1.36	0.65-2.51	1.24	0.59-2.28
14/15	Clerical work NOS	70	1.32	1.03-1.67	1.19	0.93-1.50 *
- - -						
60	Textiles	10	0.64	0.31-1.18	0.70	0.33-1.28
830	Caretakers	3	0.41	0.08-1.20	0.45	0.09-1.32
580	Postmen	2	0.30	0.04-1.09	0.32	0.04-1.15

Age 35-64 years at the beginning of each 5-year follow-up period.   Ordered by the social class adjusted SIR.
Reference: economically active population.   * Crude and/or social class adjusted SIR significant ($p<0.05$).

Workers in many high risk occupations are also exposed to solvents, and the Finnish results thus emphasize the importance of solvents as a potential cause of pancreatic cancer to be studied in more detail.

Cancer of the respiratory organs

Nose and nasal sinuses
There was a tendency towards a higher incidence of cancer of the nose and nasal sinuses in lower social classes (fig. 14). The SIRs were elevated, e.g., among men engaged in woodwork, road building and road transport (table 21). However, only the SIR_as for male horticultural managers and service station attendants were significantly elevated in this rare cancer form (149 cases in males and 84 in females).

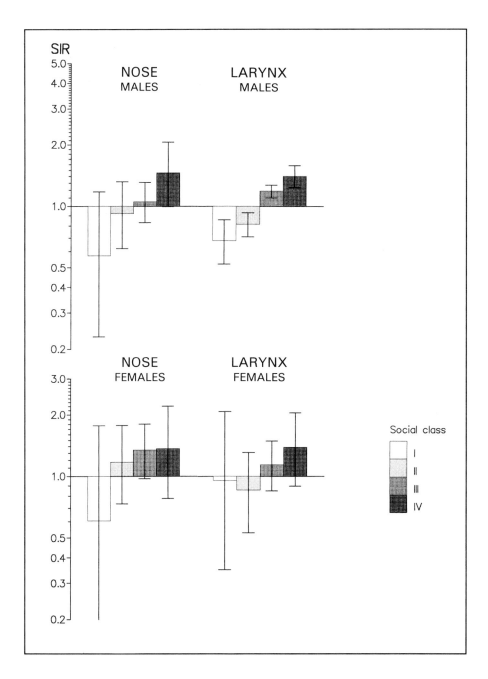

Fig. 14. Standardized incidence ratios (SIR), with 95% confidence intervals, for cancers of the nose and larynx among working-aged Finns in 1971-85, by sex and social class. Reference: economically active population.

Table 21. Cancer of the nose and sinuses, men: number of cancer cases (Obs.) and crude and social class adjusted standardized incidence ratios (SIR) with 95% confidence intervals (95% CI) for selected occupational categories in 1971-85

Occupation		Obs.	Crude		Adjusted	
			SIR	95% CI	SIR	95% CI
303	Horticultural managers	2	16.0	1.93-57.6	17.9	2.17-64.7 *
233	Service station attendants	3	14.4	2.97-42.1	15.2	3.12-44.3 *
698	Roadbuilding hands	6	3.05	1.12-6.65	2.40	0.88-5.22 *
673	Construction carpenters	11	1.89	0.94-3.38	1.85	0.92-3.31
540	Motor-vehicle and tram drivers	11	1.42	0.71-2.54	1.13	0.71-2.56
- - -						
0	Technical, humanistic, etc. work	7	0.57	0.23-1.17	0.75	0.30-1.54
300	Farmers, silviculturists	19	0.70	0.42-1.09	0.68	0.41-1.06
8	Services	3	0.59	0.12-1.72	0.59	0.12-1.71

Age 35-64 years at the beginning of each 5-year follow-up period. Ordered by the social class adjusted SIR.
Reference: economically active population.   * Crude and/or social class adjusted SIR significant (p<0.05).

Comment. The elevated risk of sinonasal cancer among woodworkers is in accordance with earlier studies and is likely to be caused by wood dust [94, 95]. Many of the other occupations with increased risks in the present study involve, e.g., gasoline exhaust. There were no cases of sinonasal cancer in shoe or leather goods manufacture in contrast to some earlier studies showing an excess risk in this occupational category [73]. Neither was this study able to confirm earlier observations of excess risks associated with refining of nickel and some other metals [73].

There has been very little evidence of non-occupational causes of sinonasal cancer. The Finnish social class pattern gives some support to the suggestions of the role of smoking as a causative factor of sinonasal cancer as proposed in several studies [96-98].

Larynx

The incidence of cancer of the larynx among men of social class IV was two times that of men of social class I (fig. 14). In all social classes the incidence was decreasing. Among women the total number of cases was only 104 and the chance variation thus larger than among males (1269 cases). The incidence of laryngeal cancer did not change by period.

Men in some travel and sales occupations and in metal industry experienced high incidences, whereas men in various technical occupations showed low rates (table 22, *appendix table C13*). The SIRs for female shoemakers (SIR_a 22.4, 95% CI 2.71-80.8) and machine shop and steel workers (7.85, 1.62-22.9) were significantly elevated but based on only 2 and 3 observed cases, respectively (*appendix table C14*).

Table 22. Cancer of the larynx, men: number of cancer cases (Obs.) and crude and social class adjusted standardized incidence ratios (SIR) with 95% confidence intervals (95% CI) for selected occupational categories in 1971-85

Occupation		Obs.	Crude		Adjusted		
			SIR	95% CI	SIR	95% CI	
148	Travel agents	2	39.0	4.72-141	48.3	5.84-174	*
612	Furriers	2	8.33	1.01-30.1	8.73	1.06-31.5	*
501	Ship pilots	4	5.04	1.37-12.9	6.31	1.72-16.2	*
560	Port traffic supervisors	3	4.62	0.95-13.5	6.00	1.24-17.5	*
91	Occupation not specified	7	2.72	1.09-5.60	2.56	1.03-5.28	*
08	Artistic and literary professions	9	1.45	0.66-2.75	2.14	0.98-4.06	
651	Fitter-assemblers etc.	14	2.01	1.10-3.37	1.86	1.02-3.12	*
693	Concrete/cement shutterers	10	1.99	0.95-3.66	1.85	0.89-3.41	
653	Sheetmetalworkers	11	1.67	0.83-2.98	1.59	0.79-2.84	
22	Sales representatives	12	1.22	0.63-2.13	1.57	0.81-2.73	
79	Labourers not classified elsewhere	25	1.95	1.26-2.88	1.53	0.99-2.26	*
231	Shop personnel	21	1.64	1.02-2.51	1.52	0.94-2.32	*
11	Corporate administration	26	0.88	0.58-1.29	1.39	0.91-2.04	
540	Motor-vehicle and tram drivers	76	1.32	1.04-1.65	1.36	1.07-1.70	*
73	Chemical process/paper making	18	1.46	0.87-2.31	1.35	0.80-2.13	
650	Turners, machinists	23	1.43	0.91-2.14	1.34	0.85-2.00	
78	Dock and warehouse work	35	1.59	1.11-2.21	1.30	0.90-1.80	*
63	Smelting, metal and foundry work	14	1.36	0.75-2.29	1.29	0.71-2.17	
83	Caretakers and cleaners	24	1.38	0.88-2.05	1.28	0.82-1.91	
680	Painters	17	1.32	0.77-2.11	1.27	0.74-2.03	
659	Machine shop/steelworkers NOS	9	1.34	0.61-2.55	1.27	0.58-2.40	
782	Warehousemen	19	1.42	0.85-2.21	1.12	0.68-1.76	
34	Forestry work	43	1.31	0.95-1.76	1.00	0.73-1.35	
- - -							
300	Farmers, silviculturists	172	0.75	0.64-0.86	0.72	0.62-0.83	*
01	Technical work	16	0.47	0.27-0.76	0.59	0.34-0.96	*
72	Food industry	4	0.51	0.14-1.31	0.49	0.13-1.24	
052	Primary school teachers	2	0.26	0.03-0.95	0.43	0.05-1.55	*
675	Bench carpenters	-	exp 4.3	0.00-0.85	exp 4.3	0.00-0.86	*

Age 35-64 years at the beginning of each 5-year follow-up period. Ordered by the social class adjusted SIR.
Reference: economically active population.   * Crude and/or social class adjusted SIR significant (p<0.05).

Comment. There are earlier observations of an increased risk of laryngeal cancer among persons exposed to asbestos or electrolysis in nickel refining as well as in occupations where extensive smoking and drinking are frequent [73]. Some of the high SIRs in the present study are likely to be accounted for by smoking and drinking (seafareres, artists, sales representatives, managers, painters) [56], but relatively many of the high risk occupations, e.g., in metal processing, may also point to direct occupational factors.

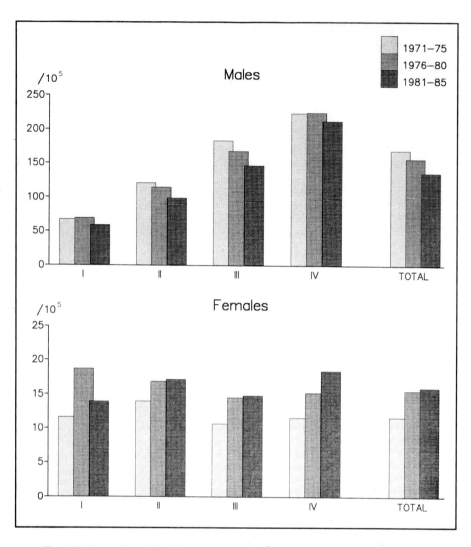

Fig. 15. Age-adjusted incidence rates per 10^5 of lung cancer among working-aged Finns in 1971-85, by sex, social class and period. *N.B. different scales for men and women.*

The social class pattern of laryngeal cancer among men corresponds to the smoking pattern; drinking seems to be less important. The incidence pattern of laryngeal cancer greatly resembles that of lip cancer: the decreasing time trends are most similar, male-female ratios exactly the same (12.2), social class patterns almost identical (somewhat larger variation in lip cancer) and even the absolute incidence rates are almost the same. Hence, the aetiological factors of these two cancers are likely to be correlated, with the exception of the additional factor of outdoor work causally associated with lip cancer only.

Lung

Lung cancer was the most common cancer among Finnish men and made up 28% of all cancer cases in 1971-85. In the age range of this study the 15,613 lung cancer cases constituted an even larger proportion of all cases, i.e., 33%. Among women lung cancer formed some 4% of the cases both in this series and in the remaining age groups.

The incidence of lung cancer in men in the present study series decreased 20% between 1971-75 and 1981-85 (from $169/10^5$ to $136/10^5$; fig. 15). However, the incidence of adenocarcinoma (11% of lung cancer cases of males) increased by one-third, at least partly due to the strong shift from the no histology category to specified histological groups (20% of all male lung cancers). The incidence of lung cancer in social class IV in 1971-75 was 3.3 times that in social class I, and the relative difference increased to 3.6 in 1981-85. The absolute difference between incidence rates of the extreme social classes, $154/10^5$, accounts for 29% of the total cancer incidence of the social class IV in 1981-85 and 100% of the difference in the total cancer incidence between social classes I and IV (cf. chapter Cancer at all sites). The relative social class risk variation was most prominent for birth cohorts born after 1930, and for lung cancers of the squamous cell carcinoma type (fig. 16) or without a histology.

In women the incidence of lung cancer in the 1970s was slightly higher in social classes I-II than in classes III-IV, but in 1981-85 the incidence turned out to be highest in social class IV (fig. 15). The social class pattern also varied by the histological type of lung cancer (fig. 16). The incidence was doubled from 1971-75 to 1981-85 for all main histological types of lung cancer among women, i.e., adenocarcinoma (30% of all cases), squamous cell carcinoma (15%) and small cell carcinoma (16%), but due to the strong decrease (—36%) in the incidence of cases without histology the total incidence of lung cancer increased only 36%.

Standardised incidence ratios (both SIR_c and SIR_a) were above 3.0 among male insulators, cutting/sewing workers, asphalt roofers and reinforced concreters (table 23, *appendix table C15*). High SIRs were also observed in all occupational categories in mining and quarrying and in many occupations involving cement or metal processing. The very lowest SIRs were obtained in occupations with exceptionally clean working conditions but also with low prevalence of smokers. Among the occupations with the highest SIRs in women there were some metal industry occupations, but many office work occupations showed high SIRs as well (table 24, *appendix table C16*). Almost all occupations with significantly low SIRs were associated with teaching or farming.

The highest occupation-specific SIRs were mostly attributable to *squamous cell* type of lung carcinoma. E.g., the SIR_a of squamous cell carcinoma among male reinforced concreters was 5.97 (95% CI 1.63-15.3), among reinforcing iron workers

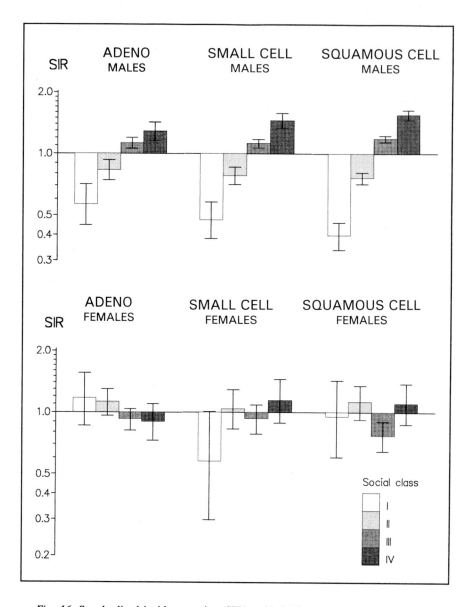

Fig. 16. Standardized incidence ratios (SIR), with 95% confidence intervals, for lung cancer among working-aged Finns in 1971-85, by sex, histologic type and social class. Reference: economically active population.

1.91 (1.09-3.10), blacksmiths 2.31 (1.52-3.36), patternmakers and cutters 2.89 (0.94-6.74), other cutting and sewing workers 4.90 (1.01-14.3) and door-to-door salesmen 2.68 (1.39-4.68). In women especially high SIR_as for squamous cell carcinoma were

Table 23. Cancer of the lung, bronchus and trachea, men: number of cancer cases (Obs.) and crude and social class adjusted standardized incidence ratios (SIR) with 95% confidence intervals (95% CI) for selected occupational categories in 1971-85

Occupation		Obs.	Crude		Adjusted		
			SIR	95% CI	SIR	95% CI	
695	Insulators	62	3.71	2.85-4.76	3.56	2.73-4.56	*
619	Cutting/sewing workers NOS	6	3.48	1.28-7.57	3.45	1.27-7.51	*
694	Asphalt roofers	18	3.50	2.07-5.53	3.25	1.92-5.13	*
086	Performing artists	9	1.56	0.71-2.96	3.18	1.46-6.04	*
691	Reinforced concreters etc.	6	3.32	1.22-7.23	3.09	1.13-6.72	*
200	Wholesalers	13	1.73	0.92-2.95	2.60	1.38-4.44	*
072	Lawyers	8	1.10	0.47-2.16	2.44	1.05-4.80	*
40	Mining and quarrying	99	2.34	1.90-2.85	2.21	1.80-2.69	*
632	Hot-rollers	11	2.36	1.18-4.23	2.19	1.09-3.92	*
080	Sculptors, painters, etc.	9	0.97	0.44-1.84	2.15	0.98-4.08	
41	Deep drilling	13	2.17	1.15-3.70	2.09	1.11-3.57	*
620	Shoemakers and cobblers	22	1.76	1.10-2.67	2.09	1.31-3.16	*
750	Basket and brush makers	9	1.67	0.76-3.17	2.05	0.94-3.89	
49	Mining and quarrying NOS	32	2.18	1.49-3.07	2.01	1.37-2.84	*
634	Blacksmiths	64	1.86	1.43-2.38	1.91	1.47-2.44	*
232	Door-to-door salesmen	24	1.41	0.90-2.10	1.79	1.15-2.67	*
501	Ship pilots	13	1.37	0.73-2.35	1.78	0.95-3.04	
591	Canal/harbour guards, ferrymen	10	1.82	0.87-3.34	1.69	0.81-3.11	
756	Stone cutters	20	1.67	1.02-2.58	1.68	1.03-2.60	*
119	Private sector managers NOS	30	0.72	0.49-1.03	1.63	1.10-2.32	*
692	Reinforcing iron workers	37	1.70	1.20-2.35	1.57	1.10-2.16	*
654	Plumbers	173	1.58	1.35-1.82	1.50	1.29-1.74	*
690	Bricklayers and tile setters	142	1.51	1.27-1.77	1.42	1.20-1.66	*
653	Sheetmetalworkers	112	1.45	1.19-1.73	1.39	1.14-1.66	*
693	Concrete/cement shutterers	89	1.48	1.19-1.82	1.39	1.11-1.71	*
890	Hotel porters	29	1.47	0.99-2.12	1.37	0.92-1.96	
734	Pulp mill workers	60	1.47	1.12-1.90	1.36	1.04-1.76	*
832	Chimney sweeps	23	1.46	0.93-2.19	1.35	0.86-2.03	
772	Construction machinery operators	137	1.35	1.13-1.59	1.33	1.12-1.56	*
680	Painters	210	1.35	1.17-1.54	1.31	1.14-1.50	*
82	Waiters	10	1.07	0.51-1.97	1.30	0.63-2.40	
659	Machine shop/steelworkers NOS	111	1.37	1.13-1.64	1.30	1.07-1.55	*
780	Dockers	93	1.44	1.17-1.77	1.29	1.04-1.58	*
699	Construction workers NOS	40	1.30	0.93-1.77	1.29	0.92-1.76	
673	Construction carpenters	801	1.36	1.27-1.46	1.27	1.19-1.36	*
51	Deck and engine-room crew	39	1.36	0.97-1.86	1.25	0.89-1.71	
79	Labourers not classified elsewhere	277	1.75	1.55-1.96	1.23	1.09-1.38	*
22	Sales representatives	104	0.92	0.76-1.11	1.21	0.99-1.45	
655	Welders and flame cutters	101	1.26	1.02-1.51	1.17	0.95-1.41	*
697	Building hands	495	1.68	1.54-1.84	1.17	1.06-1.27	*
804	Civilian guards	98	1.38	1.12-1.69	1.17	0.95-1.42	*
67	Woodwork	1,117	1.20	1.13-1.27	1.13	1.07-1.20	*
698	Roadbuilding hands	327	1.61	1.44-1.79	1.13	1.01-1.26	*
110	Corporate managers	82	0.49	0.39-0.61	1.09	0.87-1.35	*
111	Technical managers	15	0.48	0.27-0.80	1.09	0.61-1.79	*
34	Forestry work	602	1.54	1.42-1.67	1.07	0.98-1.15	*
- - -							

Table 23 (continued)

Occupation		Obs.	Crude		Adjusted	
			SIR	95% CI	SIR	95% CI
084	Journalists	12	0.49	0.25-0.86	0.99	0.51-1.74 *
004	Mechanical engineers	15	0.42	0.23-0.69	0.94	0.53-1.55 *
096	PR officers	15	0.56	0.31-0.92	0.87	0.49-1.44 *
051	Subject teachers	16	0.38	0.22-0.62	0.86	0.49-1.40 *
90	Military occupations	22	0.53	0.33-0.80	0.86	0.54-1.30 *
01	Technical work	257	0.64	0.56-0.72	0.83	0.73-0.93 *
230	Buyers, office sales staff	27	0.59	0.39-0.86	0.82	0.54-1.19 *
562	Railway traffic supervisors	19	0.57	0.34-0.89	0.81	0.49-1.27 *
027	Consultancy, agriculture	11	0.55	0.28-0.99	0.80	0.40-1.44 *
054	Vocational teachers	27	0.50	0.33-0.72	0.80	0.52-1.16 *
005	Chemotechnical engineers	4	0.34	0.09-0.88	0.78	0.21-1.99 *
300	Farmers, silviculturists	2,355	0.81	0.78-0.84	0.77	0.74-0.80 *
563	Road transport supervisors	11	0.48	0.24-0.86	0.76	0.38-1.36 *
801	Policemen	52	0.58	0.44-0.77	0.76	0.56-0.99 *
671	Timber workers	88	0.77	0.62-0.95	0.73	0.59-0.90 *
002	Electrical engineers	5	0.31	0.10-0.72	0.70	0.23-1.62 *
052	Primary school teachers	26	0.30	0.20-0.44	0.69	0.45-1.00 *
570	Post/telecommunications officials	14	0.52	0.29-0.88	0.68	0.37-1.15 *
55	Transport services	74	0.64	0.50-0.80	0.64	0.50-0.81 *
231	Shop personnel	100	0.68	0.55-0.82	0.64	0.52-0.77 *
550	Railway staff	72	0.63	0.49-0.79	0.63	0.49-0.80 *
53	Engine drivers	34	0.66	0.46-0.92	0.61	0.43-0.86 *
145	Bank clerks	6	0.37	0.14-0.81	0.61	0.22-1.33 *
007	Engineers NOS	2	0.27	0.03-0.97	0.61	0.07-2.19 *
053	Teachers of practical subjects	4	0.32	0.09-0.81	0.56	0.15-1.45 *
050	University teachers	5	0.24	0.08-0.57	0.55	0.18-1.28 *
113	Administrative managers	4	0.22	0.06-0.57	0.50	0.14-1.28 *
800	Firemen	9	0.44	0.20-0.83	0.49	0.22-0.93 *
056	Education officers	2	0.27	0.03-0.99	0.47	0.06-1.70 *
030	Medical doctors	6	0.20	0.07-0.44	0.45	0.17-0.99 *
090	Auditors	1	0.18	0.00-0.99	0.38	0.01-2.14 *
073	Solicitors	1	0.15	0.00-0.85	0.34	0.01-1.90 *
039	Medical workers NOS	3	0.36	0.07-1.04	0.32	0.07-0.95 *
020	Chemists	1	0.13	0.00-0.75	0.30	0.01-1.66 *
000	Architects	1	0.13	0.00-0.71	0.29	0.01-1.61 *
008	Surveyors	1	0.13	0.00-0.71	0.28	0.01-1.59 *
070	Barristers and judges	1	0.10	0.00-0.57	0.23	0.01-1.26 *
060	Clergy and lay preachers	2	0.07	0.01-0.27	0.14	0.02-0.51 *
031	Dentists	-	exp 5.8	0.00-0.64	exp 2.6	0.00-1.43 *
147	Social insurance clerks	-	exp 4.5	0.00-0.81	exp 3.5	0.00-1.06 *
724	Food preservation	-	exp 4.0	0.00-0.93	exp 4.2	0.00-0.87 *

Age 35-64 years at the beginning of each 5-year follow-up period. Ordered by the social class adjusted SIR.
Reference: economically active population.   * Crude and/or social class adjusted SIR significant ($p<0.05$).

Table 24. Cancer of the lung, bronchus and trachea, women: number of cancer cases (Obs.) and crude and social class adjusted standardized incidence ratios (SIR) with 95% confidence intervals (95% CI) for selected occupational categories in 1971-85

Occupation		Obs.	Crude		Adjusted	
			SIR	95% CI	SIR	95% CI
083	Authors	2	9.87	1.19-35.7	8.81	1.07-31.8 *
804	Civilian guards	3	7.45	1.54-21.8	7.84	1.62-22.9 *
129	Book-keeping workers/cashiers NOS	2	8.61	1.04-31.1	7.45	0.90-26.9 *
780	Dockers	6	5.90	2.17-12.8	6.56	2.41-14.3 *
050	University teachers	3	5.08	1.05-14.8	5.38	1.11-15.7 *
084	Journalists	7	3.51	1.41-7.24	3.68	1.48-7.59 *
581	Caretakers/messengers	5	3.35	1.09-7.81	3.62	1.18-8.46 *
650	Turners, machinists	5	3.13	1.02-7.30	3.53	1.15-8.24 *
820	Waiters in restaurants	33	3.13	2.16-4.40	3.41	2.35-4.79 *
110	Corporate managers	5	3.35	1.09-7.81	3.14	1.02-7.33 *
552	Bus/tram services	7	2.52	1.01-5.20	2.86	1.15-5.89 *
697	Building hands	21	3.08	1.91-4.71	2.79	1.72-4.26 *
77	Machinists	11	2.74	1.37-4.91	2.72	1.36-4.87 *
150	Property managers, warehousemen	7	2.88	1.16-5.93	2.54	1.02-5.22 *
70	Printing	12	1.63	0.84-2.85	1.83	0.94-3.19
782	Warehousemen	14	1.89	1.03-3.17	1.77	0.97-2.97 *
130	Private secretaries	12	1.92	0.99-3.35	1.74	0.90-3.04
76	Packing and labelling	27	1.49	0.98-2.17	1.67	1.10-2.43 *
672	Plywood makers	11	1.41	0.71-2.53	1.59	0.79-2.84
121	Office cashiers	11	1.78	0.89-3.18	1.58	0.79-2.83
13	Stenographers and typists	20	1.73	1.06-2.68	1.57	0.96-2.42 *
123	Shop and restaurant cashiers	12	1.55	0.80-2.71	1.39	0.72-2.43
159	Clerical workers NOS	12	1.56	0.80-2.72	1.38	0.71-2.41
810	Housekeepers	12	1.55	0.80-2.70	1.38	0.71-2.40
131	Typists	8	1.52	0.65-2.99	1.37	0.59-2.69
821	Waiters in cafés etc.	17	1.38	0.80-2.21	1.36	0.79-2.18
144	Office clerks	80	1.43	1.14-1.79	1.29	1.02-1.60 *
84	Hygiene and beauty services	14	1.33	0.72-2.22	1.23	0.67-2.06
831	Cleaners	122	1.27	1.06-1.51	1.17	0.98-1.39 *
- - -						
310	Agricultural workers	13	0.68	0.36-1.16	0.69	0.37-1.18
812	Kitchen assistants	15	0.69	0.39-1.14	0.63	0.35-1.03
300	Farmers, silviculturists	36	0.52	0.37-0.72	0.54	0.38-0.75 *
311	Gardeners	4	0.56	0.15-1.44	0.53	0.15-1.37
73	Chemical process/paper making	3	0.46	0.09-1.34	0.52	0.11-1.51
312	Livestock workers	74	0.45	0.35-0.56	0.46	0.36-0.58 *
570	Post/telecommunications officials	4	0.47	0.13-1.20	0.42	0.11-1.08
091	Social workers	2	0.42	0.05-1.52	0.39	0.05-1.42
051	Subject teachers	3	0.33	0.07-0.96	0.35	0.07-1.02 *
052	Primary school teachers	6	0.31	0.11-0.68	0.33	0.12-0.71 *
035	Psychiatric nurses	-	exp 4.1	0.00-0.91	exp 4.5	0.00-0.82 *

Age 35-64 years at the beginning of each 5-year follow-up period.   Ordered by the social class adjusted SIR.
Reference: economically active population.   * Crude and/or social class adjusted SIR significant (p<0.05).

obtained for waitresses in restaurants (4.73, 2.04-9.32) and building hands (4.62, 1.99-9.09).

The excess was mainly accounted for by *small cell carcinoma* in male lawyers (SIR$_a$ 6.63, 1.81-17.0), wholesalers (5.85, 1.90-13.7), performing artists (5.79, 1.19-16.9), ship pilots (3.92, 1.29-9.30), stone cutters (3.10, 1.14-6.75) and in the whole branch of mining and quarrying (2.45, 1.66-3.48).

Adenocarcinoma showed clearly the highest histology-specific SIR$_a$ for male insulators (3.96, 1.81-7.51) and plumbers (1.87, 1.23-2.72).

Comment. The social class pattern of lung cancer incidence in men in 1971-85 corresponds to the earlier noted smoking pattern by social class. Practically all Finnish men who participated in World War II, i.e., those born before the 1930s, practiced smoking. When the dangers of smoking became known in the late 1950s, highly educated men stopped smoking first. In 1968, less than 40% of men with academic professions smoked, whereas the percentage among industrial workers was still above 60% [48]. The relative social class difference in the percentage of young men who started smoking after the Second World War is likely to be even larger, and therefore the social class variation in lung cancer incidence among men born after 1930 is larger than in the older birth cohorts.

Urban women, especially those of higher social classes, were the first women to adopt the habit of smoking. Later on, working-class women also started increasingly to smoke, and today they smoke more than highly educated women. These changes are reflected in the time trend of the social class pattern of lung cancer in women. The male-female ratio of the incidence rates for adenocarcinoma was 3, for small cell carcinoma 8 and for squamous cell carcinoma 15. This, together with the observed social class trends and occupation-specific SIRs, suggests that adenocarcinoma is less dependent on smoking than the others and/or that the inducing period between smoking and onset of cancer is longest for squamous cell carcinoma.

The impact of smoking is so large in relation to lung cancer causation that weaker factors, e.g., occupational ones tend to go unnoticed. Asbestos fibres are regarded as representing an important carcinogenic hazard in the work-place and are probably the most important occupational risk ever identified [73]. Furthermore, in this series of occupations with known asbestos exposure (insulators, concreters, miners, blacksmiths, plumbers, bricklayers, cement shutlerers) also showed high SIRs for lung cancer.

Exposure to steel, nickel, and hexavalent forms of chromium has sometimes been associated with increased lung cancer risk [73]. The hypothesis of metal dust aetiology seems possible in light of the Finnish results, too. However, many workers in the metal industry and machinery may be exposed to asbestos as well. Silica dust has been shown to cause lung cancer in interaction with smoking [99], and stone cutters and miners in the present series also had high SIRs, especially of small cell carcinoma.

The association with occupational exposures seems, in general, to be strongest for squamous cell carcinoma and clearly weakest for adenocarcinoma. The two occupations with the largest excess risk of adenocarcinoma — insulators and plumbers — would deserve a more detailed inspection. E.g., the role of soldering fumes should be studied.

The low risk of engine drivers (SIR_a 0.61) is an example of the fact that asbestos exposure is strongly hazardous only in connection with smoking: until the mid-1960s, all locomotive drivers were exposed to asbestos during their training phase but smoking in the steam engines was difficult and thus rare. The locomotive drivers had an increased risk of mesothelioma but relatively low risk of lung cancer [100]. Even anthophyllite asbestos miners in Finland who have long and high levels of exposure to asbestos have a relatively low lung cancer risk if they do not smoke [101, 102].

Among women, the highest SIRs were much larger than among men. However, the reference incidence among women, i.e., the average incidence among economically active women, is only 9.3% of the reference incidence of men. Thus the age-adjusted lung cancer incidence of female university teachers ($70/10^5$) giving an SIR_c of 5.08 is not very much higher than the incidence among male university teachers ($40/10^5$) corresponding to an SIR_c of 0.24. In populations like Icelanders or Maoris in New Zealand, where the prevalence of smoking among women and men has been similar for a longer time, the incidence of lung cancer is also on the same level [103]. In the present series it seems that occupational categories with similar smoking habits in both sexes also experience a similar lung cancer incidence in men and women.

Passive smoking during working-hours should be regarded as a direct occupational risk factor, since in Finland there was before the 1990s no regulation forbidding smoking in working-rooms. This problem may explain part of the systematically high SIRs of waitresses and women working in offices, although active smoking is likely to be more important.

Primary school teachers, dentists and priests hardly ever smoke at work. They also have very low risks of lung cancer. Hence, the occupation of these workers in a way protects them against lung cancer. Similarly, smoking was generally not accepted among women in the countryside, which is likely to be the main reason for the very low SIRs of women in agricultural occupations.

Mesothelioma

Most of the mesotheliomas are located in the pleura, a small part in the peritoneum. Taking all of them together, there were 130 mesotheliomas among men and 65 among women in the age range of this study. There was a very strong relative increase in the incidence from 1971-75 to 1981-85 (men: from 0.5 to $2.0/10^5$, women: from 0.3 to $0.7/10^5$). The only significant social class-specific SIR was that of men of the first social class (SIR 1.77, 95% CI 1.10-2.71). High occupation-specific SIRs were observed, e.g., among architects, insulators, bakers and painters (table 25). The incidence of mesotheliomas among male farmers was significantly low.

Comment. Knowing the strong association between asbestos exposure and the risk of mesothelioma, one would expect the highest SIRs to be found in social class

Table 25. Mesothelioma: number of cancer cases (Obs.) and crude and social class adjusted standardized incidence ratios (SIR) with 95% confidence intervals (95% CI) for selected occupational categories in 1971-85

Occupation		Obs.	Crude		Adjusted	
			SIR	95% CI	SIR	95% CI
MEN						
099	Humanistic/scientific workers NOS	2	38.7	4.68-140	26.8	3.24-96.8 *
695	Insulators	3	15.1	3.10-44.0	13.7	2.83-40.1 *
000	Architects	2	20.6	2.50-74.5	12.0	1.45-43.3 *
04	Health-care related work	2	12.0	1.46-43.4	10.4	1.26-37.6 *
721	Bakers and pastry chiefs	2	8.65	1.05-31.2	8.28	1.00-29.9 *
68	Painting and lacquering	7	4.23	1.70-8.72	3.99	1.60-8.22 *
- - -						
2	Sales professions	3	0.49	0.10-1.43	0.56	0.12-1.64
300	Farmers, silviculturists	11	0.47	0.24-0.85	0.50	0.25-0.89 *
WOMEN						
6/7	Industrial and construction work	11	1.43	0.71-2.56	1.31	0.66-2.35
- - -						
0	Technical, humanistic, etc. work	2	0.35	0.04-1.26	0.38	0.05-1.39

Age 35-64 years at the beginning of each 5-year follow-up period. Ordered by the social class adjusted SIR.
Reference: economically active population. * Crude and/or social class adjusted SIR significant (p<0.05).

III-IV including blue-collar workers certainly exposed to asbestos. The highest incidence in social class I is thus unexpected. As mesothelioma in Finland is likely to be reimbursed as an occupational disease, the possible past asbestos exposures of mesothelioma patients have been studied in detail. A clear preceding asbestos exposure was found for some 70% of all mesotheliomas, although the current position did not necessarily point to any apparent exposure [104]. White collar patients typically had short-term asbestos exposures in their youth, for instance during their summer jobs in house-building work.

The late effects of increasing asbestos use until its carcinogenic potential was detected will be seen long after the year 2000. Part of the strongly increasing incidence of mesotheliomas may be attributable to a change in the histological terminology.

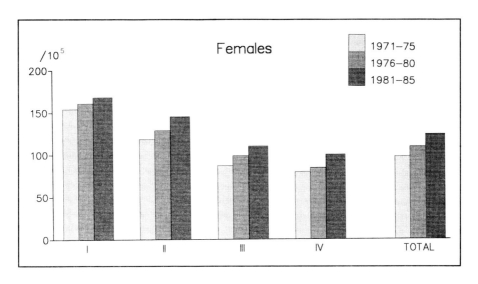

Fig. 17. Age-adjusted incidence rates per 10^5 of breast cancer among working-aged Finnish women, by social class and period.

Cancer of the breast

The 13,782 cases of breast cancer constituted up to 30% of all cancers among women in the present series. The incidence was $162/10^5$ in the highest social class and $87/10^5$ in the lowest one (fig. 17). The incidence grew in all social classes, however in social class I at a slower rate than in the others. The SIR among women of social class I born after 1930 was below 1.3, among the older ones above 1.5.

In women there were 20 three-digit occupational categories out of 311 with an SIR_a significantly (p<0.05) above 1.0 and 11 with an SIR_a significantly below 1.0 (table 26, *appendix table C18*). The incidence was high in various occupations associated with artistic work, design and printing, as well as in various clerical and technical professions. Both crude and social-class adjusted SIRs were significantly below 1.0 in all agricultural occupations except gardening and fur-farm work. Low SIRs were observed also for solicitors, commercial managers, postwomen, painters and lacquerers, launderers and in all occupational categories in glass and ceramic work.

Men had only 47 cases of breast cancer. The SIR patterns by social class (fig. 18) and by the main occupational branches roughly resembled those for women, e.g., the risk was elevated in administrative and clerical work (SIR_c 1.60, 95% CI 0.44-4.09; *appendix table C17*).

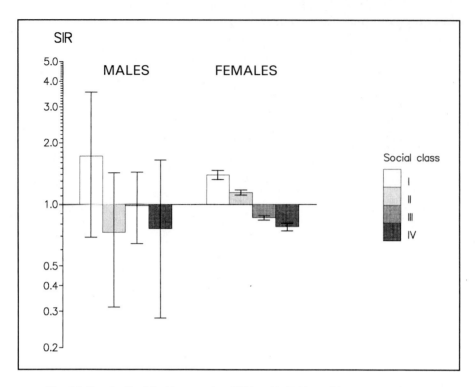

Fig. 18. Standardized incidence ratios (SIR), with 95% confidence intervals, for breast cancer among working-aged Finns in 1971-85, by sex and social class. Reference: economically active population.

Table 26. Cancer of the female breast: number of cancer cases (Obs.) and crude and social class adjusted standardized incidence ratios (SIR) with 95% confidence intervals (95% CI) for selected occupational categories in 1971-85

	Occupation	Obs.	Crude		Adjusted	
			SIR	95% CI	SIR	95% CI
90	Military occupations	3	4.46	0.92-13.0	5.08	1.05-14.9 *
664	Telephone installers and repairmen	4	4.35	1.18-11.1	5.02	1.37-12.9 *
016	Technicians NOS	6	3.61	1.32-7.85	3.01	1.11-6.56 *
081	Commercial artists	5	3.10	1.01-7.24	2.62	0.85-6.11 *
080	Sculptors, painters, etc.	12	3.93	2.03-6.86	2.59	1.34-4.53 *
709	Printing workers NOS	12	1.87	0.97-3.27	2.08	1.07-3.62 *
114	Managers of ideal organizations	6	3.20	1.18-6.97	2.06	0.75-4.47 *
562	Railway traffic supervisors	26	2.56	1.67-3.75	2.02	1.32-2.95 *
754	Photolab. workers	12	1.72	0.89-3.00	1.88	0.97-3.29
80	Watchmen, security guards	10	1.79	0.86-3.28	1.86	0.89-3.41
604	Knitters	32	1.50	1.03-2.12	1.71	1.17-2.42 *
096	PR officers	19	2.21	1.33-3.45	1.69	1.02-2.64 *

Table 26 (continued)

Occupation		Obs.	Crude		Adjusted	
			SIR	95% CI	SIR	95% CI
239	Sales staff NOS	20	1.48	0.91-2.29	1.65	1.01-2.55 *
121	Office cashiers	97	1.96	1.59-2.39	1.60	1.30-1.95 *
027	Consultancy, agriculture	33	1.98	1.37-2.79	1.59	1.09-2.23 *
622	Shoe sewers	31	1.37	0.93-1.94	1.58	1.07-2.24 *
703	Bookbinders	39	1.35	0.96-1.84	1.57	1.11-2.14 *
55	Transport services	36	1.36	0.95-1.88	1.54	1.08-2.13 *
018	Draughtsmen, survey assistants	32	1.81	1.24-2.56	1.52	1.04-2.15 *
615	Patternmakers and cutters	35	1.24	0.87-1.73	1.43	1.00-2.00
085	Industrial designers	11	2.03	1.01-3.64	1.42	0.71-2.53 *
032	Nurses	269	1.66	1.47-1.86	1.38	1.22-1.55 *
000	Architects	7	2.06	0.83-4.25	1.35	0.54-2.77
611	Dressmakers	89	1.48	1.19-1.82	1.33	1.07-1.64 *
041	Physiotherapists	14	1.56	0.85-2.62	1.31	0.72-2.20
055	Preschool teachers	24	1.52	0.98-2.27	1.27	0.81-1.89
10	Public administration	38	1.91	1.35-2.62	1.24	0.88-1.70 *
131	Typists	73	1.47	1.15-1.85	1.22	0.95-1.53 *
086	Performing artists	8	1.73	0.75-3.41	1.21	0.52-2.38
091	Social workers	65	1.58	1.22-2.01	1.20	0.92-1.52 *
038	Institutional children's nurses	51	1.37	1.02-1.80	1.14	0.85-1.51 *
130	Private secretaries	86	1.36	1.09-1.68	1.14	0.91-1.41 *
019	Laboratory assistants	54	1.37	1.03-1.78	1.14	0.85-1.48 *
146	Insurance clerks	34	1.35	0.94-1.89	1.13	0.78-1.58
159	Clerical workers NOS	86	1.39	1.11-1.71	1.13	0.90-1.40 *
053	Teachers of practical subjects	67	1.46	1.13-1.85	1.10	0.85-1.40 *
145	Bank clerks	132	1.31	1.09-1.54	1.09	0.91-1.29 *
051	Subject teachers	154	1.61	1.36-1.87	1.09	0.92-1.27 *
120	Book-keepers, accountants	159	1.33	1.13-1.55	1.08	0.92-1.25 *
034	Midwives	32	1.31	0.90-1.85	1.08	0.74-1.52
031	Dentists	29	1.59	1.07-2.29	1.04	0.70-1.50 *
- - -						
052	Primary school teachers	239	1.47	1.29-1.67	0.97	0.85-1.09 *
300	Farmers, silviculturists	304	0.74	0.66-0.82	0.83	0.74-0.93 *
310	Agricultural workers	107	0.78	0.64-0.94	0.82	0.68-0.99 *
602	Weavers	41	0.71	0.51-0.96	0.78	0.56-1.06 *
672	Plywood makers	41	0.66	0.48-0.90	0.77	0.55-1.04 *
605	Textile finishers/dyers	14	0.65	0.35-1.09	0.75	0.41-1.26
752	Plastics	14	0.65	0.35-1.08	0.75	0.41-1.25
821	Waiters in cafés etc.	78	0.74	0.59-0.93	0.74	0.59-0.93 *
312	Livestock workers	817	0.68	0.64-0.73	0.74	0.69-0.79 *
726	Dairy workers	25	0.62	0.40-0.91	0.72	0.46-1.06 *
751	Industrial rubber products	9	0.57	0.26-1.08	0.66	0.30-1.25
850	Launderers	33	0.57	0.40-0.81	0.65	0.45-0.91 *
580	Postmen	37	0.51	0.36-0.70	0.61	0.43-0.84 *
68	Painting and lacquering	9	0.51	0.23-0.97	0.59	0.27-1.12 *
71	Glass and ceramic work	10	0.43	0.20-0.78	0.49	0.24-0.91 *
220	Commercial travellers, etc.	8	0.59	0.26-1.17	0.49	0.21-0.97 *
650	Turners, machinists	5	0.41	0.13-0.96	0.48	0.15-1.11 *
54	Road transport	6	0.51	0.19-1.12	0.46	0.17-0.99 *
112	Commercial managers	-	exp 3.6	0.00-1.02	exp 5.5	0.00-0.67 *
073	Solicitors	-	exp 3.8	0.00-0.96	exp 5.9	0.00-0.62 *

Age 35-64 years at the beginning of each 5-year follow-up period. Ordered by the social class adjusted SIR.
Reference: Economically active population.   * Crude and/or social class adjusted SIR significant (p<0.05).

Comment. The most important risk factors of breast cancer are known to be hormonal and connected with reproductive behaviour. The age at menarche (lowest in high social classes) and the age at menopause (highest in high social classes) fit with the observed social class pattern of breast cancer risk (almost two-fold incidence in social class I compared to that of social class IV) whereas there is relatively little difference between social classes in the age of first birth or in the average number of children [105].

Consumption of animal fat is shown to increase the risk of breast cancer [106]. In earlier decades wealthy persons consumed more meat and animal fat than poor ones; the lower social classes increased their consumption later. This is in accordance with social class variation being especially large in women born before 1930, and also with the slower increase of breast cancer incidence in social class I than in the other classes. The similarities between the risk patterns of men and women — if not just chance findings for men — also speak for a role of non-hormonal factors, such as dietary ones, as a component in the aetiology of breast cancer.

There is some evidence that physical exercise may protect against breast cancer, especially in premenopausal age [107, 108]. Work in the low-risk occupations (painters, postwomen, launderers, rubber product workers, waitresses in cafés, housekeeping workers and workers in agriculture) typically include a lot of physical activity, and only in farming does the number of children exceed the Finnish average [57]. The low risks which appear even after adjustment for social class suggest that physically active work may protect against breast cancer. The list of low-risk occupations includes many occupations with exposures to solvents and other hazardous agents and thus confirms the earlier impression that occupational chemicals are not associated with an increased risk of breast cancer.

Many of the occupations with moderately elevated risk of breast cancer were typical sedentary occupations, including almost all administrative and clerical professions. The highest SIR_a of all (5.08) was obtained in women in military occupations. Telephone installers, technicians and security guards also had high SIRs. Women in these traditionally "male" occupations are not the most typical multichild family mothers [57], i.e., the reproductive factors are likely to increase their risk of breast cancer. Similar reasons may be also behind the high SIRs of women in various artistic jobs (sculptors and painters, commercial artists, architects, performing artists) and managerial occupations: children do not suit the careers of women in these occupations [57].

Ionizing radiation may increase the risk of breast cancer [109, 110]. Nurses had an SIR_c of 1.66, significantly higher than that of auxiliary nurses (0.92). Whether part of this excess is attributable to the X-ray nurses cannot be decided on the basis of occupational classification of the present study series.

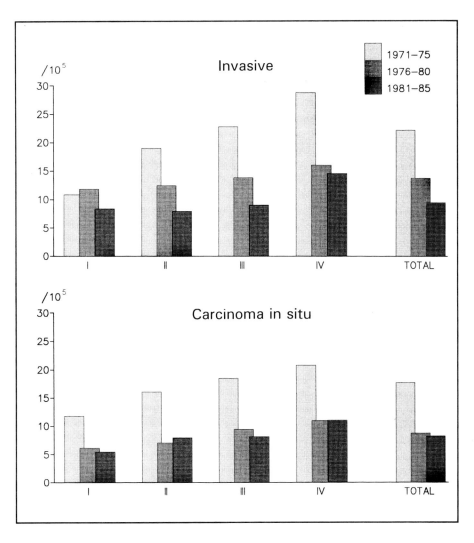

Fig. 19. Age-adjusted incidence rates per 10^5 of invasive and carcinoma in situ cancer of the cervix uteri among working-aged Finnish women, by social class and period.

Cancer of the female genital organs

Cervix uteri

The incidence of invasive cervical cancer in the age-groups of the study series decreased by one-third between 1971-75 and 1981-85 (fig. 19). This decrease was strongest in social classes II and III which meant that during the 15-year observation period the differences between social classes I-III almost disappeared. In the 1980s the

Table 27. Invasive cancer of the cervix uteri: number of cancer cases (Obs.) and crude and social class adjusted standardized incidence ratios (SIR) with 95% confidence intervals (95% CI) for selected occupational categories in 1971-85

Occupation		Obs.	Crude		Adjusted	
			SIR	95% CI	SIR	95% CI
818	Hotel/restaurant manageresses	5	3.87	1.26-9.03	4.57	1.48-10.7 *
54	Road transport	5	3.43	1.12-8.01	3.83	1.24-8.93 *
679	Woodworkers NOS	5	3.43	1.11-8.00	3.35	1.09-7.81 *
820	Waiters in restaurants	24	2.19	1.41-3.26	2.24	1.44-3.34 *
774	Greasers	7	2.94	1.18-6.07	2.20	0.89-4.54 *
611	Dressmakers	15	1.76	0.99-2.91	1.96	1.09-3.23 *
672	Plywood makers	15	1.91	1.07-3.15	1.89	1.06-3.12 *
821	Waiters in cafés etc.	19	1.48	0.89-2.31	1.52	0.91-2.37
75	Industrial work NOS	18	1.50	0.89-2.37	1.49	0.88-2.36
760	Packers and labellers	28	1.50	1.00-2.17	1.49	0.99-2.15
130	Private secretaries	9	1.28	0.58-2.43	1.48	0.68-2.81
84	Hygiene and beauty services	14	1.28	0.70-2.15	1.38	0.75-2.31
69	Construction work NOS	14	1.74	0.95-2.92	1.31	0.72-2.19
83	Caretakers and cleaners	153	1.44	1.22-1.67	1.12	0.95-1.30 *
05	Teaching	22	0.51	0.32-0.78	0.88	0.55-1.33 *
03	Medical work and nursing	44	0.71	0.51-0.95	0.79	0.57-1.06 *
312	Livestock workers	109	0.67	0.55-0.80	0.64	0.53-0.77 *
20	Wholesale and retail dealers	8	0.49	0.21-0.96	0.57	0.25-1.13 *
310	Agricultural workers	6	0.32	0.12-0.69	0.31	0.11-0.67 *

Age 35-64 years at the beginning of each 5-year follow-up period. Ordered by the social class adjusted SIR. Reference: economically active population.   * Crude and/or social class adjusted SIR significant (p<0.05).

social class IV showed a more than 1.5-fold incidence compared to the three higher ones. The highest occupation-specific SIRs were observed among women working in hotels and restaurants, road transport and in miscellaneous industrial occupations (table 27, *appendix table C19*). Among agricultural workers the SIR_a was only 0.31, and it was low also, e.g., among livestock workers, nurses and teachers.

Carcinoma in situ lesions of the cervix uteri are also registered by the Finnish Cancer Registry, although they not included in the regular cancer statistics. Among women of this study series, 1,374 in situ carcinomas of the cervix were diagnosed. The incidence decreased even more than that of the invasive cancer; the decrease from the period 1971-75 to 1976-80 was 54% in all social classes. All the time women of the lowest social class had about a two-fold incidence of in situ carcinoma compared to the rate of the highest class. The relative social class variation in incidence was smallest in the age-group 45-49 years (fig. 20).

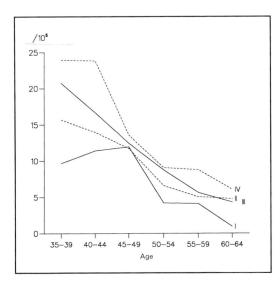

Fig. 20. Incidence of carcinoma in situ among Finnish women in 1971-85, by social class and age.

High occupation-specific SIRs for in situ carcinoma of the cervix uteri were obtained, e.g., among performing artists, chemical process workers, building hands and waitresses (table 28). Nurses, teachers and livestock workers had significantly low SIRs.

Comment. In Finland there has been a nation-wide screening programme since the mid-1960s aiming at detecting precancerous lesions of cervical cancer. Every woman is invited to a free-of-charge Pap-smear test at least at the ages of 35, 40, 45 and 50. This screening accounts for a great deal of the reduction in the incidence [111]. It is also known that in recent years women in the highest and lowest social classes do participate in the organised screening less frequently than women of the middle classes [112, 113]. Although wealthy women compensate the nonparticipation by more frequent private smears, the effect of this nonsystematic testing seems not to be comparable with that of the organised programme.

Sexual habits, especially human papillomavirus infections associated with the number of sexual partners, are a well-established risk factor in cervical cancer, whereas direct occupational exposures are not [73, 114]. Smoking may play some role in the aetiology of cervical cancer. The list of occupations with the highest risks of cervical cancer is headed by many of those which — at least in theory — typically allow frequent sexual partners. A number of the very low SIRs belong to occupations in which the women are traditionally thought to be strictly monogamous or are well informed about the risk factors in cervical cancer. However, only anecdotal evidence (but no facts) exists about the typical sexual behaviour of persons in various occupations; thus no scientific conclusions can be drawn on the association between the number of sexual partners and risk of cervical cancer. The elevated risks of woodworkers, plywood makers, dressmakers and spinners are not likely to be

Table 28. Carcinoma in situ of the cervix uteri: number of cancer cases (Obs.) and crude and social class adjusted standardized incidence ratios (SIR) with 95% confidence intervals (95% CI) for selected occupational categories in 1971-85

Occupation		Obs.	Crude		Adjusted	
			SIR	95% CI	SIR	95% CI
086	Performing artists	4	7.07	1.93-18.1	11.6	3.16-29.7 *
624	Sole fitters etc.	3	12.1	2.50-35.5	11.3	2.33-33.0 *
64	Precision mechanical work	3	5.33	1.10-15.6	5.13	1.06-15.0 *
573	Telegraphists	4	3.85	1.05-9.85	4.55	1.24-11.6 *
739	Chemical process workers NOS	6	3.81	1.40-8.30	3.53	1.30-7.68 *
659	Machine shop/steelworkers NOS	14	3.61	1.98-6.06	3.35	1.83-5.62 *
606	Textile quality controllers	5	3.59	1.17-8.39	3.31	1.07-7.72 *
820	Waiters in restaurants	24	2.40	1.54-3.58	2.27	1.45-3.38 *
69	Construction work NOS	15	2.62	1.47-4.33	2.12	1.19-3.50 *
821	Waiters in cafés etc.	23	1.97	1.25-2.96	1.93	1.22-2.90 *
201	Retailers	16	1.56	0.89-2.54	1.87	1.07-3.03 *
76	Packing and labelling	32	1.96	1.34-2.76	1.79	1.23-2.53 *
159	Clerical workers NOS	10	1.52	0.73-2.80	1.79	0.86-3.30
840	Hairdressers and barbers	12	1.63	0.84-2.85	1.78	0.92-3.10
75	Industrial work NOS	15	1.46	0.82-2.41	1.36	0.76-2.24
831	Cleaners	92	1.51	1.22-1.85	1.20	0.97-1.47 *
- - -						
052	Primary school teachers	7	0.39	0.16-0.80	0.72	0.29-1.49 *
300	Farmers, silviculturists	22	0.74	0.46-1.11	0.67	0.42-1.02
051	Subject teachers	4	0.33	0.09-0.83	0.64	0.17-1.63 *
310	Agricultural workers	8	0.63	0.27-1.24	0.61	0.26-1.19
036	Auxiliary nurses	17	0.61	0.36-0.98	0.56	0.33-0.90 *
312	Livestock workers	59	0.51	0.39-0.66	0.48	0.37-0.62 *
032	Nurses	5	0.24	0.08-0.57	0.29	0.09-0.67 *

Age 35-64 years at the beginning of each 5-year follow-up period. Ordered by the social class adjusted SIR. Reference: economically active population. * Crude and/or social class adjusted SIR significant (p<0.05).

attributable to sexual habits or smoking (only woodworkers experienced an elevated risk of lung cancer). It is feasible — in contrast to what has been concluded from earlier studies — that occupational exposures in the wood and textile industries could increase the risk of cervical cancer.

The substantial decrease in the incidence of in situ carcinoma of the cervix uteri in the mid-1970s is partly due to the high proportion of screen-detected cases associated with the increasing screening activity up to the early 1970s. There was also a shift in the terminology of cervical lesions from carcinoma in situ to *dysplasia gravis* which may have caused an artificial decrease in the incidence of in situ cancers. The lack of social class differences around the age of 50 is likely to be associated with diagnostic activity among women. In young and old ages wealthy women tend to visit their gynaecologists more regularly than the poorer ones, whereas at the age of menopause everybody will be examined.

There were great similarities in the occupational SIRs for in situ carcinomas and invasive cancer of the cervix. It seems that the aetiological background of the in situ lesions is not much different from that of invasive cancer.

Corpus uteri

Cancer of the corpus uteri — the second most common cancer among women in the study series with 3,842 cases — was in 1971-75 a cancer of affluence with a 64% higher incidence in social class I than in class IV (fig. 21). By 1985 this difference had almost disappeared. The social class difference diminished towards younger birth cohorts (fig. 22). Among women born in the 1910s the incidence ratio between social classes I and IV in 1981-85 was still 2.5.

There was relatively little occupational variation in the SIRs of endometrial cancer. SIRs above 2.0 were obtained among biologists, wooden surface finishers, shoe sewers, journalists and cashiers (table 29, *appendix table C20*). In electrical work the risk of endometrial cancer seemed to be very small.

Comment. Despite the large number of endometrial cancer cases in the study series the extreme SIRs were mainly based on small numbers of cases. Most of the occupations with a high SIR_a are likely to have nothing to do with hazardous agents in the work environment. Similar occupations were found at both ends of the list, e.g., subject teachers (SIR_a 1.27) vs. primary school teachers (0.69), or nurses (1.27) vs. psychiatric nurses (0.47). All this speaks — in agreement with earlier observations — for the interpretation that the occupational SIR pattern seen for endometrial cancer is due to confounding or merely a collection of chance findings. Many low-risk occupations deal with taking care of small children (midwives, children's nurses, primary school teachers). One may speculate whether there is a selection of women with a special "child-lowing" hormonal function to these occupations. How electrical work or operating telephone/switchboard could be associated with a low risk of endometrial cancer, remains unclear.

The strong social class variation in the incidence of endometrial cancer among women born before 1920 but not among the later-born ones needs more detailed study. The explanation may lay, e.g., in social class differences in reproductive behaviour, or it may be related to hormonal aspects at menopause whose effects to the cancer incidence do not come up before the age of about 60. It is known that for instance estrogen replacement therapy at menopause increases the risk of endometrial cancer [115, 116].

The prevalence of women who have undergone a hysterectomy in Finland in 1989 was about 20% in all age-groups between 50 and 64, and in women with only primary school education the prevalence was 6-9 percent units larger than among women with a higher educational status [117]. During the period of the present study the percentages were on average one-third lower, but still the incidence rates of endometrial cancer presented here would be some 10% higher and the social class differences slightly smaller if they would have been calculated per corpus-years

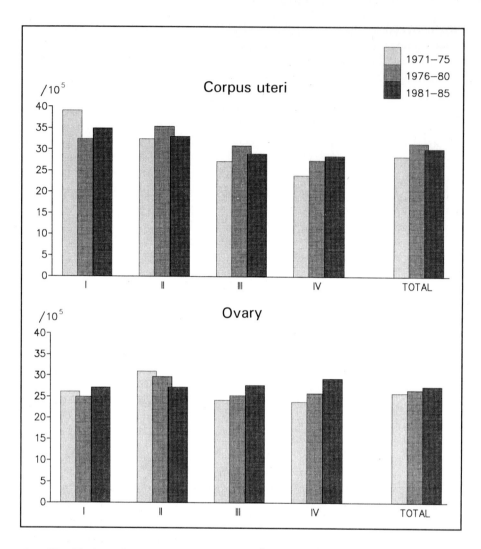

Fig. 21. Age-adjusted incidence rates per 10^5 of cancers of the corpus uteri and ovary among working-aged Finnish women in 1971-85, by social class and period.

instead of women-years. (Correspondingly, the social class variation for cervical cancer should actually be even larger than presented in the previous chapter.)

Ovary

The incidence of ovarian cancer was almost the same in all social classes (fig. 21). There was a slight decrease in the incidence in social class II and an increase in classes III and IV during the study period, but no consistent trend by birth cohort or

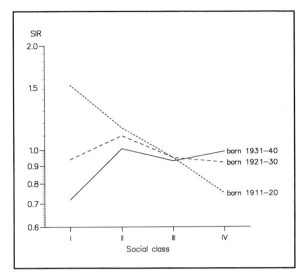

Fig. 22. Standardized incidence ratios (SIR) of endometrial cancer among Finnish women in 1971-85, by birth cohort and social class. Reference: economically active population.

age. All occupations in the branch of printing and many occupations dealing with chemicals showed relatively high SIRs (table 30, *appendix table C21*). Only woodworkers and livestock workers had significantly low SIRs.

Comment. Although ovarian cancer is supposed to have a similar hormonal aetiology as breast cancer or endometrial cancer, the socioeconomic pattern is somewhat different. On the other hand, there were relatively many occupations with low SIRs of both endometrial and ovarian cancers (institutional children's nurses, midwives, pharmacists, launderers, electrical workers, livestock workers), which speaks for a similar aetiology. There were also numerous high-risk occupations such as bookbinders, patternmakers and cutters, insurance clerks, etc. common in endometrial and ovarian cancers. The proportion of women with one or both ovaries removed in the present series is some 5% [117], i.e., the effect of oophorectomies is small.

There are almost no earlier observations of occupational risk factors for ovarian cancer. However, the high prevalence of occupations with apparent chemical exposure on the list of high-risk occupations of the present study gives a strong hint that chemical agents, possibly solvents, may have a role in the causation of ovarian cancer. Paper dust and glues exist commonly in many of the high-risk occupations, and rubber and plastics workers also seem to have some excess cases of ovarian cancer.

Other female genitals

The incidence of cancers of other female genitals did not vary much by social class. However, social class patterns for the two main specific sites within this rubric

Table 29. Cancer of the corpus uteri: number of cancer cases (Obs.) and crude and social class adjusted standardized incidence ratios (SIR) with 95% confidence intervals (95% CI) for selected occupational categories in 1971-85

Occupation		Obs.	Crude		Adjusted		
			SIR	95% CI	SIR	95% CI	
026	Biologists	2	15.7	1.90-56.7	14.2	1.72-51.3	*
678	Wooden surface finishers	6	3.04	1.12-6.62	3.24	1.19-7.06	*
622	Shoe sewers	11	1.88	0.94-3.37	2.01	1.00-3.59	*
084	Journalists	10	2.32	1.11-4.27	2.00	0.96-3.67	*
121	Office cashiers	27	2.07	1.37-3.02	1.75	1.15-2.54	*
774	Greasers	7	1.38	0.56-2.85	1.59	0.64-3.27	
146	Insurance clerks	10	1.82	0.87-3.35	1.58	0.76-2.91	
06	Religious professions	8	1.77	0.76-3.49	1.51	0.65-2.98	
145	Bank clerks	34	1.64	1.13-2.29	1.44	1.00-2.01	*
131	Typists	19	1.64	0.99-2.56	1.41	0.85-2.20	
615	Patternmakers and cutters	9	1.34	0.61-2.54	1.41	0.64-2.67	
054	Vocational teachers	12	1.63	0.84-2.84	1.39	0.72-2.43	
703	Bookbinders	10	1.31	0.63-2.40	1.39	0.66-2.55	
814	Communal home-help services	14	1.30	0.71-2.19	1.34	0.73-2.25	
616	Garment workers	59	1.25	0.95-1.61	1.32	1.01-1.70	*
032	Nurses	52	1.48	1.11-1.94	1.27	0.95-1.67	*
051	Subject teachers	28	1.37	0.91-1.98	1.27	0.84-1.83	
031	Dentists	7	1.53	0.61-3.15	1.16	0.47-2.39	
- - -							
831	Cleaners	149	0.77	0.65-0.89	0.91	0.77-1.07	*
036	Auxiliary nurses	46	0.82	0.60-1.09	0.86	0.63-1.15	
312	Livestock workers	282	0.83	0.73-0.93	0.86	0.76-0.97	*
310	Agricultural workers	32	0.82	0.56-1.16	0.84	0.57-1.19	
58	Postal services/couriers	17	0.73	0.42-1.16	0.81	0.47-1.30	
052	Primary school teachers	34	0.82	0.57-1.15	0.69	0.48-0.97	*
571	Telephone operators	11	0.72	0.36-1.29	0.61	0.30-1.09	
034	Midwives	4	0.66	0.18-1.69	0.56	0.15-1.45	
035	Psychiatric nurses	5	0.55	0.18-1.29	0.47	0.15-1.10	
038	Institutional children's nurses	4	0.50	0.14-1.28	0.44	0.12-1.12	
572	Switchboard operators	3	0.47	0.10-1.36	0.40	0.08-1.16	
71	Glass and ceramic work	2	0.31	0.04-1.11	0.33	0.04-1.19	
66	Electrical work	2	0.25	0.03-0.91	0.26	0.03-0.95	*

Age 35-64 years at the beginning of each 5-year follow-up period. Ordered by the social class adjusted SIR. Reference: economically active population. * Crude and/or social class adjusted SIR significant (p<0.05).

differed: the incidence of cancer of the *vulva* (274 cases) in social class II was somewhat higher than in the others, whereas cancer of the *vagina* (106 cases) showed a tendency towards higher incidence rates in the lower social classes (fig. 23). The incidence of cancer of the vagina was especially high among women of the lowest social class born in the 1920s (combined SIR 1.98, 95% CI 1.22-3.02).

Table 30. Cancer of the ovary: number of cancer cases (Obs.) and crude and social class adjusted standardized incidence ratios (SIR) with 95% confidence intervals (95% CI) for selected occupational categories in 1971-85

Occupation		Obs.	Crude		Adjusted	
			SIR	95% CI	SIR	95% CI
319	Agricultural workers NOS	3	9.68	2.00-28.3	10.3	2.11-30.0 *
702	Lithographers	3	5.31	1.09-15.5	5.44	1.12-15.9 *
621	Shoe cutters etc.	4	3.59	0.98-9.20	3.71	1.01-9.50 *
700	Typographers etc.	8	3.19	1.38-6.29	3.30	1.42-6.50 *
709	Printing workers NOS	5	3.19	1.04-7.45	3.26	1.06-7.62 *
751	Industrial rubber products	9	2.33	1.06-4.42	2.41	1.10-4.57 *
615	Patternmakers and cutters	11	1.69	0.84-3.03	1.73	0.87-3.10
146	Insurance clerks	10	1.79	0.86-3.29	1.69	0.81-3.11
73	Chemical process/paper making	20	1.62	0.99-2.50	1.68	1.03-2.59 *
121	Office cashiers	21	1.75	1.08-2.67	1.61	0.99-2.45 *
019	Laboratory assistants	15	1.68	0.94-2.77	1.58	0.89-2.61
580	Postmen	27	1.48	0.97-2.15	1.55	1.02-2.25 *
605	Textile finishers/dyers	8	1.49	0.64-2.94	1.55	0.67-3.04
840	Hairdressers and barbers	27	1.64	1.08-2.39	1.54	1.01-2.24 *
703	Bookbinders	10	1.42	0.68-2.61	1.47	0.70-2.70
092	Librarians, museum officials	10	1.59	0.76-2.92	1.46	0.70-2.68
752	Plastics	7	1.35	0.54-2.79	1.39	0.56-2.86
811	Chefs, cooks etc.	48	1.30	0.96-1.72	1.35	0.99-1.79
120	Book-keepers, accountants	42	1.46	1.05-1.97	1.34	0.97-1.81 *
571	Telephone operators	20	1.44	0.88-2.22	1.32	0.80-2.03
76	Packing and labelling	45	1.25	0.91-1.67	1.29	0.94-1.73
- - -						
72	Food industry	35	0.77	0.54-1.07	0.80	0.55-1.11
850	Launderers	11	0.76	0.38-1.35	0.79	0.39-1.41
032	Nurses	29	0.81	0.54-1.16	0.77	0.51-1.10
312	Livestock workers	222	0.73	0.64-0.83	0.75	0.65-0.85 *
66	Electrical work	5	0.65	0.21-1.51	0.66	0.22-1.55
038	Institutional children's nurses	5	0.61	0.20-1.43	0.59	0.19-1.37
04	Health-care related work	10	0.61	0.29-1.11	0.56	0.27-1.03
67	Woodwork	17	0.53	0.31-0.84	0.54	0.32-0.87 *

Age 35-64 years at the beginning of each 5-year follow-up period. Ordered by the social class adjusted SIR.
Reference: economically active population. * Crude and/or social class adjusted SIR significant (p<0.05).

Women in "health care related work" (including mainly pharmacists) had an SIR$_a$ of 4.28 (95% CI 1.19-8.54) for cancer of the vulva, physiotherapists even 13.6 (1.64-49.0). Building hands had an SIR$_a$ of 3.46 (1.12-8.54). The lowest SIRs among occupations with at least five expected cases were those of teachers (SIR$_a$ 0.23, 0.01-1.26), women in medical work and nursing (0.63, 0.21-1.48) and women in housekeeping and domestic work (0.64, 0.24-1.40).

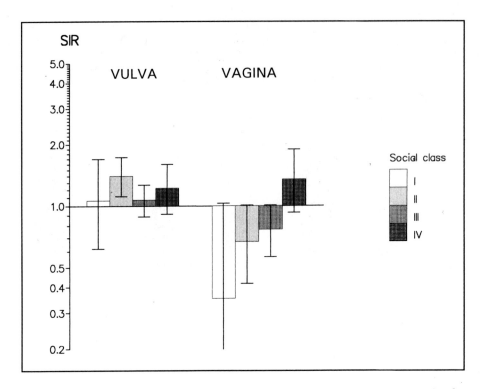

Fig. 23. Standardized incidence ratios (SIR), with 95% confidence intervals, for cancers of the vulva and vagina among working-aged Finnish women in 1971-85, by social class. Reference: economically active population.

Kitchen assistants had a significantly high SIR_c (3.59, 95% CI 1.16-8.37) for cancer of the vagina which somewhat diminished after adjusting for the social class (SIR_a 2.73, 0.89-6.37). The SIR_a was lowest among women in farming and animal husbandry (SIR_a 0.56, 0.22-1.14).

Comment. Knowledge about the risk factors of cancers of the "other female genitals" is limited. Cancers of the vulva and vagina showed different social class patterns, vaginal cancer being associated with low social class. The relative risk of vaginal cancer was highest among women of the lowest social class who were around 20 years of age at the time of World War II. There is no data, e.g., about the sexual behaviour of these young women during the wartime. The small numbers of cases did not allow proper analyses by occupation, but the low-risk occupations suggest that a high hygienic standard may be protective against cancer of the vulva.

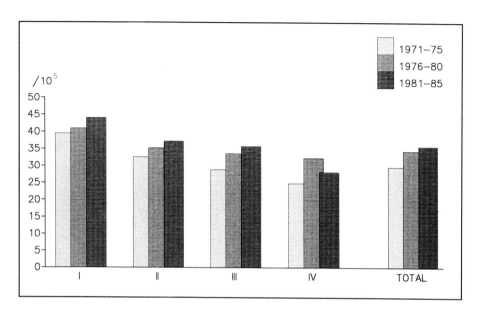

Fig. 24. Age-adjusted incidence rates per 10^5 of cancer of the prostate among working-aged Finnish men in 1971-85, by social class and period.

Cancer of male genital organs

Prostate

Because of the exceptionally high mean age of patients at the diagnosis of cancer of the prostate (in Finland 72 years) and the relatively low maximal age limit of the present study (69 years at the end of each 5-year observation period), a major part of the cases of prostatic cancer were not included in the study. Still, the number of included cases (3,270) was the third largest of all sites among men. The incidence of prostatic cancer in this age range was increasing during the study period, and in all periods and all birth cohorts the incidence was largest among men of the highest social classes (fig. 24).

The list of high-risk occupations included occupations with exposures to various possibly hazardous agents but also many technical, clerical and managerial professions (table 31, *appendix table C22*). The only SIR_a significantly below 1.0 was that of forestry workers. Low SIRs were also obtained, e.g., among physicians and food industry workers.

Comment. The variation in the incidence of prostatic cancer has often been explained by differences in the diagnostic activity, i.e., frequency of thin-needle biopsies. This kind of screening artefact is usually connected with cancer of very old men, but it may also have something to do with the higher incidence among high

Table 31. Cancer of the prostate: number of cancer cases (Obs.) and crude and social class adjusted standardized incidence ratios (SIR) with 95% confidence intervals (95% CI) for selected occupational categories in 1971-85

Occupation		Obs.	Crude		Adjusted		
			SIR	95% CI	SIR	95% CI	
121	Office cashiers	4	5.74	1.56-14.7	5.53	1.51-14.2	*
631	Hardeners, temperers, etc.	3	5.19	1.07-15.2	5.27	1.09-15.4	*
621	Shoe cutters etc.	4	4.57	1.24-11.7	4.64	1.26-11.9	*
311	Gardeners	10	1.89	0.91-3.48	2.19	1.05-4.02	*
60	Textiles	18	2.00	1.18-3.16	2.02	1.20-3.19	*
563	Road transport supervisors	11	2.12	1.06-3.80	1.92	0.96-3.43	*
699	Construction workers NOS	12	1.76	0.91-3.07	1.76	0.91-3.07	
665	Linemen	9	1.63	0.74-3.09	1.65	0.75-3.13	
119	Private sector managers NOS	18	1.93	1.14-3.04	1.58	0.94-2.50	*
04	Health-care related work	8	1.74	0.75-3.44	1.56	0.67-3.08	
500	Ship's masters and mates	9	1.77	0.81-3.35	1.54	0.71-2.93	
674	Boatbuilders etc.	8	1.54	0.67-3.04	1.54	0.67-3.04	
210	Insurance salesmen	9	1.59	0.73-3.01	1.52	0.70-2.89	
70	Printing	18	1.50	0.89-2.37	1.52	0.90-2.41	
71	Glass and ceramic work	10	1.51	0.72-2.77	1.52	0.73-2.80	
655	Welders and flame cutters	23	1.48	0.94-2.22	1.49	0.95-2.24	
739	Chemical process workers NOS	8	1.43	0.62-2.81	1.44	0.62-2.84	
672	Plywood makers	9	1.38	0.63-2.63	1.40	0.64-2.66	
001	Civil engineers	8	1.69	0.73-3.34	1.39	0.60-2.74	
013	Mechanical technicians	30	1.34	0.90-1.91	1.30	0.87-1.85	
07	Legal professions	13	1.55	0.83-2.65	1.28	0.68-2.20	
10	Public administration	26	1.54	1.01-2.26	1.26	0.82-1.85	*
80	Watchmen, security guards	62	1.22	0.94-1.57	1.22	0.93-1.56	
90	Military occupations	10	1.35	0.65-2.49	1.20	0.58-2.21	
- - -							
698	Roadbuilding hands	36	0.74	0.52-1.02	0.85	0.60-1.18	
34	Forestry work	47	0.57	0.42-0.76	0.66	0.48-0.88	*
72	Food industry	12	0.58	0.30-1.02	0.59	0.30-1.03	
030	Medical doctors	3	0.46	0.09-1.35	0.38	0.08-1.10	
562	Railway traffic supervisors	3	0.39	0.08-1.15	0.36	0.07-1.05	

Age 35-64 years at the beginning of each 5-year follow-up period. Ordered by the social class adjusted SIR. Reference: economically active population. * Crude and/or social class adjusted SIR significant (p<0.05).

social class men of the present study series. On other hand, medical doctors had a very low risk of prostatic cancer.

Cadmium is virtually the only occupational agent which has been connected with prostatic cancer [118]. Some of the workers in high incidence occupations (hardeners, glass and ceramic workers, welders) may be exposed to cadmium but also to numerous other chemicals. The results of the present study suggest that occupational factors

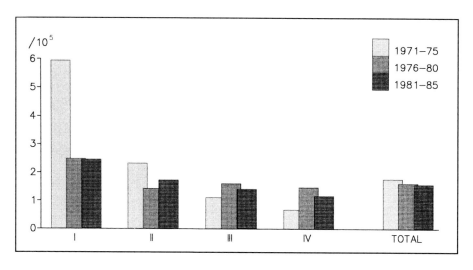

Fig. 25. Age-adjusted incidence rates per 10^5 of testicular cancer among working-aged Finnish men in 1971-85, by social class and period.

included, e.g., in many industrial occupations and gardening may have a role in the causation of prostatic cancer in the ages below 70.

Testis

The incidence of testicular cancer slightly decreased with time. In 1971-75, the age-adjusted incidence in social class I was 11-fold compared to that of class IV, but ten years later only two-fold (fig. 25). The highest birth cohort-specific SIRs were observed in the 1970s among men of social class I born in 1916-20 (SIR 6.36, 95% CI 2.56-13.1). The age trend for testicular cancer — decreasing incidence by age from 35-39 years onwards — is unique among all invasive cancers included in this study. There was only one occupation with more than one observed case and both SIR_c and SIR_a significantly above 1.0, namely university teachers: 3 cases, SIR_c 9.43 (2.57-24.1), SIR_a 4.99 (1.36-12.8).

Comment. The reason for the extreme social class difference in the incidence of testicular cancer in the early 1970s and the diminishing of the difference after that is unknown. Once again, one could speculate whether some exposure associated with World War II may play a role: the incidence was highest among men who were around 20 years of age during the war and were exposed to the special conditions (e.g., exceptional cold) at the front.

Risk factors like tight clothing, bicycling, hormonal disturbances and especially chryptorchidism have been suggested to be associated with testicular cancer [73, 119]. Lately, the quality of semen has been suspected to be associated with the incidence of testicular cancer. It is known that, e.g., Danish men have a lower sperm count than Finns, and they have about a fivefold incidence of testicular cancer [103]. Smoking of mothers may be one factor worsening the quality of semen [120]. Women in the highest social class were almost the only women in Finland who smoked before the 1950s, and young men of social class I had by far the highest incidence of testicular cancer especially in the 1950s. Some occupational agents, most convincingly lead, are known to reduce the sperm count [121], but no excess attributable to these agents was seen in the occupation-specific SIRs of testicular cancer. The elevated risk of university teachers has not been reported in other studies.

Other male genitals

Almost all cancers of "other male genitals" are in the *penis* (107 cases in the present study series). In the *scrotum* there were only four cancers in the age range of this study. There was very little difference between social classes in the incidence of penile cancer. The only occupation-specific SIR_a significantly different from 1.0 was that for medical doctors (2 cases; SIR_a 8.62, 95% CI 1.04-31.1). Nonsignificantly increased SIR_as were obtained among railway traffic supervisors (7.49, 0.91-27.1), miners (3.64, 0.44-13.1), construction workers (1.34, 0.54-2.76) and woodworkers (1.31, 0.60-2.48).

Comment. This study did not bring any light to the unknown aetiology of cancer of the penis [71]. Cancer of the scrotum was analysed as a separate entity solely for historical reasons. The first observation that contact with materials in the work environment could cause a malignant disease was that of an unusually high frequency of scrotal cancer among London chimney sweeps [8]. None of the four cases of scrotal cancer in the present study series was among chimney sweeps or in other occupations with an elevated risk in earlier studies, i.e., persons exposed to polycyclic hydrocarbors or mineral oils [39, 73].

Cancer of the urinary organs

Kidney and renal pelvis

Cancer of the kidney especially among men was positively associated with high social class in the 1970s (fig. 26). The incidence among men of social class I was in 1971-80 more than two-fold that in social class IV. With the rapid increase of incidence in the lowest social class — a 50% increase in both sexes from 1976-80 to 1981-85 — the social class difference disappeared. The increase in social class IV in both sexes was strongest in ages around 60.

The list of high-SIR occupations of men started with two sales occupations followed by, e.g., relatively many traffic occupations (table 32, *appendix tables C23-24*). The risk was rather low, e.g., in agricultural occupations. In women the SIRs for sauna attendants and chocolate makers were significantly elevated, and none of the occupations showed an SIR significantly below 1.0.

In the study series there were 174 cases of cancer of the *renal pelvis* (included also in the figures of total kidney cancer). Women of social class I had a high incidence of cancer of the renal pelvis (SIR 3.24, 95% CI 1.62-5.80). There was a miscellaneous collection of significantly elevated SIRs but no SIRs significantly below 1.0 (table 33).

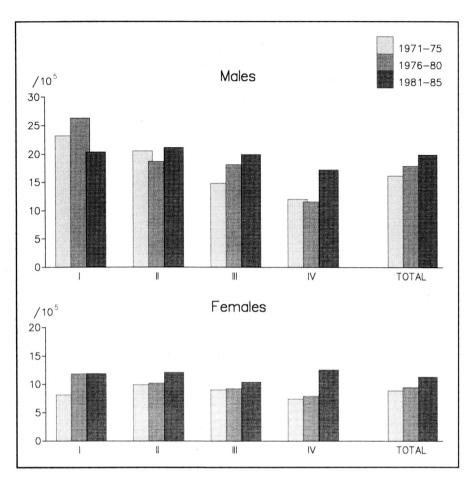

Fig. 26. Age-adjusted incidence rates per 10^5 of kidney cancer among working-aged Finns in 1971-85, by sex, social class and period.

Comment. A wide range of natural and man-made chemicals induce renal cancer experimentally but to date no chemical has been associated unequivocally with renal cancer in humans [73]. However, workers in petroleum-related and dry-cleaning industries have shown an increased risk of renal cancer [122], and lately the observation of kidney cancer following gasoline exposure has been extended from male rats [123] to men [124].

In the present study launderers had the lowest SIR_a of all female workers (0.20), i.e., chemical agents used for instance in dry-cleaning appear not be very hazardous. While the majority of the epidemiological studies found no link between gasoline exposure and renal cell cancer [125], a recent Danish study reported significantly elevated risks for truck drivers and other persons exposed to gasoline [126]. Elevated

Table 32. Cancer of the kidney: number of cancer cases (Obs.) and crude and social class adjusted standardized incidence ratios (SIR) with 95% confidence intervals (95% CI) for selected occupational categories in 1971-85

Occupation		Obs.	Crude		Adjusted	
			SIR	95% CI	SIR	95% CI
MEN						
211	Real estate/stockbrokers	6	7.02	2.58-15.3	6.25	2.30-13.6 *
221	Sales agents	5	3.70	1.20-8.63	3.29	1.07-7.68 *
050	University teachers	12	4.02	2.08-7.02	3.18	1.64-5.55 *
670	Round-timber workers	7	2.53	1.02-5.21	2.60	1.05-5.36 *
500	Ship's masters and mates	8	2.73	1.18-5.37	2.23	0.96-4.39 *
699	Construction workers NOS	9	2.23	1.02-4.23	2.22	1.01-4.21 *
653	Sheetmetalworkers	18	1.60	0.95-2.53	1.62	0.96-2.56
697	Building hands	46	1.17	0.86-1.56	1.59	1.16-2.12 *
735	Paper and board mill workers	12	1.53	0.79-2.68	1.58	0.81-2.75
70	Printing	12	1.42	0.73-2.48	1.45	0.75-2.54
773	Operators of stationary engine	16	1.40	0.80-2.27	1.44	0.82-2.34
540	Motor-vehicle and tram drivers	144	1.45	1.23-1.70	1.40	1.18-1.64 *
53	Engine drivers	10	1.38	0.66-2.53	1.39	0.67-2.56
110	Corporate managers	38	1.74	1.23-2.39	1.34	0.95-1.84 *
23	Sales work	48	1.35	0.99-1.79	1.31	0.97-1.74
680	Painters	27	1.27	0.84-1.85	1.28	0.84-1.86
030	Medical doctors	7	1.58	0.64-3.27	1.28	0.51-2.63
01	Technical work	76	1.31	1.03-1.64	1.17	0.93-1.47 *
00	Technical professions	25	1.35	0.87-1.99	1.12	0.72-1.65
- - -						
310	Agricultural workers	12	0.63	0.33-1.10	0.73	0.38-1.28
34	Forestry work	30	0.55	0.37-0.78	0.73	0.49-1.04 *
300	Farmers, silviculturists	241	0.68	0.59-0.76	0.70	0.61-0.79 *
698	Roadbuilding hands	12	0.47	0.25-0.83	0.65	0.33-1.13 *
052	Primary school teachers	4	0.29	0.08-0.75	0.25	0.07-0.63 *
665	Linemen	-	exp 3.7	0.00-1.00	exp 3.6	0.00-1.02 *
210	Insurance salesmen	-	exp 3.5	0.00-1.06	exp 3.9	0.00-0.95 *
WOMEN						
843	Sauna attendants etc.	6	6.02	2.21-13.1	6.29	2.31-13.7 *
722	Chocolate and confectionery makers	4	4.08	1.11-10.4	4.21	1.15-10.8 *
84	Hygiene and beauty services	12	1.76	0.91-3.08	1.66	0.86-2.89
310	Agricultural workers	16	1.31	0.75-2.13	1.32	0.75-2.14
- - -						
20	Wholesale and retail dealers	7	0.66	0.27-1.36	0.59	0.24-1.21
580	Postmen	3	0.47	0.10-1.38	0.50	0.10-1.45
09	Humanistic and social work etc.	3	0.45	0.09-1.32	0.42	0.09-1.23
850	Launderers	1	0.20	0.00-1.09	0.20	0.01-1.12

Age 35-64 years at the beginning of each 5-year follow-up period. Ordered by the social class adjusted SIR.
Reference: economically active population. * Crude and/or social class adjusted SIR significant (p<0.05).

Table 33. Cancer of the renal pelvis: number of cancer cases (Obs.) and crude and social class adjusted standardized incidence ratios (SIR) with 95% confidence intervals (95% CI) for selected occupational categories in 1971-85

Occupation		Obs.	Crude		Adjusted	
			SIR	95% CI	SIR	95% CI
MEN						
655	Welders and flame cutters	4	5.72	1.56-14.6	4.99	1.36-12.8 *
680	Painters	6	5.11	1.87-11.1	4.49	1.65-9.76 *
540	Motor-vehicle and tram drivers	9	1.67	0.76-3.18	1.61	0.74-3.05
- - -						
300	Farmers, silviculturists	13	0.65	0.35-1.11	0.62	0.33-1.07
0	Technical, humanistic, etc. work	4	0.45	0.12-1.16	0.55	0.15-1.40
WOMEN						
053	Teachers of practical subjects	3	22.6	4.66-66.0	15.1	3.11-44.1 *
570	Post/telecommunications officials	2	9.90	1.20-35.7	10.1	1.22-36.5 *
831	Cleaners	7	2.57	1.03-5.30	2.23	0.90-4.60 *
- - -						
31	Farming, animal husbandry	2	0.38	0.05-1.38	0.44	0.05-1.58

Age 35-64 years at the beginning of each 5-year follow-up period.   Ordered by the social class adjusted SIR.
Reference: economically active population.   * Crude and/or social class adjusted SIR significant (p<0.05).

SIRs of motor-vehicle drivers and some other persons who drive much in their work (e.g., sales agents) in the present study suggest that gasoline-related agents may be carcinogenic. Solvents seem to be a potential cause of renal cancer, as e.g. printers and painters had slightly elevated SIRs.

The best determinant for socioeconomic and occupational variation in the incidence of kidney cancer may be obesity [122], or simply a diet including much meat. The social class pattern of kidney cancer resembles that of colon cancer and could similarly be associated with meat or animal fat consumption. In earlier decades meat consumption used to be highest among the rich but later on became popular among poorer people. Obesity does not prevent persons from working in most of the high risk occupations as it may do in many of the low risk occupations (linemen, postmen, forestry workers etc.). People of low social class born in the 1910s, who had to live the years of economic recession and war but had good times in terms of food availability in the 1960s, showed first a low incidence of kidney cancer and then, around 1980, an exceptionally strong increase. This might well speak for the obesity and meat consumption theory.

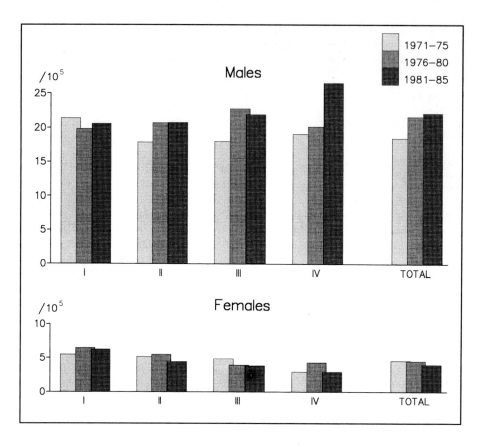

Fig. 27. Age-adjusted incidence rates per 10^5 of cancer of the bladder, ureter and urethra among working-aged Finns in 1971-85, by sex, social class and period.

Cancers of the renal pelvis were studied separately because they are usually urothelial carcinomas, as in the bladder. The significantly elevated SIRs of painters, cleaners and welders — although based on small numbers of cases — point towards a possible solvent aetiology. The social class patterns do not imply that smoking would be a very important risk factor in kidney cancer, although this has been argued for both cancer of the renal pelvis [127] and renal adenocarcinoma [128].

Bladder, ureter and urethra

There was almost no difference between social classes in the incidence of cancer of the bladder (including ureter and urethra) in men, but a downward trend towards lower social classes among women (fig. 27). The variation by calendar time and by birth cohort was weak and inconsistent.

Table 34. Cancer of the bladder, ureter and urethra: number of cancer cases (Obs.) and crude and social class adjusted standardized incidence ratios (SIR) with 95% confidence intervals (95% CI) for selected occupational categories in 1971-85

Occupation		Obs.	Crude		Adjusted		
			SIR	95% CI	SIR	95% CI	
MEN							
120	Book-keepers, accountants	9	2.34	1.07-4.45	2.37	1.08-4.49	*
119	Private sector managers NOS	13	2.16	1.15-3.69	2.13	1.14-3.65	*
220	Commercial travellers, etc.	24	1.52	0.98-2.27	1.61	1.03-2.40	*
76	Packing and labelling	9	1.58	0.72-3.01	1.58	0.72-3.00	
804	Civilian guards	15	1.55	0.87-2.56	1.55	0.87-2.56	
773	Operators of stationary engine	18	1.46	0.86-2.30	1.46	0.86-2.30	
655	Welders and flame cutters	18	1.45	0.86-2.28	1.43	0.85-2.26	
653	Sheetmetalworkers	16	1.39	0.80-2.26	1.38	0.79-2.25	
659	Machine shop/steelworkers NOS	16	1.36	0.78-2.21	1.36	0.78-2.21	
550	Railway staff	22	1.34	0.84-2.04	1.35	0.85-2.05	
690	Bricklayers and tile setters	18	1.33	0.79-2.11	1.34	0.80-2.12	
201	Retailers	31	1.31	0.89-1.86	1.33	0.90-1.89	
110	Corporate managers	32	1.33	0.91-1.88	1.33	0.91-1.88	
40	Mining and quarrying	8	1.31	0.56-2.58	1.31	0.56-2.58	
63	Smelting, metal and foundry work	23	1.28	0.81-1.92	1.28	0.81-1.92	
651	Fitter-assemblers etc.	15	1.23	0.69-2.03	1.22	0.69-2.02	
654	Plumbers	20	1.22	0.75-1.88	1.21	0.74-1.88	
69	Construction work NOS	130	1.24	1.04-1.46	1.19	1.00-1.41	*
- - -							
01	Technical work	47	0.78	0.58-1.04	0.82	0.60-1.09	
300	Farmers, silviculturists	322	0.79	0.71-0.88	0.79	0.71-0.88	*
31	Farming, animal husbandry	21	0.82	0.51-1.25	0.79	0.49-1.21	
05	Teaching	24	0.70	0.45-1.04	0.72	0.46-1.08	
677	Woodworking machine operators etc.	5	0.68	0.22-1.60	0.68	0.22-1.60	
734	Pulp mill workers	4	0.67	0.18-1.72	0.67	0.18-1.72	
735	Paper and board mill workers	4	0.50	0.14-1.28	0.50	0.14-1.27	
656	Plate/constructional steel workers	-	exp 3.7	0.00-0.99	exp 3.7	0.00-0.99	*
WOMEN							
773	Operators of stationary engine	2	28.1	3.39-101	27.3	3.30-98.6	*
21	Real estate, services, securities	2	13.2	1.59-47.6	11.9	1.43-42.8	*
550	Railway staff	2	11.7	1.41-42.1	11.5	1.39-41.5	*
729	Food-product workers NOS	2	10.6	1.28-38.2	10.2	1.23-36.8	*
780	Dockers	3	9.32	1.92-27.2	9.42	1.94-27.5	*
131	Typists	6	3.92	1.44-8.52	3.85	1.41-8.38	*
61	Cutting/sewing etc.	20	1.64	1.00-2.53	1.55	0.95-2.40	*
201	Retailers	7	1.33	0.54-2.75	1.27	0.51-2.62	
76	Packing and labelling	7	1.29	0.52-2.65	1.22	0.49-2.51	
- - -							
300	Farmers, silviculturists	16	0.72	0.41-1.16	0.78	0.44-1.26	
312	Livestock workers	32	0.63	0.43-0.88	0.64	0.44-0.90	*
12	Clerical work	4	0.43	0.12-1.10	0.41	0.11-1.06	

Age 35-64 years at the beginning of each 5-year follow-up period. Ordered by the social class adjusted SIR.
Reference: economically active population. * Crude and/or social class adjusted SIR significant (p<0.05).

In men, there were only some occupations with significantly elevated SIRs, and the 95% confidence intervals of them all included 1.15, i.e., the increases in this fourth common cancer form of men in this study series were not convincingly strong (table 34, *appendix table C25*). The collection of high incidence occupations looked more or less like a random selection of white and blue-collar occupations. However, there was a cluster of metal work occupations with moderately elevated SIRs (1.2-1.4). Paper and pulp manufacturing, instead, was associated with low SIRs. The highest occupation-specific SIRs among women were higher than those among men (table 34, *appendix table C26*), partly because of the 75% lower reference incidence level. Also in women it is difficult to find any common features in the high risk occupations. All occupational categories in agriculture in both sexes showed SIR_as at least one-fifth below the Finnish average.

Comment. Occupation, besides smoking, has been traditionally implicated as major factor in bladder cancer, thanks to early observations in the dye and rubber industry which led to the identification of a number of carcinogenic aromatic amines [39]. Excess risks have been reported in the leather, painting and other industries using organic chemicals as well as among locomotive drivers and painters [129, 130]. The SIR_as of bladder cancer for all these occupations in the present study were 0.93-1.11, i.e., this study does not confirm earlier observations. Neither was this study convincing about the importance of smoking in the causation of bladder cancer, since both the social class pattern and list of high-risk occupations are rather dissimilar to those for lung cancer and also do not otherwise fit with what is known about smoking in different population subgroups in Finland.

Many of the occupations showing elevated risks of bladder cancer among women also had an SIR above 1.0 in men (operators of stationary engines, railway staff, packers and labellers, retailers). All of these are not likely to be due to chance. Occupational agents in the metal industry also seem to be associated with an intermediate risk.

Cancer of the skin

Melanoma
In 1971-75, there was a ratio of 2.5 between men of social classes I and IV in the incidence of skin melanoma. The difference somewhat diminished with time due to the more rapid increase in lower social classes, but it was still in 1981-85 almost twofold (fig. 28). In women there was very little difference between social classes in the incidence of skin melanoma in the early 1970s but, due to the increase in classes I-III, ten years later women also had a social class gradient similar to that of men.

Eleven percent of skin melanomas of men were located in the head and neck, 22% in limbs and 62% in trunk. The ratio between the incidence rates of skin melanoma of the extreme social classes I and IV in the limbs was four, in the trunk two, but in the head and neck less than 1.5 (fig. 29). In women, 12% of the cases

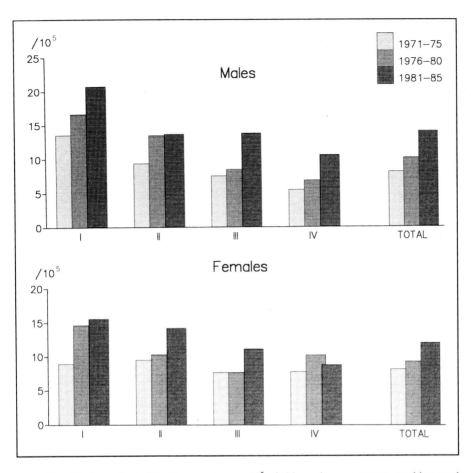

Fig. 28. Age-adjusted incidence rates per 10^5 of skin melanoma among working-aged Finns in 1971-85, by sex, social class and period.

were in the head and neck, 53% in limbs, and 31% in trunk. The social class gradient was similar to that of men only for melanomas of the trunk, whereas in other parts of the body the pattern was inconsistent.

There were almost no occupations with similarly high or low SIRs in both sexes (table 35, *appendix tables C27-28*). The only significantly high SIR_as based on more than one observed case were those of male shop personnel and female furriers. Men in forestry and log floating and in public sector management, and female subject teachers were the only ones showing significantly low SIR_as.

None of the occupations among men showed an SIR for skin melanoma in the head and neck significantly different from 1.0. Female teachers had an SIR_c of 2.51 (95% CI 1.08-4.95) and SIR_a of 1.66 (0.72-3.28). The incidence of skin melanoma in the trunk was highest among male veterinary surgeons, university teachers and

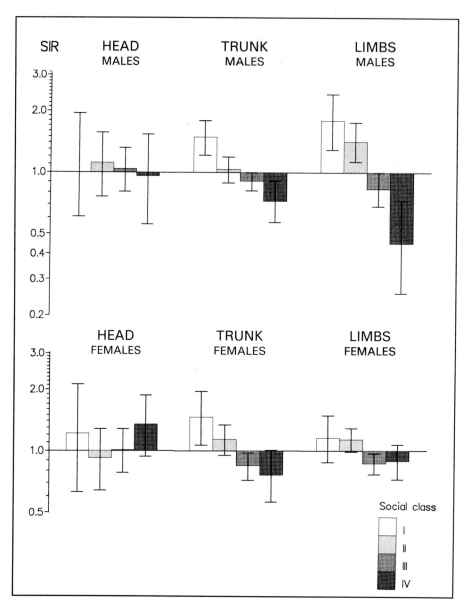

Fig. 29. Standardized incidence ratios (SIR), with 95% confidence intervals, for skin melanoma among working-aged Finns in 1971-85, by subsite, sex and social class. Reference: economically active population.

painters, and female office cashiers and post/telecommunication officials. Low SIRs were observed, e.g., among male forestry workers and postmen/couriers. The SIR_as of

Table 35. Melanoma of the skin: number of cancer cases (Obs.) and crude and social class adjusted standardized incidence ratios (SIR) with 95% confidence intervals (95% CI) for selected occupational categories in 1971-85

Occupation		Obs.	Crude		Adjusted	
			SIR	95% CI	SIR	95% CI
MEN						
025	Veterinary surgeons	3	6.86	1.41-20.0	4.66	0.96-13.6 *
050	University teachers	7	3.14	1.26-6.46	2.11	0.85-4.34 *
653	Sheetmetalworkers	13	1.60	0.85-2.74	1.69	0.90-2.89
09	Humanistic and social work etc.	16	2.20	1.26-3.57	1.65	0.95-2.68 *
231	Shop personnel	25	1.47	0.95-2.16	1.56	1.01-2.31 *
660	Electricians (indoors)	21	1.44	0.89-2.21	1.54	0.95-2.36
68	Painting and lacquering	22	1.46	0.92-2.21	1.54	0.96-2.33
830	Caretakers	19	1.31	0.79-2.05	1.42	0.85-2.21
772	Construction machinery operators	16	1.32	0.76-2.15	1.35	0.77-2.20
801	Policemen	11	1.49	0.74-2.66	1.35	0.67-2.41
051	Subject teachers	10	1.96	0.94-3.60	1.33	0.64-2.45
013	Mechanical technicians	16	1.47	0.84-2.39	1.33	0.76-2.15
052	Primary school teachers	19	1.89	1.14-2.95	1.28	0.77-1.99 *
14/15	Clerical work NOS	33	1.35	0.93-1.90	1.20	0.83-1.69
110	Corporate managers	22	1.70	1.07-2.58	1.10	0.69-1.66 *
- - -						
20	Wholesale and retail dealers	9	0.68	0.31-1.30	0.61	0.28-1.16
34	Forestry work	15	0.41	0.23-0.67	0.59	0.33-0.98 *
201	Retailers	8	0.64	0.27-1.25	0.57	0.25-1.13
652	Machine and motor repairers	11	0.54	0.27-0.96	0.56	0.28-1.01 *
58	Postal services/couriers	3	0.45	0.09-1.31	0.48	0.10-1.41
56	Traffic supervisors	2	0.38	0.05-1.39	0.31	0.04-1.10
10	Public administration	2	0.34	0.04-1.24	0.22	0.03-0.80 *
WOMEN						
612	Furriers	3	5.72	1.18-16.7	6.04	1.24-17.6 *
07	Legal professions	3	5.87	1.21-17.2	4.76	0.98-13.9 *
035	Psychiatric nurses	8	2.38	1.03-4.69	2.02	0.87-3.97 *
121	Office cashiers	10	2.25	1.08-4.13	1.85	0.89-3.41 *
69	Construction work NOS	8	1.54	0.67-3.04	1.74	0.75-3.44
812	Kitchen assistants	19	1.29	0.77-2.01	1.46	0.88-2.29
57	Post and telecommunications	25	1.69	1.10-2.50	1.42	0.92-2.10 *
310	Agricultural workers	15	1.26	0.70-2.08	1.31	0.73-2.16
145	Bank clerks	15	1.52	0.85-2.51	1.30	0.73-2.15
09	Humanistic and social work etc.	11	1.31	0.65-2.34	1.08	0.54-1.93
052	Primary school teachers	20	1.39	0.85-2.14	1.05	0.64-1.63
- - -						
82	Waiters	13	0.73	0.39-1.25	0.76	0.40-1.30
60	Textiles	10	0.65	0.31-1.20	0.74	0.35-1.35
201	Retailers	8	0.81	0.35-1.60	0.64	0.28-1.27
76	Packing and labelling	7	0.52	0.21-1.08	0.60	0.24-1.24
123	Shop and restaurant cashiers	3	0.47	0.10-1.37	0.39	0.08-1.15
051	Subject teachers	3	0.34	0.07-0.99	0.27	0.05-0.78 *
65	Machine shop/steelworkers	1	0.19	0.00-1.04	0.21	0.01-1.18

Age 35-64 years at the beginning of each 5-year follow-up period. Ordered by the social class adjusted SIR.
Reference: economically active population. * Crude and/or social class adjusted SIR significant ($p<0.05$).

skin melanoma in limbs were significantly high among male concrete/cement shutterers (5.07, 1.65-11.8) and railway staff (3.10, 1.14-6.75), and significantly low among machinists (0.15, 0.004-0.85). Among women SIR_as of melanoma in limbs were high among furriers (11.0, 2.26-32.0), corporate managers (6.44, 1.33-18.8), medical doctors (4.93, 1.02-14.4) and social insurance clerks (4.90, 1.01-14.3), each of them however based on three observed cases only.

Comment. Sunburns are known to increase the risk of skin melanoma [131]. Especially repeated burning of the skin in childhood seems to be hazardous for Nordic people [132]. People from higher social classes started some thirty years ago travelling to the south, mainly to the Mediterranean, which later on became popular in lower social classes as well. This may be one reason for the levelling-off in the social class differences in the incidence of skin melanoma.

The residual occupational variation after adjustment for social class is small. If anything, one may conclude that there are almost no outdoor occupations with increased SIRs. In the early 1970s, persons working all year indoors tended to be at a high risk for skin melanoma, whereas outdoor workers had a low risk. This difference seems to have disappeared with time, maybe with the changing fashion of tanned skin. Yet there are examples where indoor workers have higher risks than their colleagues who work regularly outdoors. E.g., female telecommunication officials had an SIR_a of 1.46 and telephone operators an SIR_a of 1.30, but the SIR_a among postwomen carrying post to the customers was only 0.72.

The analyses by subsite further speak for the strong role of sunshine on white skin in the causation of skin melanoma. Most people regularly get small amounts of sun exposure on the head and neck, women also on the limbs, and there is very little social class variation in the incidence of melanoma in these skin areas. The trunk of indoor workers is exposed to sunshine only during short holiday periods and — as far as the fashion of tanned skin continues — sunburns in the upper trunk are frequent among Finns of higher social classes, and their risk of getting skin melanoma on the trunk is therefore fourfold compared to that of lowest social class. The traditional swimming suit fashion may explain the high male-female ratio (2.2) in the incidence of skin melanoma of the trunk.

Also the occupation-specific risks by subsite of the skin seem to point to the role of sunburns in the aetiology of skin melanoma. Almost all high-risk occupations of skin melanoma of the trunk were typical indoor occupations and many of the significantly low ones included regular outdoor activities. The patterns for other parts of the skin were less inconsistent. No signs of the role of occupational carcinogens were apparent.

Non-melanoma skin cancer
There were no trends by social class or by time in the incidence of non-melanoma skin cancer among men (fig. 30). This cancer category (usually referred as "other skin") consists mainly of squamous cell carcinomas; basal cell carcinomas are

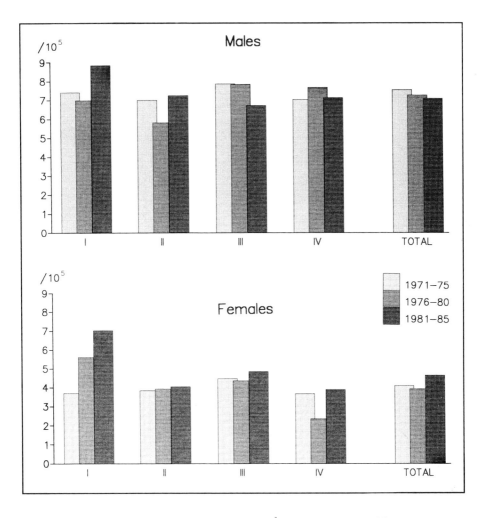

Fig. 30. Age-adjusted incidence rates per 10^5 of non-melanoma skin cancer among working-aged Finns in 1971-85, by sex, social class and period.

excluded. In women the incidence in social class I was increasing due to the high SIRs (1.5-2.1) in the two oldest age-groups in the two latter periods.

About 60% of the non-melanoma skin cancers in both sexes were located in the head and neck, 14% in the trunk and 22% in the limbs. Only in the trunk was there some indication of a consistent social class trend, the men of the highest social class showing a 3.6-fold incidence compared to men of social class IV; in women the difference was 1.6-fold. However, the numbers of cases in social classes I and IV were only around 10 and the random variation large (appendix table B).

Table 36. Non-melanoma skin cancer, excluding basalioma: number of cancer cases (Obs.) and crude and social class adjusted standardized incidence ratios (SIR) with 95% confidence intervals (95% CI) for selected occupational categories in 1971-85

Occupation		Obs.	Crude		Adjusted	
			SIR	95% CI	SIR	95% CI
MEN						
093	Community planning professions	2	10.6	1.28-38.2	9.88	1.20-35.7 *
670	Round-timber workers	5	4.68	1.52-10.9	4.64	1.51-10.8 *
659	Machine shop/steelworkers NOS	10	2.38	1.14-4.38	2.37	1.14-4.36 *
772	Construction machinery operators	11	1.93	0.96-3.45	1.95	0.97-3.48
052	Primary school teachers	9	1.85	0.84-3.51	1.60	0.73-3.04
302	Forestry managers	8	1.51	0.65-2.97	1.60	0.69-3.15
73	Chemical process/paper making	12	1.54	0.80-2.69	1.53	0.79-2.67
14/15	Clerical work NOS	20	1.35	0.82-2.08	1.42	0.87-2.19
30	Agricultural/forestry management	172	1.12	0.96-1.30	1.13	0.97-1.31

11	Corporate administration	14	0.76	0.42-1.28	0.69	0.38-1.16
697	Building hands	10	0.67	0.32-1.22	0.68	0.32-1.24
660	Electricians (indoors)	4	0.54	0.15-1.39	0.54	0.15-1.38
201	Retailers	4	0.48	0.13-1.22	0.51	0.14-1.30
58	Postal services/couriers	-	exp 3.9	0.00-0.95	exp 3.9	0.00-0.94 *
WOMEN						
114	Managers of ideal organizations	2	30.5	3.69-110	20.5	2.48-74.1 *
843	Sauna attendants etc.	3	6.87	1.42-20.1	7.68	1.58-22.5 *
036	Auxiliary nurses	12	1.69	0.87-2.95	1.61	0.83-2.81
14/15	Clerical work NOS	30	1.27	0.86-1.82	1.33	0.90-1.90
312	Livestock workers	55	1.22	0.92-1.59	1.22	0.92-1.59

23	Sales work	20	0.82	0.50-1.27	0.80	0.49-1.23
57	Post and telecommunications	2	0.37	0.04-1.33	0.39	0.05-1.42

Age 35-64 years at the beginning of each 5-year follow-up period. Ordered by the social class adjusted SIR. Reference: economically active population. * Crude and/or social class adjusted SIR significant (p<0.05).

There were only a few occupations with a significantly high or low SIR (table 36, *appendix tables C29-30*). In some of the occupations in farming and forestry the SIRs for non-melanoma skin cancer were — in contrast to most other sites — above 1.0. The excess among male farmers was seen only in cancer of the head and neck (both SIR_a and SIR_c 1.28, 95% CI 1.06-1.52) but not in the trunk or limbs, whereas that of female livestock workers was attributable to limbs only (SIR_a 1.90, 1.13-3.01).

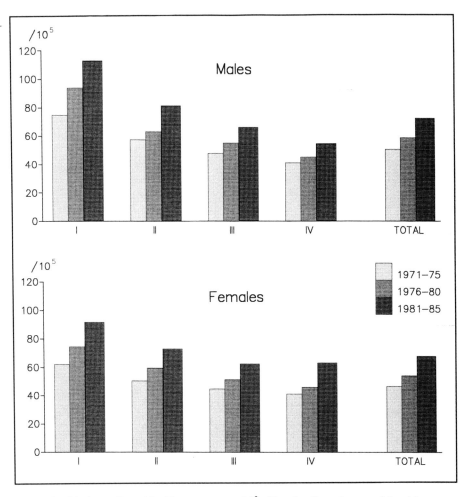

Fig. 31. Age-adjusted incidence rates per 10^5 of basal cell carcinoma of the skin among working-aged Finns in 1971-85, by sex, social class and period.

Among men there were also significantly high subsite-specific SIR_as based on at least three observed cases in the head and neck among round timber workers (6.55, 1.78-16.8) and machine shop/steelworkers (2.93, 1.18-6.04), in the trunk among construction machinery operators (5.65, 1.84-13.2) and in the limbs among forestry consultants (9.62, 1.98-28.1) and miners (5.24, 1.08-15.3). In women there were no significantly elevated SIRs for non-melanoma skin cancer in any of the subsites.

Comment. The somewhat increased SIRs for forestry managers, farmers and agricultural workers are in line with the hypothesis that cumulative UV-radiation would be a risk factor in non-melanoma skin cancer. Even teachers may have been heavily exposed to sun radiation during their three-month summer holidays. Knowing that the farmers in former times always used long-sleeved clothing, the subsite distribution of male farmers — all excess risk in the head and neck — further supports this hypothesis. Cumulative UV-radiation increases with age and its effects are likely to be seen predominantly in advanced ages, maybe mainly in ages above the age range of this study. Many of the low-risk occupations of skin melanoma (retailers, postal service workers, civil engineering technicians, waiters etc.) also had a low risk of non-melanoma skin cancer. This is as expected, since those indoor workers who do not burn their skin in the sun are not likely to get large cumulative doses of UV-radiation, either. The occupation with the highest SIR_a of non-melanoma skin cancer among men, community planning, also showed a significantly high SIR_a for skin melanoma (table 35). This is likely to be one of the chance findings necessarily existing in studies with a huge number of comparisons.

There is some evidence that certain exposures on the skin might increase the risk of non-melanoma skin cancer [39]. In the light of the present results, metal dusts and maybe mineral oils seem to be potential carcinogenic agents for non-melanoma skin cancer.

Basal cell carcinoma

Basal cell carcinomas of the skin are registered in the data base of the Finnish Cancer Registry although not calculated in official cancer statistics. In the study series there were 13,481 basaliomas. The incidence in both sexes and in all social classes increased by some 45% from 1971-75 to 1981-85 (fig. 31). Men in the highest social class had a 50% higher incidence than those in the lowest class. In women the trend was similar but slightly weaker.

Some occupations showed high SIRs in both sexes, e.g., insurance clerks, medical doctors and primary school teachers (tables 37-38, *appendix tables C31-32*). Men working on ships and locomotives had consistently high SIRs, and so had women in most clerical occupations.

Comment. The registration of basal cell carcinomas may not be as complete as that for other malignancies [133]. However, the possible undercoverage of registration is not likely to be associated with occupation. Evidently persons with a high level of education are most likely go to the doctor with their skin lesions and to get their basaliomas removed. On the top of the list there also seem to be a cluster of occupations with regular compulsory health controls like chocolate makers, engine drivers and ship personnel. Possible occupational risks may go unnoticed because of the strong diagnostic bias.

Cancer of the eye and nervous system

Eye

There were 352 cancers of the eye in the study series; 90% of them were melanomas. No consistent trends over time or by social class were observed. Goldsmiths had two cases of cancer of the eye (SIR_a 13.5, 95% CI 1.63-48.6), plumbers six (3.82, 1.40-8.29) and auxiliary nurses six (2.94, 1.08-6.40). The only significantly low SIR_a was that for female livestock workers (0.35, 0.11-0.82).

Table 37. Basal cell carcinoma of the skin, men: number of cancer cases (Obs.) and crude and social class adjusted standardized incidence ratios (SIR) with 95% confidence intervals (95% CI) for selected occupational categories in 1971-85

Occupation		Obs.	Crude		Adjusted		
			SIR	95% CI	SIR	95% CI	
037	Technical nursing assistants	3	11.7	2.41-34.2	12.7	2.62-37.1	*
602	Weavers	6	3.08	1.13-6.71	3.18	1.17-6.91	*
083	Authors	4	4.34	1.18-11.1	2.83	0.77-7.25	*
146	Insurance clerks	12	3.24	1.67-5.65	2.57	1.33-4.48	*
014	Chemotechnicians	13	2.60	1.39-4.45	2.36	1.26-4.04	*
017	Cartographers	10	2.05	0.98-3.77	1.86	0.89-3.42	
510	Deck crew	17	1.68	0.98-2.69	1.82	1.06-2.92	*
672	Plywood makers	24	1.68	1.08-2.50	1.82	1.16-2.70	*
890	Hotel porters	14	1.62	0.88-2.72	1.75	0.96-2.93	
71	Glass and ceramic work	20	1.51	0.92-2.34	1.63	0.99-2.51	
053	Teachers of practical subjects	14	2.20	1.20-3.70	1.61	0.88-2.70	*
502	Chief engineers in ships	14	1.74	0.95-2.92	1.59	0.87-2.67	
012	Teletechnicians	15	1.70	0.95-2.80	1.55	0.87-2.55	
096	PR officers	24	1.96	1.26-2.92	1.54	0.99-2.30	*
144	Office clerks	35	1.67	1.16-2.33	1.53	1.07-2.13	*
011	Power technicians	27	1.67	1.10-2.42	1.51	0.99-2.20	*
53	Engine drivers	33	1.36	0.94-1.91	1.49	1.02-2.09	*
50	Ship's officers	39	1.75	1.24-2.39	1.46	1.03-1.99	*
735	Paper and board mill workers	34	1.29	0.89-1.80	1.40	0.97-1.95	
111	Technical managers	31	2.11	1.43-3.00	1.39	0.94-1.97	*
030	Medical doctors	31	2.07	1.41-2.94	1.36	0.92-1.93	*
70	Printing	36	1.26	0.88-1.74	1.35	0.95-1.88	
013	Mechanical technicians	74	1.44	1.13-1.81	1.31	1.03-1.65	*
500	Ship's masters and mates	17	1.72	1.00-2.76	1.29	0.75-2.07	*
21	Real estate, services, securities	30	1.48	1.00-2.12	1.28	0.86-1.83	*
052	Primary school teachers	85	1.88	1.50-2.32	1.23	0.98-1.52	*
050	University teachers	18	1.77	1.05-2.80	1.16	0.69-1.84	*
07	Legal professions	25	1.63	1.05-2.40	1.11	0.72-1.63	*
110	Corporate managers	123	1.67	1.39-1.98	1.10	0.91-1.30	*
- - -							
698	Roadbuilding hands	65	0.77	0.59-0.98	0.99	0.77-1.27	*
34	Forestry work	128	0.70	0.58-0.82	0.92	0.77-1.09	*
697	Building hands	91	0.69	0.56-0.85	0.91	0.73-1.12	*
79	Labourers not classified elsewhere	45	0.67	0.49-0.90	0.88	0.64-1.18	*
540	Motor-vehicle and tram drivers	273	0.82	0.73-0.92	0.83	0.73-0.93	*
310	Agricultural workers	41	0.64	0.46-0.87	0.74	0.53-1.01	*
773	Operators of stationary engine	25	0.65	0.42-0.96	0.70	0.45-1.04	*
330	Fishermen	7	0.53	0.21-1.09	0.57	0.23-1.18	
40	Mining and quarrying	9	0.47	0.21-0.89	0.50	0.23-0.95	*
563	Road transport supervisors	4	0.39	0.11-1.00	0.31	0.08-0.78	*

Age 35-64 years at the beginning of each 5-year follow-up period.   Ordered by the social class adjusted SIR.
Reference: economically active population.   * Crude and/or social class adjusted SIR significant ($p < 0.05$).

Table 38. Basal cell carcinoma of the skin, women: number of cancer cases (Obs.) and crude and social class adjusted standardized incidence ratios (SIR) with 95% confidence intervals (95% CI) for selected occupational categories in 1971-85

Occupation		Obs.	Crude		Adjusted	
			SIR	95% CI	SIR	95% CI
702	Lithographers	4	3.89	1.06-9.96	4.38	1.19-11.2 *
140	Computer book-keepers	5	3.70	1.20-8.63	3.19	1.04-7.44 *
722	Chocolate and confectionery makers	14	2.46	1.35-4.13	2.74	1.50-4.59 *
122	Bank and post office cashiers	20	2.43	1.49-3.76	2.11	1.29-3.26 *
774	Greasers	15	1.72	0.96-2.83	1.98	1.11-3.26 *
030	Medical doctors	13	2.38	1.27-4.07	1.61	0.86-2.75 *
146	Insurance clerks	18	1.75	1.03-2.76	1.52	0.90-2.40 *
159	Clerical workers NOS	43	1.49	1.08-2.00	1.27	0.92-1.71 *
032	Nurses	96	1.45	1.18-1.77	1.26	1.02-1.53 *
034	Midwives	15	1.44	0.81-2.37	1.24	0.69-2.05
57	Post and telecommunications	104	1.40	1.14-1.68	1.19	0.98-1.43 *
120	Book-keepers, accountants	76	1.38	1.08-1.72	1.17	0.92-1.47 *
052	Primary school teachers	124	1.68	1.40-1.99	1.15	0.96-1.36 *
051	Subject teachers	63	1.66	1.28-2.13	1.13	0.87-1.44 *
- - -						
580	Postmen	24	0.67	0.43-0.99	0.75	0.48-1.12 *
850	Launderers	18	0.62	0.37-0.99	0.68	0.40-1.07 *
201	Retailers	47	0.79	0.58-1.05	0.67	0.49-0.89 *
622	Shoe sewers	4	0.38	0.10-0.98	0.43	0.12-1.09 *

Age 35-64 years at the beginning of each 5-year follow-up period.   Ordered by the social class adjusted SIR.
Reference: economically active population.   * Crude and/or social class adjusted SIR significant (p<0.05).

Comment. The aetiology of cancer of the eye is unclear and has not thought to include occupational factors [71]. In light of the results of the present study, the possible role of metal exposure cannot be fully excluded, and the high SIR of goldsmiths repairing watches may also be associated with radium dials: radium dial painters have been found to have an increased risk of cancer at several sites [109, 134].

Nervous system

There were 3,447 nervous system tumours in the study series, 90% of them in the brain. The category of nervous system tumours is a miscellaneous collection of very different cancers. Glial tumours made up 47% of all nervous system tumours in men and 31% in women, i.e., the majority of malignant nervous system tumours. Benign brain tumours have been traditionally included in the category of nervous system cancer, because benign tumours may also behave aggressively. The most

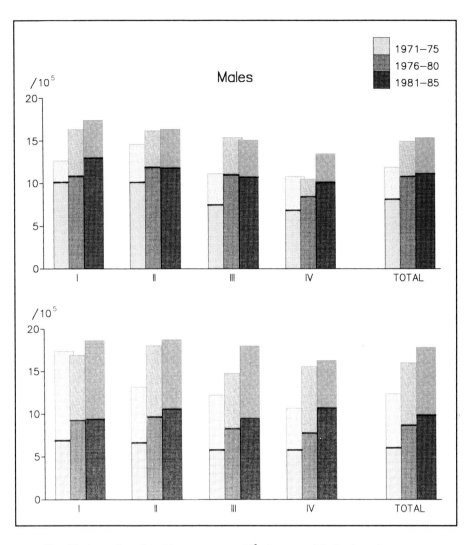

Fig. 32. Age-adjusted incidence rates per 10^5 of cancer of the brain and nervous system among working-aged Finns in 1971-85, by sex, social class and period. The upper part of each bar (above the cross line) indicates the incidence of *benign* tumours.

common benign tumour type is meningeoma, which constituted 23% of the nervous system tumours of the present study series among men and 43% among women.

Among women, there used to be a consistent social class gradient in the incidence of nervous system tumours: in 1971-75 the incidence was 61% higher in social class I than in social class IV (fig. 32). This difference almost disappeared by the mid-1980s together with an increase of the incidence in lower social classes. The social class pattern among men was similar but less consistent. The social class difference existed mainly in the oldest age-groups. Most of the social class variation in the 1970s can be accounted for by the benign brain tumours of women over 55 years of age. That is why the slope of the social class trend for benign tumours is steeper than for malignant tumours (fig. 32).

The highest occupation-specific SIR_a in men for all nervous system tumours taken together was observed among distillers and in women among cigarette makers (table 39, *appendix tables C33-34*). Persons in medical work and nursing also generally showed SIRs above 1.0, and so did men in the military and the police force as well as women in the food industry and in hygiene and beauty services. The only SIR_as significantly below 1.0 were those for labourers, primary school teachers and indoor electricians, all of them in males only.

If only gliomas were included in the analysis, the SIR_a of female cigarette makers increased to 24.5 (95% CI, 2.97-88.7), sauna attendants to 6.97 (1.44-20.4), garment workers to 1.84 (1.01-3.09), auxiliary nurses to 1.66 (0.95-2.70) and nurses to 1.60 (0.83-2.80). In men, shoemakers had an SIR_a of 9.44 (1.14-34.1) and food preservation workers 8.88 (1.07-32.1). The only significantly low SIR_a was that of male labourers (0.17, 0.004-0.95).

Although most of the SIR_as deviating from 1.0 were attributable to malignant nervous system tumours, for instance the high SIR for male painters was attributable to benign tumours only. The risk of meningeomas in men was significantly elevated among male medical workers NOS (SIR_a 10.0, 95% CI 1.21-36.2) and agricultural consultants (5.40, 1.11-15.8), and among female vocational teachers (3.62, 1.45-7.45) and social workers (3.15, 1.44-5.98).

Comment. Diagnostic level affects the incidence of cancer of the nervous system. Probably the waning away of the social class differences after the mid-1970s can be accounted for by the increasing availability of new diagnostic methods such as computerised tomography for all patients.

Earlier studies have reported increased risks of nervous system tumours in workers exposed to various chemicals in the vinyl chloride, petrochemical and rubber industries, in laboratories, and among anatomists, but most of these associations have not been properly confirmed in other studies [73]. Observations of the present study suggest that chemical exposures may be important in the causation of cancer of the nervous system. Diagnostic differences may explain the elevated SIRs of medical personnel, but they are not likely to explain the high risks of distillers and other chemical process workers, cigarette makers, shoe and leather workers, painters or gardeners.

Electrical workers other than telephone installers and repairmen showed SIRs below 1.0, indoor electricians even significantly low (SIR_a 0.50). This is not in accordance with the hypotheses put forward about the role of low frequency electrical and magnetic fields in the causation of brain tumours [135, 136].

Table 39. Cancer of the brain and nervous system: number of cancer cases (Obs.) and crude and social class adjusted standardized incidence ratios (SIR) with 95% confidence intervals (95% CI) for selected occupational categories in 1971-85

Occupation		Obs.	Crude		Adjusted		
			SIR	95% CI	SIR	95% CI	
MEN							
730	Distillers	2	9.87	1.19-35.7	9.95	1.20-35.9	*
755	Musical instrument makers etc.	2	8.59	1.04-31.0	8.42	1.02-30.4	*
085	Industrial designers	3	7.43	1.53-21.7	6.79	1.40-19.9	*
735	Paper and board mill workers	16	2.27	1.30-3.69	2.30	1.31-3.73	*
664	Telephone installers and repairmen	9	1.74	0.80-3.30	1.76	0.80-3.33	
03	Medical work and nursing	13	1.77	0.94-3.03	1.68	0.89-2.87	
112	Commercial managers	18	1.72	1.02-2.72	1.59	0.94-2.51	*
78	Dock and warehouse work	36	1.23	0.86-1.71	1.39	0.97-1.92	
801	Policemen	14	1.52	0.83-2.56	1.38	0.75-2.31	
00	Technical professions	26	1.46	0.96-2.14	1.33	0.87-1.95	
22	Sales representatives	23	1.40	0.89-2.11	1.33	0.84-1.99	
680	Painters	23	1.31	0.83-1.97	1.31	0.83-1.96	
90	Military occupations	10	1.32	0.63-2.43	1.27	0.61-2.33	
- - -							
83	Caretakers and cleaners	13	0.61	0.33-1.05	0.63	0.33-1.07	
310	Agricultural workers	9	0.51	0.23-0.97	0.55	0.25-1.04	*
660	Electricians (indoors)	9	0.49	0.23-0.94	0.50	0.23-0.94	*
052	Primary school teachers	6	0.48	0.18-1.04	0.45	0.16-0.97	*
580	Postmen	2	0.34	0.04-1.24	0.35	0.04-1.26	
50	Ship's officers	2	0.37	0.04-1.34	0.34	0.04-1.23	
79	Labourers not classified elsewhere	3	0.20	0.04-0.58	0.24	0.05-0.69	*
WOMEN							
742	Cigarette makers	3	11.3	2.33-33.0	11.4	2.35-33.3	*
727	Prepared foods	4	3.59	0.98-9.18	3.68	1.00-9.43	*
10	Public administration	8	3.06	1.32-6.04	2.57	1.11-5.06	*
091	Social workers	13	2.41	1.28-4.13	2.16	1.15-3.69	*
159	Clerical workers NOS	16	1.96	1.12-3.19	1.80	1.03-2.92	*
58	Postal services/couriers	16	1.48	0.84-2.40	1.58	0.90-2.56	
130	Private secretaries	13	1.55	0.83-2.65	1.47	0.78-2.51	
62	Shoes and leather	11	1.43	0.71-2.56	1.45	0.72-2.59	
032	Nurses	31	1.45	0.99-2.06	1.37	0.93-1.95	
036	Auxiliary nurses	40	1.30	0.93-1.78	1.33	0.95-1.81	
84	Hygiene and beauty services	15	1.32	0.74-2.18	1.24	0.69-2.04	
- - -							
76	Packing and labelling	13	0.67	0.35-1.14	0.68	0.36-1.17	
60	Textiles	14	0.61	0.34-1.03	0.62	0.34-1.05	
310	Agricultural workers	11	0.61	0.31-1.10	0.62	0.31-1.11	
67	Woodwork	9	0.52	0.24-0.99	0.54	0.24-1.02	*
051	Subject teachers	7	0.57	0.23-1.17	0.50	0.20-1.03	
038	Institutional children's nurses	2	0.41	0.05-1.49	0.39	0.05-1.42	

Age 35-64 years at the beginning of each 5-year follow-up period.   Ordered by the social class adjusted SIR.
Reference: economically active population.   * Crude and/or social class adjusted SIR significant (p<0.05).

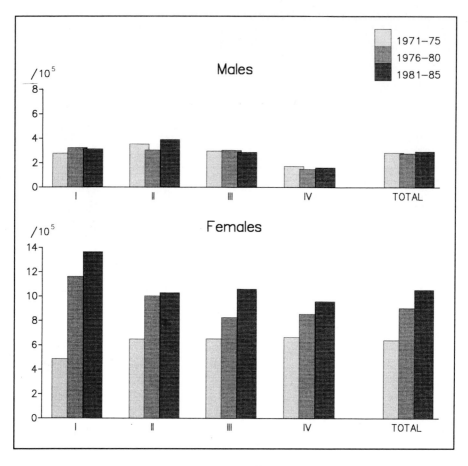

Fig. 33. Age-adjusted incidence rates per 10^5 of thyroid cancer among working-aged Finns in 1971-85, by sex, social class and period.

Cancer of the endocrine glands

Thyroid

The age-adjusted incidence rate of thyroid cancer among women in 1971-75 was 2.2 times that of men; this ratio increased to 3.6 in 1981-85 (fig. 33). Among men, the incidence in social class IV was significantly lower than in other classes, mainly due to an especially low incidence of non-localised papillary carcinoma (SIR in social class IV 0.21, 95% CI 0.03-0.77). Among women, the incidence of follicular carcinoma (24% of all cases) slightly decreased with time and towards higher social classes (fig. 34). The opposite was true for papillary carcinoma (60% of all cases). The trends were stronger for localised than for non-localised tumours.

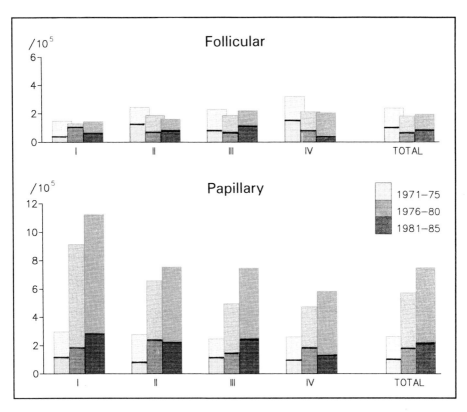

Fig. 34. Age-adjusted incidence rates per 10^5 of thyroid cancer among working-aged Finnish women, by histological type, social class and period. The upper part of each bar (above the cross line) indicates the incidence of tumours at *localized stage* at diagnosis.

The only significantly low SIR was the SIR_c for men in farming and animal husbandry (table 40). Male lithographers, plate workers, engine drivers and public sector managers, as well as female textile workers and patternmakers, had SIR_as above 3.5. These SIRs were mainly attributable to the dominating papillary type of thyroid carcinoma. The risk of follicular carcinoma was significantly increased among male teachers of practical subjects (SIR_a 21.1, 95% CI 2.55-76.3), and turners and machinists (3.92, 1.07-10.0), and among female metal platers (26.3, 3.19-95.1) and hairdressers (3.77, 1.03-9.65).

Comment. Almost nothing is known about the association between lifestyle factors and the risk of thyroid cancer. Part of the social class variation in the incidence of localised papillary carcinoma can be accounted for by differences in diagnostic activity. There might also be a temporal shift from follicular to papillary carcinoma in the case of ground-glass type of tumours [137] which may partly explain

Table 40. Cancer of the thyroid: number of cancer cases (Obs.) and crude and social class adjusted standardized incidence ratios (SIR) with 95% confidence intervals (95% CI) for selected occupational categories in 1971-85

Occupation		Obs.	Crude		Adjusted	
			SIR	95% CI	SIR	95% CI
MEN						
702	Lithographers	2	12.6	1.53-45.6	12.7	1.54-46.0 *
656	Plate/constructional steel workers	4	6.43	1.75-16.5	6.25	1.70-16.0 *
53	Engine drivers	5	4.33	1.41-10.1	3.95	1.28-9.22 *
10	Public administration	6	3.90	1.43-8.48	3.55	1.30-7.73 *
652	Machine and motor repairers	10	1.98	0.95-3.65	1.91	0.92-3.51
80	Watchmen, security guards	8	1.67	0.72-3.29	1.56	0.68-3.08
14/15	Clerical work NOS	10	1.58	0.76-2.90	1.38	0.66-2.54
- - -						
34	Forestry work	4	0.43	0.12-1.10	0.75	0.20-1.91
66	Electrical work	4	0.61	0.17-1.57	0.59	0.16-1.51
2	Sales professions	9	0.64	0.29-1.21	0.58	0.26-1.10
31	Farming, animal husbandry	-	exp 4.5	0.00-0.82	exp 3.5	0.00-1.06 *
WOMEN						
609	Textile workers NOS	5	5.73	1.86-13.4	5.88	1.91-13.7 *
615	Patternmakers and cutters	9	4.06	1.86-7.70	4.10	1.87-7.77 *
201	Retailers	12	1.48	0.77-2.59	1.48	0.76-2.58
840	Hairdressers and barbers	8	1.48	0.64-2.91	1.47	0.64-2.90
032	Nurses	19	1.40	0.84-2.18	1.41	0.85-2.20
310	Agricultural workers	13	1.32	0.70-2.26	1.34	0.71-2.29
- - -						
82	Waiters	10	0.67	0.32-1.23	0.67	0.32-1.24
72	Food industry	9	0.66	0.30-1.25	0.67	0.31-1.27
67	Woodwork	5	0.52	0.17-1.21	0.53	0.17-1.24

Age 35-64 years at the beginning of each 5-year follow-up period. Ordered by the social class adjusted SIR. Reference: economically active population. * Crude and/or social class adjusted SIR significant (p<0.05).

the decreasing trend in follicular carcinoma and increasing trend in papillary carcinoma.

Enhanced risks of papillary carcinoma have been obtained in iodine-rich areas, whereas the follicular type is more common in areas of endemic goiter, possibly due to iodine deficiency [73]. Salt with added potassium chloride is one of the main sources of iodine intake. Persons in higher social classes were likely to start using iodine-rich salt earlier than other people. The different social class patterns of follicular and papillary carcinomas of the thyroid thus fit with the iodine hypothesis. Since the incidence of thyroid cancer is increasing, the magnitude of the possible protective effect of iodine on follicular carcinoma causation seems to be smaller than the risk increasing effect on the causation of papillary carcinoma.

Occupational exposure to radiation is known to increase the risk of thyroid cancer [71, 110]. Some of the risk difference between nurses (SIR_a 1.41) and auxiliary nurses (SIR_a 1.00) might be accounted for by radiation. The occupational classification used in this study did not allow the separation of X-ray nurses from other nurses. There is a broad selection of possibly harmful agents in the working environment of many of the occupations with a high SIR, but it is difficult to point out any specific potential occupation-related risk factors on the basis of this study.

Other endocrine glands

The incidence of cancers of endocrine glands other than the thyroid was low ($1.1/10^5$ in males and $0.6/10^5$ in females), but it was increasing with time in both sexes. There was no consistent trend by social class.

Five of the 111 male patients were painters (SIR_a 3.44, 95% CI 1.12-8.03) and four were civil engineering technicians (SIR_a 4.44, 1.21-11.4). One female civil engineering technician also had an endocrine cancer, 150 times more than expected (Exp_a). The other significantly high SIR_a among women was that of social workers (3 observed cases, SIR_a 11.7, 2.41-34.1).

Comment. The heterogeneous category "cancer of other endocrine glands" consists of a number of small groups of cancer, probably with different aetiologies. There are problems in defining malignancy, in diagnostics and in registration, e.g., in the case of phaeochromocytoma and thymoma. Hereditary aspects like MEN syndromes might also complicate the interpretation of the results. The cancers among civil engineering technicians and painters might be worth studying case by case, to search for common carcinogenic exposures in their work histories.

Cancer of the bone and connective tissue

Bone

There was no consistent social class trend (fig. 35) and no change with time in the incidence of bone cancer in the study series. The highest SIR_as were obtained among male auxiliary nurses (SIR_a 77.0, 95% CI 1.95-429), pharmacists (17.3, 2.80-62.6) and boat builders (8.86, 1.07-32.0), but the numbers of cases were very small (1, 2 and 2, respectively). Female midwives had a significantly high incidence (2 cases; SIR_a 10.5, 1.27-38.0) and cleaners a significantly low incidence (no observed cases; 95% CI for the SIR_a 0-0.98).

Comment. Radiation and viruses possibly cause osteosarcoma [71, 73, 134], and this might be associated with the high SIRs of bone cancer obtained in mainly health-care related occupations.

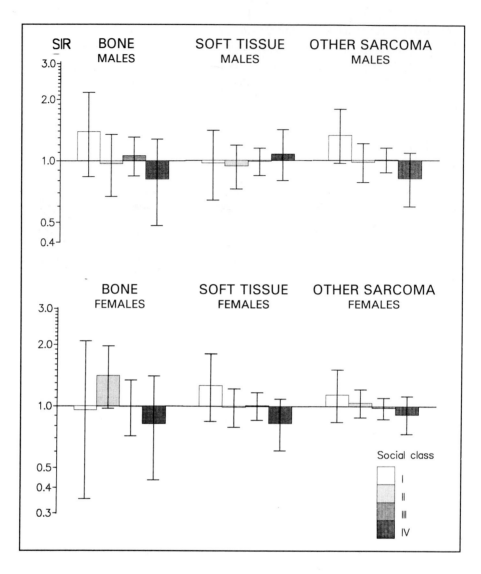

Fig. 35. Standardized incidence ratios (SIR), with 95% confidence intervals, for cancers of the bone and soft tissue and sarcoma in other organs among working-aged Finns in 1971-85, by sex and social class. Reference: economically active population.

Soft tissue

The incidence of soft tissue sarcoma among women of social class I was 25% above and in class IV 19% below the average (fig. 35). In men the incidence was the same in all social classes. The social class patterns in both sexes were inconsistent over time but the incidence among the total population remained stable.

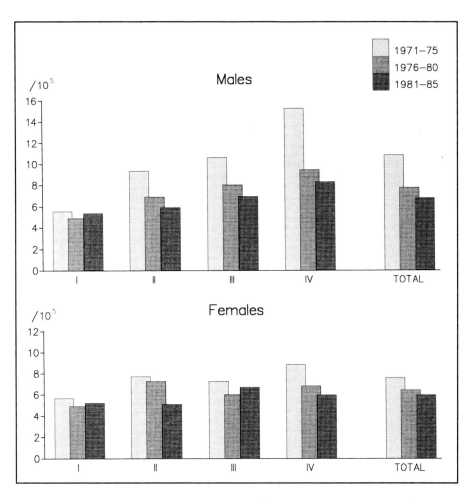

Fig. 36. Age-adjusted incidence rates per 10^5 of cancer of unspecified organs among working-aged Finns in 1971-85, by sex, social class and period.

In males, the highest occupation-specific SIRs were those of dentists (2 cases; SIR_a 12.9, 95% CI 1.56-46.6), commercial travellers (8 cases; 2.91, 1.26-5.73) and corporate managers (8 cases; 2.59, 1.12-5.10). Male farmers had an SIR_a of 0.82 (0.60-1.09), whereas both occupations with a significantly enhanced incidence among women were in agriculture: farmers had an SIR_a of 1.84 (1.09-2.90) based on 18 observed cases and livestock workers an SIR_a of 1.44 (1.02-1.97) based on 39 cases.

Comment. Farmers have earlier been found to have an increased risk of soft tissue sarcoma which has been explained by agricultural chemicals [138]. The high risk among female agricultural workers was also clearly seen in the present study, although the number of soft tissue cancers of women in the whole series was only

Table 41. Cancer of unspecified organs: number of cancer cases (Obs.) and crude and social class adjusted standardized incidence ratios (SIR) with 95% confidence intervals (95% CI) for selected occupational categories in 1971-85

Occupation		Obs.	Crude		Adjusted	
			SIR	95% CI	SIR	95% CI
MEN						
580	Postmen	7	2.86	1.15-5.89	2.76	1.11-5.69 *
052	Primary school teachers	8	1.65	0.71-3.24	2.37	1.02-4.66 *
655	Welders and flame cutters	10	2.17	1.04-4.00	2.15	1.03-3.95 *
11	Corporate administration	17	0.86	0.50-1.38	1.39	0.81-2.23
79	Labourers not classified elsewhere	15	1.69	0.95-2.79	1.24	0.69-2.04
697	Building hands	25	1.54	1.00-2.27	1.15	0.74-1.70
34	Forestry work	30	1.38	0.93-1.97	1.05	0.71-1.49
698	Roadbuilding hands	16	1.42	0.81-2.31	1.04	0.60-1.69
- - -						
650	Turners, machinists	6	0.56	0.20-1.22	0.55	0.20-1.20
72	Food industry	2	0.38	0.05-1.36	0.38	0.05-1.36
WOMEN						
201	Retailers	13	1.79	0.95-3.07	1.81	0.96-3.10
310	Agricultural workers	13	1.56	0.83-2.67	1.55	0.83-2.65
300	Farmers, silviculturists	46	1.45	1.07-1.94	1.42	1.04-1.90 *
61	Cutting/sewing etc.	20	1.18	0.72-1.82	1.18	0.72-1.83
- - -						
81	Housekeeping, domestic work, etc.	25	0.72	0.47-1.06	0.68	0.44-1.01
231	Shop personnel	23	0.68	0.43-1.02	0.68	0.43-1.02
12	Clerical work	4	0.31	0.08-0.79	0.32	0.09-0.83 *

Age 35-64 years at the beginning of each 5-year follow-up period. Ordered by the social class adjusted SIR. Reference: economically active population. * Crude and/or social class adjusted SIR significant (p<0.05).

321. There is no evidence of an effect in animals, nor did male farmers of the present study (who have probably been more exposed to these chemicals than women) show an increased risk. It may be that the increased risk of soft tissue sarcomas is attributable to other factors than chemicals associated with farming like animal transmitted viruses. In Finland, women have traditionally taken care of animal husbandry. The viral aetiology may also explain the high risk among, e.g., dentists.

Cancer at unspecified sites

There was a strong tendency towards a higher incidence in lower social classes in the incidence of cancer at unspecified sites (fig. 36; excludes the few cancers classified to ICD-7 199.0: "Cancer of other specific organs"). The incidence among men in the lowest class was more than twofold that of class I. However, the incidence strongly decreased with time in classes II-IV. The incidence among women in social classes II-IV was lower than that of men, but the decrease with time was slower. Thus, both the social class variation and the male-female difference were disappearing.

In men, high SIRs were observed in some occupations of affluence but especially among unskilled workers (table 41). Postmen had the highest SIR among all occupations (SIR_c 2.86) whereas other male workers in transport and communication had a significantly low incidence of cancer at unspecified sites (SIR_c for the rest of the branch 0.65, 95% CI 0.46-0.89). Men in agricultural occupations had SIRs slightly below 1.0 on contrary to agricultural women who showed high SIRs. Many of the low-incidence occupations of women were in the housekeeping branch.

Comment. It looks like the incidence of cancer at unspecified sites in both sexes and in all social classes would decrease towards a value of about 5 per 10^5, i.e., 0.8% of the total cancer incidence of the age range of this study. Maybe this is close to the proportion of cancers in which it is impossible to define the site of origin, not even when the best possible procedures of diagnostics could be applied. The occupational variation in incidence gives an impression that there are two types of persons with an excess of unspecified cancers: persons with a low level of awareness about cancer may go to the doctor with an already advanced stage of disease and get less specialised medical care and their diagnosis is therefore delayed, and persons with predominantly a high living standard purposely do not want to have their cancer diagnosed.

Haematological cancers

Non-Hodgkin's lymphoma
There were 2,377 non-Hodgkin's lymphomas in the study series, 690 of them classified to have their origin in organs other than the lymph nodes. (The extranodal lymphomas were not included in the organ-specific results in the previous chapters.) The incidence was increasing in both sexes, in women more than in men (fig. 37). Almost all of the increase in males was attributable to extranodal cases (76% increase from 1971-75 to 1981-85) whereas in women the incidence of both nodal and extranodal lymphoma increased by some 70%. There was a gradient of higher risks in higher social classes in 1971-75 which disappeared by the early 1980s. By far the greatest social class variation was obtained among men of the oldest age-group (incidence $41/10^5$ in social class I and $17/10^5$ in class IV).

The variation in occupation-specific SIRs of extranodal lymphoma was small and did not show any apparent consistency. The only SIR_as significantly different from 1.0 were those of male clerical workers (SIR_a 1.88, 95% CI 1.08-3.06) and men in sales professions (0.53, 0.26-0.98). For most of the occupations, also the incidence

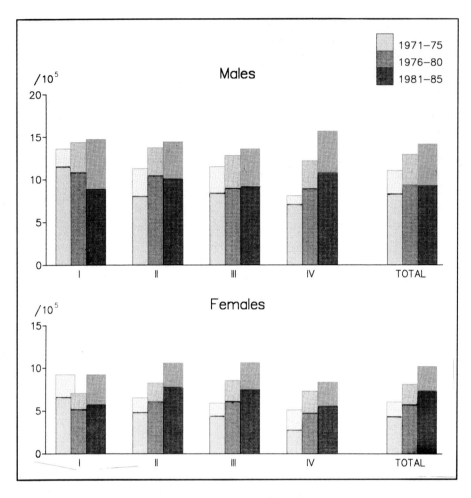

Fig. 37. Age-adjusted incidence rates per 10^5 of non-Hodgkin's lymphoma among working-aged Finns in 1971-85, by sex, social class and period. The upper part of each bar (above the cross line) indicates the incidence of *extranodal* lymphomas.

of *nodal non-Hodgkin's lymphoma* was rather close to the average. All managerial workers except corporate managers had significantly high SIRs, and some metal and machine worker categories showed elevated SIRs (table 42, *appendix tables C35-36*). Shop personnel and clerical workers typically had low SIRs.

Comment. According to present knowledge only a modest effect of environmental factors can be associated with non-Hodgkin's lymphoma. Occasional clusters have been ascribed to viral and chemical exposures, such as phenoxy acids, chlorophenols, organic solvents, pesticides and herbicides, however, without definitive confirmation [73]. The present results weakly suggest that there might be this type of

Table 42. Non-Hodgkin's lymphoma (nodal only): number of cancer cases (Obs.) and crude and social class adjusted standardized incidence ratios (SIR) with 95% confidence intervals (95% CI) for selected occupational categories in 1971-85

Occupation		Obs.	Crude		Adjusted	
			SIR	95% CI	SIR	95% CI
MEN						
657	Metal platers and coaters	3	8.15	1.68-23.8	8.38	1.73-24.5*
114	Managers of ideal organizations	4	3.97	1.08-10.2	3.39	0.92-8.69*
781	Freight handlers	7	2.62	1.05-5.40	2.59	1.04-5.34*
111	Technical managers	6	2.81	1.03-6.11	2.56	0.94-5.58*
804	Civilian guards	9	2.25	1.03-4.27	2.38	1.09-4.52*
773	Operators of stationary engine	12	2.14	1.11-3.74	2.21	1.14-3.87*
054	Vocational teachers	9	2.29	1.05-4.34	2.14	0.98-4.06*
112	Commercial managers	13	2.17	1.16-3.71	2.01	1.07-3.43*
655	Welders and flame cutters	11	1.66	0.83-2.98	1.71	0.86-3.07
698	Roadbuilding hands	20	1.63	0.99-2.52	1.66	1.02-2.57*
63	Smelting, metal and foundry work	13	1.58	0.84-2.70	1.62	0.86-2.78
550	Railway staff	11	1.53	0.76-2.74	1.58	0.79-2.83
772	Construction machinery operators	12	1.48	0.77-2.59	1.50	0.77-2.61
- - -						
67	Woodwork	43	0.74	0.53-1.00	0.76	0.55-1.03*
34	Forestry work	21	0.77	0.48-1.18	0.76	0.47-1.16
830	Caretakers	8	0.67	0.29-1.31	0.69	0.30-1.36
231	Shop personnel	7	0.61	0.25-1.26	0.63	0.25-1.30
680	Painters	6	0.57	0.21-1.24	0.58	0.21-1.27
22	Sales representatives	5	0.56	0.18-1.32	0.53	0.17-1.24
08	Artistic and literary professions	2	0.38	0.05-1.37	0.35	0.04-1.26
WOMEN						
713	Glass and ceramics decorators	2	9.67	1.17-34.9	8.91	1.08-32.2*
147	Social insurance clerks	3	7.34	1.51-21.5	6.95	1.43-20.3*
061	Deacons and social workers	3	5.48	1.13-16.0	5.31	1.09-15.5*
73	Chemical process/paper making	7	2.85	1.15-5.87	2.64	1.06-5.45*
60	Textiles	16	1.84	1.05-2.99	1.71	0.98-2.78*
821	Waiters in cafés etc.	8	1.63	0.71-3.22	1.58	0.68-3.12
- - -						
231	Shop personnel	26	0.79	0.52-1.16	0.74	0.48-1.08
144	Office clerks	12	0.53	0.27-0.92	0.51	0.26-0.89*
310	Agricultural workers	3	0.43	0.09-1.25	0.42	0.09-1.23

Age 35-64 years at the beginning of each 5-year follow-up period. Ordered by the social class adjusted SIR.
Reference: economically active population. * Crude and/or social class adjusted SIR significant (p<0.05).

occupational background behind some of the elevated risks in industry. Agricultural or horticultural chemicals seem, however, not to be important since the SIR_a for agricultural workers was close to 1.0 and for forestry workers even below it. A recent

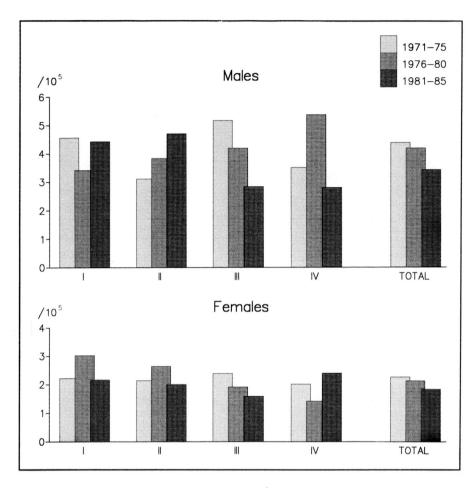

Fig. 38. Age-adjusted incidence rates per 10^5 of Hodgkin's disease among working-aged Finns in 1971-85, by sex, social class and period.

specific Finnish study of cancer risk among pesticide sprayers did not show any excess risk, either [139].

The cluster of high risk among managers is odd, and so is the more than twofold difference in the incidence of nodal lymphoma between about 65 years-old men of social classes I and IV. The development of immunohistochemical methods (e.g., lymphomas in the brain were earlier classified as microgliomas) may explain the steep increase of the incidence of extranodal lymphoma, but diagnostic differences are not likely to cause differences between population subgroups in the incidence of nodal lymphoma.

Table 43. Hodgkin's disease: number of cancer cases (Obs.) and crude and social class adjusted standardized incidence ratios (SIR) with 95% confidence intervals (95% CI) for selected occupational categories in 1971-85

Occupation		Obs.	Crude		Adjusted	
			SIR	95% CI	SIR	95% CI
MEN						
025	Veterinary surgeons	3	19.4	4.00-56.7	16.8	3.46-49.0 *
803	Prison guards	3	5.01	1.03-14.6	5.10	1.05-14.9 *
665	Linemen	4	4.40	1.20-11.3	4.45	1.21-11.4 *
201	Retailers	10	2.20	1.05-4.04	2.27	1.09-4.17 *
05	Teaching	15	1.64	0.92-2.70	1.52	0.85-2.51
652	Machine and motor repairers	11	1.46	0.73-2.61	1.50	0.75-2.68
80	Watchmen, security guards	10	1.48	0.71-2.73	1.49	0.72-2.75
77	Machinists	17	1.36	0.79-2.18	1.38	0.81-2.21
31	Farming, animal husbandry	9	1.29	0.59-2.46	1.29	0.59-2.45
- - -						
01	Technical work	8	0.53	0.23-1.05	0.54	0.23-1.07
23	Sales work	4	0.41	0.11-1.05	0.42	0.11-1.07
11	Corporate administration	4	0.36	0.10-0.93	0.34	0.09-0.87 *
WOMEN						
5	Transport and communications	9	1.71	0.78-3.24	1.60	0.73-3.04
30	Agricultural/forestry management	11	1.32	0.66-2.37	1.40	0.70-2.50
03	Medical work and nursing	13	1.33	0.71-2.28	1.25	0.67-2.14
- - -						
81	Housekeeping, domestic work, etc.	7	0.64	0.26-1.32	0.72	0.29-1.48
2	Sales professions	12	0.75	0.39-1.31	0.70	0.36-1.21

Age 35-64 years at the beginning of each 5-year follow-up period. Ordered by the social class adjusted SIR. Reference: economically active population. * Crude and/or social class adjusted SIR significant (p<0.05).

Hodgkin's disease

The incidence of Hodgkin's disease (689 cases in this study series) in both sexes decreased by about 20% from 1971-75 to 1981-85. The patterns by social class was inconsistent (fig. 38). Significantly high SIRs were observed for male veterinary surgeons, prison guards, linemen and retailers (table 43). Male teachers, female farmers (i.e., "agricultural management") and medical workers had SIRs non-significantly above 1.0. Low SIRs were obtained, e.g., among sales workers.

Comment. Some of the high risks were observed in occupations with frequent contacts with human beings (hospital patients, prisoners) or animals. The results are thus in line with the hypothesis of an infectious aetiology of Hodgkin's disease. Low risk persons, rather, handle papers or goods in their work. Similar SIRs for Hodgkin's

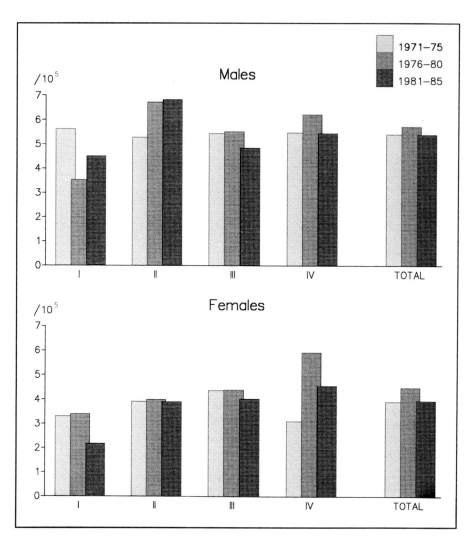

Fig. 39. Age-adjusted incidence rates per 10^5 of multiple myeloma among working-aged Finns in 1971-85, by sex, social class and period.

disease and non-Hodgkin's lymphoma in some occupations (low among office clerks and shop personnel, high among machinists and motor repairers) suggests that the aetiologies of these two forms of lymphoma are partly the same.

Multiple myeloma

The incidence of multiple myeloma did not change with time. Especially among women it was markedly lower in social class I than in the others (fig. 39). Most of

Table 44. Multiple myeloma: number of cancer cases (Obs.) and crude and social class adjusted standardized incidence ratios (SIR) with 95% confidence intervals (95% CI) for selected occupational categories in 1971-85

Occupation		Obs.	Crude		Adjusted	
			SIR	95% CI	SIR	95% CI
MEN						
831	Cleaners	2	13.9	1.68-50.2	13.4	1.62-48.5 *
01	Technical work	31	1.85	1.26-2.63	1.59	1.08-2.26 *
00	Technical professions	6	1.17	0.43-2.55	1.51	0.55-3.28
31	Farming, animal husbandry	11	1.54	0.77-2.75	1.49	0.75-2.67
78	Dock and warehouse work	15	1.41	0.79-2.33	1.40	0.78-2.31
80	Watchmen, security guards	12	1.38	0.71-2.40	1.26	0.65-2.20
- - -						
68	Painting and lacquering	4	0.59	0.16-1.51	0.60	0.16-1.54
697	Building hands	6	0.51	0.19-1.12	0.50	0.18-1.08
WOMEN						
697	Building hands	7	3.85	1.55-7.92	3.16	1.27-6.51 *
830	Caretakers	8	2.69	1.16-5.30	2.79	1.21-5.50 *
57	Post and telecommunications	8	1.54	0.66-3.02	1.60	0.69-3.16
300	Farmers, silviculturists	29	1.53	1.03-2.20	1.50	1.00-2.15 *
812	Kitchen assistants	9	1.55	0.71-2.95	1.30	0.59-2.46
- - -						
2	Sales professions	17	0.61	0.35-0.97	0.61	0.36-0.98 *
61	Cutting/sewing etc.	5	0.47	0.15-1.09	0.48	0.16-1.12
036	Auxiliary nurses	3	0.45	0.09-1.33	0.46	0.10-1.36
813	Domestic servants	3	0.52	0.11-1.53	0.46	0.10-1.36

Age 35-64 years at the beginning of each 5-year follow-up period. Ordered by the social class adjusted SIR. Reference: economically active population. * Crude and/or social class adjusted SIR significant (p<0.05).

the occupations with a high SIR in one sex showed a non-elevated risk in the other; building hands are on the very top of the SIR list for women but on the bottom of the list for men (table 44, *appendix tables C37-38*). Agricultural and technical work categories tended to have SIRs above 1.0.

Comment. The present Finnish results are in line with earlier case-control studies consistently reporting an increased risk associated with farming or agricultural work. The reason for this association has remained unknown [73]. Radiation and a range of chemicals, mainly solvents, have been suspected to be associated with multiple myeloma, but these suspicions have mainly been unconfirmed. The occupational pattern of the present study series does not point to an important role of these factors in the causation of multiple myeloma in the working-aged population.

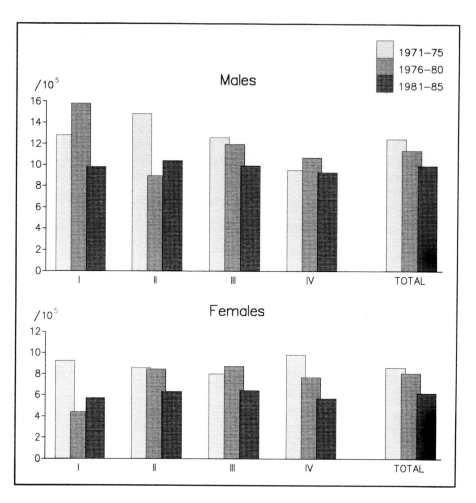

Fig. 40. Age-adjusted incidence rates per 10^5 of leukaemia among working-aged Finns in 1971-85, by sex, social class and period.

Leukaemia

The incidence of leukaemia decreased by one-fifth in ten years in both sexes (fig. 40). This decrease was somewhat slower in the acute myelocytic type of leukaemia (AML; 34% of the leukaemia cases in this study series) than in chronic lymphocytic leukaemia (CLL; 31% of leukaemias) or other types of leukaemia. The social class variation in incidence of all of the leukaemia types was rather small.

Policemen, non-commissioned officers and freighthandlers as well as female packers and institutional children's nurses had significantly high SIRs (table 45, *appendix tables C39-40*). Non-commissioned officers were at a high risk of both AML (SIR_a 5.30, 95% CI 1.44-13.6) and CLL (5.65, 1.16-16.5), and the risk among

Table 45. Leukaemia: number of cancer cases (Obs.) and crude and social class adjusted standardized incidence ratios (SIR) with 95% confidence intervals (95% CI) for selected occupational categories in 1971-85

Occupation		Obs.	Crude		Adjusted	
			SIR	95% CI	SIR	95% CI
MEN						
52	Air traffic	2	10.5	1.27-37.8	9.84	1.19-35.6 *
239	Sales staff NOS	4	3.77	1.03-9.65	3.71	1.01-9.49 *
901	Non-commissioned officers	7	2.94	1.18-6.06	3.14	1.26-6.48 *
781	Freight handlers	8	2.44	1.05-4.80	2.66	1.15-5.25 *
801	Policemen	17	2.41	1.41-3.87	2.42	1.41-3.88 *
4	Mining and quarrying	11	1.92	0.96-3.44	1.89	0.94-3.39
804	Civilian guards	7	1.33	0.54-2.75	1.42	0.57-2.93
09	Humanistic and social work etc.	9	1.45	0.66-2.74	1.37	0.62-2.59
150	Property managers, warehousemen	16	1.39	0.79-2.25	1.36	0.78-2.21
110	Corporate managers	18	1.37	0.81-2.16	1.29	0.76-2.04
310	Agricultural workers	14	1.17	0.64-1.97	1.25	0.69-2.10
- - -						
302	Forestry managers	4	0.48	0.13-1.23	0.48	0.13-1.22
70	Printing	2	0.38	0.05-1.37	0.37	0.05-1.35
00	Technical professions	4	0.35	0.10-0.90	0.33	0.09-0.84 *
WOMEN						
06	Religious professions	4	3.68	1.00-9.41	3.63	0.99-9.29 *
038	Institutional children's nurses	6	3.10	1.14-6.76	2.96	1.09-6.44 *
76	Packing and labelling	18	2.00	1.18-3.15	1.97	1.17-3.12 *
811	Chefs, cooks etc.	15	1.54	0.86-2.55	1.53	0.86-2.52
310	Agricultural workers	14	1.53	0.83-2.56	1.52	0.83-2.56
57	Post and telecommunications	15	1.54	0.86-2.53	1.45	0.81-2.39
300	Farmers, silviculturists	41	1.30	0.93-1.76	1.32	0.95-1.79
84	Hygiene and beauty services	7	1.33	0.54-2.74	1.27	0.51-2.62
036	Auxiliary nurses	16	1.22	0.70-1.98	1.17	0.67-1.89
- - -						
61	Cutting/sewing etc.	13	0.66	0.35-1.12	0.64	0.34-1.09
032	Nurses	5	0.58	0.19-1.35	0.57	0.19-1.33
201	Retailers	3	0.38	0.08-1.12	0.36	0.07-1.05

Age 35-64 years at the beginning of each 5-year follow-up period.   Ordered by the social class adjusted SIR.
Reference: economically active population.   * Crude and/or social class adjusted SIR significant (p<0.05).

watchmen and security guards (including policemen) was elevated in all subcategories of leukaemia: the SIR_a for AML was 1.52 (0.66-2.99), for CLL 1.78 (0.89-3.18) and for other leukaemia 1.53 (0.70-2.90). Female agricultural workers had a high incidence of AML (SIR_a 2.50, 1.15-4.75), whereas the other types of leukaemia were increased among female farmers (SIR_a for non-AML 1.58, 1.07-2.24). CLL was found in excess among male air traffic personnel (SIR_a 36.3, 4.39-131) and miners (4.11, 1.33-9.58).

Comment. The aetiology of leukaemia has been studied extensively in relation to how rare it is (e.g., 2.3% of the cases of the present study series). Still, ionizing radiation is almost the only known external factor proved to be associated with leukaemia, and its effect is so small that it is difficult to confirm in traditional epidemiological studies [140]. The two cases of leukaemia among air traffic personnel in the present study, giving an SIR_a of 9.84 could in principle be accounted for by the increased radiation in the planes during the flight. However, according to the theoretical estimates the maximal risk ratio among pilots in relation to the doses should not exceed 1.5 [141]. Several international and national studies on radiation-associated cancer risk among pilots and cabin crew have already been started.

A Finnish exercise based on grouping of occupational categories by the probability of being occupationally exposed to electromagnetic radiation produced a significantly increasing trend of leukaemia by increasing probability [136], and a recent Swedish study showed a strong association between CLL and occupational exposure to electromagnetic fields [135]. However, no definite evidence for an aetiological role of electromagnetic field is available and present series did not show any excess risk among electrical workers.

Chemical-related cases are estimated to be less than 1% of the total leukaemia [73]. The present study did not point to chemicals, either, although the slightly elevated risk among motor vehicle drivers (SIR_a 1.15) or significantly elevated risks among freight handlers and policemen could be associated with benzene exposure [39].

Cancer at all sites

The age-adjusted incidence of cancer at all sites among men decreased by 5% from 1971-75 to 1981-85. The incidence was 375 per 10^5 in the highest social class and 528 per 10^5 in the lowest one (fig. 41). Due to the slowest decrease in social class IV the social class difference increased with time. The social class pattern was roughly the same in all birth cohorts: men of the lowest social class always had some 30% higher incidence of overall cancer than men of the highest social class. The incidence of cancer among women increased by 9% from 1971-75 to 1981-85. The social class pattern was opposite to that of men. The average incidence during the whole follow-up period was almost 20% higher in social class I (426 per 10^5) than in the lowest class (346 per 10^5). However, the incidence in the lower social classes increased more than in class I and the risk difference was thus diminishing. The relative risk differences were smaller the later the women were born.

Out of the 273 three-digit occupational categories with at least five expected cases among men and 206 categories among women there were about ten occupations

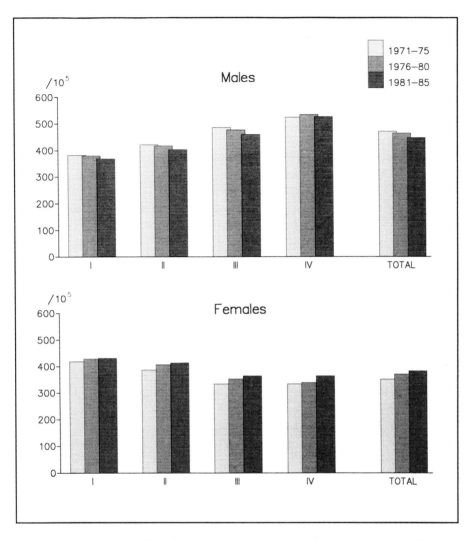

Fig. 41. Age-adjusted incidence rates per 10^5 of cancer of all sites among working-aged Finns in 1971-85, by sex, social class and period.

with both social class adjusted and crude SIRs greater than 2.0 or less than 0.5 both in both sexes, and the number of statistically significant SIRs was much larger than would be expected on the basis of chance variation only (*appendix tables C41-42*). Highest SIRs were observed among male knitters and miscellaneous cutting/sewing workers, asphalt roofers, insulators and glass and ceramics decorators (table 46). The highest SIR of all two-digit occupational categories among men was in the tobacco industry. Low rates were obtained, e.g., among physiotherapists, surveyors, auditors, chemists, dentists, religious workers, solicitors, barristers and judges.

Female auditors also had a very low cancer incidence (table 47). Other low SIRs were obtained among women in the fishing, glass and ceramic industries, and in some occupations of other industrial branches. Telephone installers, miscellaneous agricultural workers, wholesalers and sculptors/painters had the highest SIRs for overall cancer among women.

Comment. "Overall cancer" is a combination of numerous cancer diseases with different aetiologies. Therefore the occupation-specific SIRs for total cancer — as risk ratios for total cancer defined by any risk determinant — are difficult to explain in terms of possible causative factors. Anyhow, the increased or decreased incidences of total cancer in many occupations clearly indicate, that high risks of certain cancers in these occupations are not always compensated by low risks of some other cancers or vice versa.

Among occupations with the highest SIRs in men there were many occupations with known or strongly suspected occupational exposures such as asphalt roofers (SIR_a 2.07), insulators (1.85), miners (1.61), hairdressers (1.58), blacksmiths (1.46) and distillers (1.40). Many occupations typically associated with an exhausting way of life (various artistic professions, certain commercial workers etc.) also had total cancer incidence of some 40% to 70% above the average of their social class. At the bottom of the list sorted by the SIR_a for total cancer of males there are occupations with a presumable exceptionally healthy way of life (or at least with the best knowledge about what is healthy) such as physiotherapists, sports coaches, deacons and priests and many medical professions.

In women, the top of the list is more mixed. There were are industrial occupations with relatively high SIRs, e.g., glass and ceramics decorators (also high in males), welders, shoe sewers and various occupations in printing. However, many occupations in administration and technical work also showed high SIRs. The collection of occupations with a low overall cancer risk is also quite a mixture, with a likely underrepresentation of occupations with a high degree of education. Clearly the pattern of occupational cancer risks among women reveals — assuming that adjustment for social class controls for the non-occupational factors in a similar way in both sexes — that cancer cases directly attributable to occupational factors are fewer than among men.

The overall cancer incidence among men increased and among women decreased towards the lower social classes. This is due to the different primary site distributions in men and women: in women cancers of the breast, corpus uteri and ovary — all associated with a high standard of living — constitute 45% of all cases in the study series, whereas the two most common cancer types in men (cancers of the lung and stomach; 42% of all cancers of men) are typically cancers of the lower social classes. The male-female difference in total cancer pattern is further strengthened by smoking-related cancers, since the prevalence of smoking around the 1950s used to be most common among women of higher social classes but among men of lower classes.

Table 46. Cancer of all sites, men: number of cancer cases (Obs.) and crude and social class adjusted standardized incidence ratios (SIR) with 95% confidence intervals (95% CI) for selected occupational categories in 1971-85

Occupation		Obs.	Crude		Adjusted		
			SIR	95% CI	SIR	95% CI	
604	Knitters	9	2.34	1.07-4.45	2.31	1.06-4.39	*
694	Asphalt roofers	36	2.12	1.49-2.94	2.07	1.45-2.86	*
619	Cutting/sewing workers NOS	11	2.03	1.01-3.63	2.02	1.01-3.62	*
713	Glass and ceramics decorators	15	2.01	1.13-3.32	1.97	1.10-3.24	*
74	Tobacco industry	10	2.01	0.96-3.70	1.96	0.94-3.60	
695	Insulators	107	1.88	1.54-2.25	1.85	1.52-2.22	*
088	Film and radio producers	13	1.44	0.77-2.46	1.71	0.91-2.92	
657	Metal platers and coaters	30	1.74	1.17-2.48	1.70	1.15-2.43	*
840	Hairdressers and barbers	14	1.49	0.81-2.50	1.58	0.86-2.65	
612	Furriers	14	1.54	0.84-2.59	1.57	0.86-2.63	
211	Real estate/stockbrokers	30	1.42	0.96-2.03	1.54	1.04-2.19	*
086	Performing artists	24	1.27	0.81-1.89	1.50	0.96-2.23	
750	Basket and brush makers	23	1.39	0.88-2.09	1.48	0.94-2.23	
634	Blacksmiths	151	1.44	1.22-1.68	1.46	1.23-1.70	*
085	Industrial designers	13	1.25	0.66-2.13	1.44	0.77-2.47	
080	Sculptors, painters, etc.	35	1.18	0.82-1.65	1.42	0.99-1.97	
730	Distillers	8	1.44	0.62-2.84	1.40	0.60-2.76	
232	Door-to-door salesmen	68	1.29	1.00-1.63	1.39	1.08-1.76	*
632	Hot-rollers	22	1.42	0.89-2.15	1.38	0.87-2.09	
831	Cleaners	17	1.47	0.85-2.35	1.30	0.76-2.08	
890	Hotel porters	82	1.33	1.06-1.65	1.29	1.03-1.61	*
699	Construction workers NOS	124	1.29	1.07-1.53	1.28	1.07-1.52	*
670	Round-timber workers	86	1.31	1.05-1.62	1.28	1.03-1.58	*
511	Engine-room crew	41	1.31	0.94-1.77	1.27	0.91-1.73	
654	Plumbers	459	1.27	1.15-1.38	1.24	1.13-1.36	*
653	Sheetmetalworkers	325	1.26	1.13-1.40	1.24	1.11-1.38	*
692	Reinforcing iron workers	88	1.25	1.00-1.54	1.21	0.97-1.49	
756	Stone cutters	44	1.19	0.86-1.60	1.19	0.87-1.60	
710	Glass formers	36	1.22	0.85-1.69	1.19	0.83-1.64	
672	Plywood makers	120	1.22	1.01-1.44	1.18	0.98-1.40	*
63	Smelting, metal and foundry work	477	1.20	1.10-1.31	1.18	1.08-1.29	*
804	Civilian guards	266	1.24	1.10-1.39	1.17	1.04-1.32	*
701	Printers	69	1.20	0.93-1.52	1.17	0.91-1.48	
680	Painters	589	1.18	1.09-1.28	1.17	1.07-1.26	*
655	Welders and flame cutters	335	1.19	1.07-1.33	1.17	1.04-1.29	*
772	Construction machinery operators	405	1.16	1.05-1.28	1.16	1.05-1.27	*
693	Concrete/cement shutterers	225	1.17	1.03-1.33	1.15	1.00-1.30	*
781	Freight handlers	159	1.26	1.07-1.47	1.12	0.95-1.30	
697	Building hands	1,172	1.26	1.19-1.33	1.11	1.05-1.17	*
030	Medical doctors	73	0.72	0.57-0.91	0.86	0.67-1.08	*
054	Vocational teachers	134	0.75	0.63-0.88	0.85	0.71-1.00	*
052	Primary school teachers	191	0.64	0.56-0.74	0.77	0.67-0.89	*
562	Railway traffic supervisors	69	0.67	0.52-0.85	0.74	0.58-0.94	*
06	Religious professions	60	0.64	0.49-0.83	0.74	0.56-0.95	*
031	Dentists	12	0.61	0.31-1.06	0.71	0.37-1.24	
070	Barristers and judges	17	0.57	0.33-0.90	0.67	0.39-1.08	*
035	Psychiatric nurses	19	0.62	0.37-0.97	0.67	0.40-1.05	*
073	Solicitors	12	0.55	0.28-0.95	0.65	0.34-1.14	*
020	Chemists	13	0.54	0.29-0.92	0.65	0.34-1.11	*
753	Tanners and pelt dressers	12	0.54	0.28-0.94	0.53	0.27-0.92	*
090	Auditors	7	0.39	0.16-0.81	0.46	0.19-0.95	*
008	Surveyors	8	0.32	0.14-0.63	0.38	0.16-0.75	*
041	Physiotherapists	1	0.14	0.00-0.80	0.16	0.00-0.87	*

Age 35-64 years at the beginning of each 5-year follow-up period. Ordered by the social class adjusted SIR. Reference: Economically active population. * Crude and/or social class adjusted SIR significant (p<0.05).

Table 47. Cancer of all sites, women: number of cancer cases (Obs.) and crude and social class adjusted standardized incidence ratios (SIR) with 95% confidence intervals (95% CI) for selected occupational categories in 1971-85

Occupation		Obs.	Crude		Adjusted	
			SIR	95% CI	SIR	95% CI
664	Telephone installers and repairmen	7	2.45	0.99-5.05	2.63	1.06-5.42 *
319	Agricultural workers NOS	9	2.21	1.01-4.19	2.37	1.08-4.50 *
200	Wholesalers	6	2.77	1.02-6.04	2.35	0.86-5.12 *
080	Sculptors, painters, etc.	24	2.46	1.58-3.67	2.09	1.34-3.11 *
80	Watchmen, security guards	32	1.69	1.16-2.39	1.72	1.18-2.43 *
114	Managers of ideal organizations	11	1.85	0.92-3.31	1.55	0.77-2.77
550	Railway staff	17	1.45	0.84-2.32	1.52	0.89-2.44
081	Commercial artists	8	1.64	0.71-3.23	1.48	0.64-2.92
713	Glass and ceramics decorators	19	1.37	0.83-2.15	1.48	0.89-2.31
816	Pursers, stewardesses	14	1.54	0.84-2.58	1.43	0.78-2.40
622	Shoe sewers	95	1.33	1.08-1.63	1.43	1.15-1.74 *
085	Industrial designers	26	1.64	1.07-2.40	1.42	0.93-2.08 *
050	University teachers	29	1.66	1.11-2.38	1.42	0.95-2.04 *
581	Caretakers/messengers	45	1.31	0.95-1.75	1.41	1.03-1.88 *
612	Furriers	26	1.34	0.88-1.96	1.38	0.90-2.02
027	Consultancy, agriculture	80	1.53	1.21-1.91	1.37	1.08-1.70 *
703	Bookbinders	115	1.25	1.03-1.49	1.34	1.11-1.60 *
70	Printing	232	1.23	1.08-1.40	1.32	1.16-1.49 *
626	Saddlers, leather sewers, etc.	50	1.28	0.95-1.69	1.31	0.98-1.73
56	Traffic supervisors	59	1.48	1.13-1.91	1.30	0.99-1.68 *
615	Patternmakers and cutters	103	1.22	1.00-1.47	1.30	1.06-1.56 *
150	Property managers, warehousemen	85	1.46	1.17-1.81	1.30	1.04-1.60 *
754	Photolab. workers	26	1.24	0.81-1.82	1.29	0.85-1.90
086	Performing artists	20	1.47	0.90-2.27	1.28	0.78-1.97
843	Sauna attendants etc.	45	1.21	0.88-1.62	1.27	0.92-1.70
121	Office cashiers	223	1.42	1.24-1.61	1.27	1.11-1.44 *
774	Greasers	69	1.17	0.91-1.48	1.25	0.98-1.59
159	Clerical workers NOS	273	1.39	1.23-1.56	1.24	1.10-1.39 *
74	Tobacco industry	23	1.13	0.72-1.70	1.22	0.77-1.82
018	Draughtsmen, survey assistants	67	1.32	1.03-1.68	1.21	0.94-1.54 *
096	PR officers	35	1.36	0.95-1.89	1.20	0.84-1.68
820	Waiters in restaurants	318	1.14	1.02-1.27	1.20	1.07-1.33 *
032	Nurses	609	1.30	1.20-1.41	1.18	1.09-1.28 *
146	Insurance clerks	93	1.28	1.03-1.56	1.16	0.94-1.42 *
019	Laboratory assistants	147	1.27	1.07-1.48	1.15	0.97-1.35 *
110	Corporate managers	48	1.38	1.02-1.83	1.14	0.84-1.51 *
084	Journalists	70	1.29	1.00-1.63	1.12	0.88-1.42 *
840	Hairdressers and barbers	262	1.22	1.07-1.37	1.12	0.99-1.26 *
131	Typists	182	1.23	1.06-1.42	1.11	0.96-1.28 *
091	Social workers	159	1.26	1.07-1.46	1.11	0.94-1.29 *
030	Medical doctors	48	1.26	0.93-1.68	1.07	0.79-1.42
- - -						
312	Livestock workers	3,183	0.80	0.77-0.83	0.83	0.80-0.86 *
671	Timber workers	65	0.76	0.59-0.97	0.82	0.63-1.05 *
680	Painters	29	0.74	0.50-1.07	0.79	0.53-1.14
605	Textile finishers/dyers	51	0.72	0.54-0.95	0.78	0.58-1.03 *
304	Livestock breeders	21	0.72	0.45-1.10	0.76	0.47-1.17
606	Textile quality controllers	30	0.70	0.47-1.00	0.76	0.51-1.08
850	Launderers	138	0.72	0.61-0.85	0.75	0.63-0.88 *
711	Potters	15	0.62	0.35-1.02	0.66	0.37-1.10
142	Data storage assistants	18	0.67	0.40-1.06	0.63	0.37-0.99 *
4	Mining and quarrying	4	0.48	0.13-1.22	0.51	0.14-1.30
710	Glass formers	6	0.37	0.13-0.80	0.40	0.15-0.86 *
112	Commercial managers	5	0.45	0.15-1.06	0.39	0.13-0.90 *
33	Fishing	3	0.35	0.07-1.02	0.38	0.08-1.10

Age 35-64 years at the beginning of each 5-year follow-up period. Ordered by the social class adjusted SIR. Reference: Economically active population.   * Crude and/or social class adjusted SIR significant (p<0.05).

V. Cancer profiles of selected occupations

Physicians

Medical doctor is one of the occupational categories which has been used in very many epidemiological studies, partly because medical doctors are believed to be more interested in taking part in these studies and the response rate and accuracy are thus believed to be good. The cancer profile of medical doctors was selected for this presentation in order to give clues about possible incidence variation caused by diagnostic differences.

Male physicians had 73 malignant cancer cases (SIR_a 0.9, 95% CI 0.7-1.1) and female ones 48 cases (1.1, 0.8-1.4), i.e., their cancer incidence was close to the average of social class I. Male doctors had a significantly low SIR_a for lung cancer 0.4 (0.2-1.0) as a consequence of their exceptionally low prevalence of smoking [142]. Also the SIR_a of prostatic cancer was low (0.4, 0.1-1.1), whereas the two cases of penile cancer corresponded to a significantly high SIR_a (8.6, 1.0-31). The risk of bladder cancer was elevated in both sexes (combined SIR_a 1.9, 0.9-3.5). The only SIR significantly different from 1.0 among female physicians was in the SIR_c for basal cell carcinomas of the skin (2.4, 1.3-4.1). Male doctors also had a significantly high SIR_c for skin basalioma (2.1, 1.4-2.9).

The number of cancer cases among working-aged Finnish physicians was too small to reveal possible weak associations between cancer and occupational hazards such as viruses, radiation or some chemicals. Basal cell carcinoma of the skin was the only cancer type with a clear indication of a diagnostic difference between physicians and the rest of the population.

Teachers and labourers

Teachers are a large occupational category with a high educational level, whereas most labourers have only a basic education. The number of cancer cases of men in both these occupations is around 600 but the cancer profiles are almost complementary to each other (fig. 42). The SIR_c of cancers of the oesophagus, lip, lung, larynx and stomach is significantly higher among labourers than among teachers. The SIR_c of testicular cancer, skin melanoma and cancer of the nervous system is clearly higher among teachers, but the difference is statistically significant only for nervous system tumours.

The differences between the social class adjusted SIRs were much smaller (fig. 42), i.e., the different occupational cancer profiles can be in great part accounted for by the general social class variation between the social class adjusted SIRs. The only

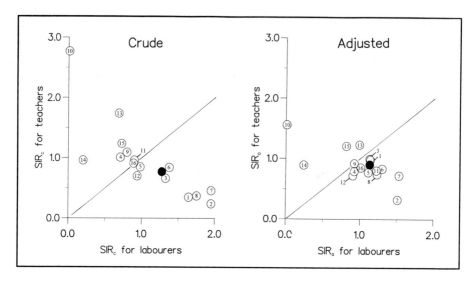

Fig. 42. Correlation between site-specific standardized incidence ratios (SIR$_c$: crude; SIR$_a$: adjusted for social class) of male teachers and labourers. ●: all sites, 1: lip, 2: oesophagus, 3: stomach, 4: colon, 5: rectum, 6: liver, 7: larynx, 8: lung, 9: prostate, 10: testis, 11: kidney, 12: bladder, 13: skin melanoma, 14: nervous system, 15: non-Hodgkin's lymphoma, 16: leukaemia.

social class adjusted SIR significantly higher for male labourers than for teachers was that of lung cancer (SIR$_a$s 1.23 and 0.74, respectively), indicating low smoking of teachers and high smoking of labourers even in comparison to other men of their own social classes I and IV, respectively.

Tobacco industry workers

The small branch of the tobacco industry showed the highest SIR for total cancer of all occupational branches among men (SIR$_c$ 2.0, 95% CI 1.0-3.7; SIR$_a$ 2.0, 0.9-3.6). One easily interprets this as expected, taking into account the easy access to cigarettes for the workers in tobacco factories. The SIR$_a$ decreased from 2.5 in 1971-75 to 1.2 in the 1980s, most likely as a consequence of a reduced amount of free cigarettes given to the workers. However, the SIR$_a$ for cancers other than lung cancer was larger than that for lung cancer (table 48). There were cancer cases in urinary organs, the liver and the nervous system in both sexes, all of these cancer sites sometimes connected with occupational exposures. It seems that it is not only hazardous to smoke tobacco but also to work in tobacco industry.

Table 48. Number of cancer cases (Obs.) and social class adjusted standardized incidence ratios (SIR$_a$) with 95% confidence intervals (95% CI) for selected primary sites among working-aged tobacco industry workers in Finland in 1971-85

Primary site	Obs	SIR$_a$	95% CI
MEN			
Colon	1	5.6	0.1-31
Liver	1	16	0.4-87
Pancreas	1	4.9	0.1-27
Lung, trachea	3	1.8	0.4-5.1
Prostate	1	2.7	0.1-15
Kidney	1	5.1	0.1-28
Bladder, ureter, urethra	1	4.5	0.1-25
Brain, nervous system	1	6.3	0.2-35
All sites	10	2.0	0.9-3.6
WOMEN			
Stomach	1	0.9	0.0-4.9
Small intestine	1	15	0.4-81
Colon	1	1.2	0.0-6.9
Liver	1	6.6	0.2-37
Mesothelioma	1	30	0.8-168
Breast	7	1.3	0.5-2.7
Corpus uteri	2	1.2	0.2-4.4
Bladder, ureter, urethra	2	7.6	0.9-28
Brain, nervous system	4	5.0	1.4-13
Thyroid	2	4.7	0.6-17
All sites	23	1.2	0.8-1.8

Reference: economically active population. Primary sites without cases excluded.

Economically inactive persons

The proportion of economically inactive men of the total 35-64 year-old male population at the time of the 1970 Population Census was 8%, including a great proportion of men unable to work. The large category of economically inactive women (38% of the total 35-64 year-old female population on January 1, 1971) included housewives and farmers' spouses not taking part in farm work and was thus less biased in terms of health status than that of males. The unemployment rate in 1970 was 2.7% among men and 1.1% among women [143], but most of the unemployed persons were classified as economically active according to their latest occupation.

Table 49. Economically inactive men: number of cancer cases (Obs.) and crude and social class adjusted standardized incidence ratios (SIR) with 95% confidence intervals (95% CI) for selected primary sites

Primary site	Obs.	Crude		Adjusted	
		SIR	95% CI	SIR	95% CI
ALL SITES	7,952	1.38	1.35-1.41	1.34	1.31-1.37
Lip	172	1.36	1.17-1.57	1.24	1.06-1.43
Tongue	28	1.72	1.14-2.48	1.66	1.11-2.40
Oral cavity	36	2.14	1.50-2.96	2.12	1.48-2.93
Pharynx excl. nasopharynx	63	2.69	2.06-3.44	2.79	2.15-3.57
Oesophagus	155	2.29	1.94-2.66	2.17	1.85-2.53
Stomach	695	1.20	1.11-1.29	1.15	1.07-1.24
Colon	227	1.15	1.00-1.30	1.23	1.08-1.40
Rectum	217	1.01	0.88-1.15	1.03	0.90-1.18
Liver	149	1.95	1.65-2.27	1.96	1.66-2.29
Gallbladder, biliary tract	56	1.47	1.11-1.90	1.44	1.09-1.87
Pancreas	285	1.20	1.06-1.34	1.18	1.05-1.32
Nose, nasal sinuses	21	1.41	0.87-2.15	1.32	0.82-2.02
Larynx	254	1.76	1.55-1.98	1.67	1.47-1.88
Lung, trachea	3,328	1.73	1.67-1.78	1.59	1.54-1.65
adenocarcinoma	*253*	*1.34*	*1.18-1.51*	*1.28*	*1.13-1.45*
small cell carcinoma	*395*	*1.37*	*1.24-1.51*	*1.26*	*1.14-1.39*
squamous cell carcinoma	*1,079*	*1.65*	*1.55-1.75*	*1.50*	*1.41-1.59*
Prostate	513	0.97	0.89-1.06	0.99	0.91-1.08
Testis	16	1.37	0.79-2.23	1.60	0.91-2.60
Penis	12	1.07	0.55-1.86	1.07	0.56-1.88
Kidney	206	0.97	0.84-1.11	1.04	0.90-1.18
renal pelvis	*22*	*1.74*	*1.09-2.64*	*1.76*	*1.10-2.66*
Bladder, ureter, urethra	341	1.31	1.18-1.45	1.32	1.18-1.46
Skin melanoma	88	0.86	0.69-1.06	0.93	0.74-1.14
head and neck	*18*	*1.59*	*0.94-2.52*	*1.65*	*0.98-2.60*
trunk	*39*	*0.61*	*0.43-0.83*	*0.64*	*0.46-0.88*
limbs	*23*	*1.05*	*0.67-1.58*	*1.24*	*0.78-1.85*
Other skin	107	1.08	0.89-1.30	1.08	0.89-1.30
Brain, nervous system	150	1.05	0.89-1.23	1.09	0.93-1.28
Thyroid	28	0.88	0.59-1.28	0.95	0.63-1.37
Bone	20	1.31	0.80-2.02	1.38	0.84-2.13
Soft tissue	31	0.91	0.62-1.29	0.88	0.60-1.25
Unspecified	172	1.51	1.29-1.74	1.42	1.21-1.64
Non-Hodgkin's lymphoma	168	1.20	1.03-1.39	1.22	1.04-1.41
Hodgkin's disease	39	0.87	0.62-1.19	0.85	0.60-1.16
Multiple myeloma	71	1.02	0.80-1.29	1.02	0.80-1.29
Leukaemia	149	1.04	0.88-1.22	1.07	0.90-1.24
Not included above:					
Skin, basal cell carcinoma	686	0.96	0.89-1.03	1.01	0.93-1.09

Reference: economically active men.

Table 50. Economically inactive women: number of cancer cases (Obs.) and crude and social class adjusted standardized incidence ratios (SIR) with 95% confidence intervals (95% CI) for selected primary sites

Primary site	Obs.	Crude		Adjusted	
		SIR	95% CI	SIR	95% CI
ALL SITES	18,935	0.99	0.97-1.00	0.99	0.98-1.01
Lip	43	1.41	1.02-1.89	1.56	1.13-2.10
Tongue	52	0.87	0.65-1.14	0.87	0.65-1.14
Salivary glands	60	1.31	1.00-1.68	1.36	1.04-1.75
Oral cavity	55	1.06	0.80-1.38	1.01	0.76-1.31
Pharynx excl. nasopharynx	49	1.20	0.89-1.59	1.30	0.96-1.72
Oesophagus	219	1.11	0.97-1.27	1.15	1.00-1.31
Stomach	1,237	1.13	1.07-1.19	1.15	1.09-1.22
Small intestine	61	1.08	0.83-1.39	1.06	0.81-1.36
Colon	814	0.92	0.86-0.99	0.93	0.87-1.00
Rectum	695	1.05	0.97-1.13	1.06	0.98-1.14
Liver	177	1.25	1.08-1.44	1.26	1.09-1.46
Gallbladder, biliary tract	390	1.42	1.28-1.56	1.47	1.33-1.62
Pancreas	619	1.09	1.00-1.18	1.11	1.03-1.20
Nose, nasal sinuses	41	1.68	1.21-2.28	1.79	1.29-2.43
Larynx	48	1.25	0.92-1.65	1.32	0.97-1.74
Lung, trachea	763	0.94	0.88-1.01	0.97	0.91-1.04
adenocarcinoma	*219*	*0.98*	*0.85-1.11*	*1.00*	*0.87-1.14*
small cell carcinoma	*121*	*0.94*	*0.78-1.12*	*1.00*	*0.83-1.18*
squamous cell carcinoma	*130*	*0.85*	*0.71-1.00*	*0.87*	*0.73-1.03*
Breast	5,059	0.91	0.88-0.93	0.90	0.88-0.93
Cervix uteri	790	0.95	0.89-1.02	0.96	0.90-1.03
Corpus uteri	1,527	0.97	0.92-1.01	0.96	0.92-1.01
Ovary	1,238	0.86	0.81-0.91	0.86	0.81-0.91
Vulva	141	1.43	1.21-1.68	1.56	1.31-1.83
Vagina	34	0.60	0.42-0.84	0.62	0.43-0.86
Kidney	557	1.11	1.02-1.21	1.12	1.03-1.21
renal pelvis	*30*	*1.26*	*0.85-1.80*	*1.29*	*0.87-1.84*
Bladder, ureter, urethra	227	0.87	0.76-0.99	0.83	0.72-0.94
Skin melanoma	453	0.93	0.85-1.02	0.95	0.86-1.04
Other skin	241	1.03	0.90-1.16	1.00	0.88-1.13
Eye	74	1.05	0.83-1.32	1.07	0.84-1.34
Brain, nervous system	800	1.11	1.03-1.19	1.09	1.02-1.17
Thyroid	428	1.07	0.97-1.18	1.07	0.97-1.17
follicular	*116*	*1.30*	*1.07-1.55*	*1.34*	*1.11-1.59*
papillary	*236*	*0.97*	*0.85-1.10*	*0.97*	*0.85-1.09*
Bone	41	1.19	0.85-1.61	1.28	0.92-1.73
Soft tissue	127	0.97	0.81-1.14	0.96	0.80-1.13
Unspecified	397	1.03	0.94-1.14	1.04	0.94-1.15
Non-Hodgkin's lymphoma	432	1.04	0.95-1.14	1.04	0.94-1.14
Hodgkin's disease	103	0.96	0.79-1.16	0.94	0.77-1.13
Multiple myeloma	238	1.06	0.93-1.20	1.08	0.95-1.22
Leukaemia	423	1.08	0.98-1.18	1.09	0.99-1.20
Not included above:					
Cervix uteri, carcinoma in situ	465	0.93	0.85-1.02	0.95	0.87-1.04
Skin, basal cell carcinoma	3,090	1.06	1.03-1.10	1.06	1.02-1.10

Reference: economically active men.

The total cancer incidence among economically inactive men was 38% larger than the incidence among economically active men, whereas there was no difference between the economically active and inactive women (table 49). The relative proportion of economically inactive men increased from social class I to class IV, and the prevalence of economically inactive women at the time of the 1970 Population Census was highest in social class I and lowest in class II. Still, adjustment for social class did not markedly change the SIR patterns.

High and statistically significant site-specific SIR_as among economically inactive men were obtained for cancer of the pharynx other than nasopharynx (2.79), oesophagus (2.17), oral cavity (2.12), liver (1.96), larynx (1.67), renal pelvis (1.66) and lung (1.59), all of these cancers associated with smoking or drinking. The elevated SIR_a of 1.44 among economically inactive men and 1.47 among women for cancer of the gallbladder might be accounted for by obesity which is likely to be more common among economically inactive men than among economically active ones.

Economically inactive women also had elevated SIRs for alcohol-related cancers (table 50), but the excesses were smaller than those of men. The risks are diluted because the proportion of women with alcohol abuse among economically inactive women is much smaller than that among men. Among women the risk of gallbladder cancer was also elevated (SIR_a 1.47). The high SIR_a of lip cancer (1.56) is probably attributable to the high proportion of farmer's spouses, or the reasons may be similar as those behind the high risk of lip cancer among cooks (table 7).

Cancer of the vulva showed a significant excess (SIR_a 1.56) in contrast to cancer of the vagina (SIR_a 0.62). The reasons for this deviation as well as the reasons for significantly elevated SIR_as of cancers of the nose (1.79) and salivary glands (1.36), and of follicular thyroid carcinoma cannot be anticipated on the basis of current aetiological knowledge. Economically inactive women have a high average number of children [57] and this is reflected as significantly low SIRs for cancers of the breast and ovary.

VI. General discussion

Quality of the data sources

Population Census 1970
Census 1970 was the first census in Finland which was computerised. This was the practical reason why that census was used for this study, even if the earlier ones might have been more relevant because cancer normally has a long latent period between exposure and outcome.

Although the average undercoverage of the 1970 Population Census in the age range of the study was only 2.3 percent, it might in theory be so strongly associated with cancer risk factors cancer that it could cause a bias in the social class or occupational category-specific results. The occupational distribution of a random sample of cancer patients missing from the 1970 Population Census was studied by using the information on occupation in the Cancer Registry records, and the distribution was similar to that of the general population [144]. The undercoverage of the Census thus does not have any major effect on the observed occupational cancer risk pattern.

The prevalence of missing census records by primary site, however, indicates that there is some selection. The highest percentages of missing census data (table 6) were obtained among persons who later got cancer of the larynx (4.8%), the pharynx other than nasopharynx (3.9%), the oesophagus (3.5%) or the liver (3.1%), i.e., cancers associated with alcohol abuse. The percentage of undercoverage of the Population Census among cancer patients slightly increased towards the younger birth cohorts.

Record linkage and follow-up for death
Sometimes the Population Register Center changes the personal identification number (PID) for a person, mainly because of an error in the originally registered date of birth. These changes — made now and then even after the death of the person — existed to some extent in the first years after the introduction of the PID system in 1967, but their frequency has since then been reduced to a very minimum.

Changes in personal identification numbers since 1971 have been taken into account in the Cancer Registry files and partially in annual death files of Statistics Finland but not in the file of the 1970 Population Census. Follow-up for death and cancer morbidity for some of those whose person-numbers have been changed between the last day of 1970 and the last day of 1985 may have failed, but the magnitude of PID changes in the present study series is so small that it has no effect on the observed cancer risk estimates [145]. In the routine record linkages between the Cancer Registry and the Central Population Registry, only 48 changed person-numbers have been revealed among some 500,000 linked cancer patients by the end of 1993.

The automatised record linkage based on PID, has proved to be very accurate in comparison to the best manual linkage procedures. The routine follow-up system for death of the Finnish Cancer Registry provides an example of both manual and automatised record linkage. Until 1975, follow-up was done manually by comparing alphabetical lists of cancer patients with annual alphabetical lists of deceased persons. Since 1976 the same procedure has been fully computerised. In the early 1990s it was possible to check the success of these linkages when the whole cancer register was matched with the population register to identify possible imaginary persons, changes in PIDs, and missing dates of death or emigration. It was discovered that there were some 1% failures in the manual linkage, whereas in the period of automatised linkages the only missing deaths were those few who were registered after the time of record linkage [145].

The follow-up for death was done for the 1970 Population Census cohort to avoid the bias caused by different general mortality in different social classes and occupational categories. Since the mortality in the age groups of this study in 1971-85 varied from $2/10^5$ to $40/10^5$, and the difference between extreme socioeconomic classes was about twofold [46], the maximal effect on the SIR variation because of differences in the general mortality was only some 0.2%-4%, depending on the age group. In the calculations of absolute incidence rates, the numbers of exact person-years are more necessary than in SIR calculations, and they are essential if the analysis is extended to older age-groups. The coverage and accuracy of the annual death and emigration files at Statistics Finland are known to be high, i.e., the lack of follow-up information is not a source of any bias in numbers of person-years.

Cancer Registry

The completeness and accuracy of the Finnish Cancer Registry are very high. Various check-ups have shown that the Registry covers more than 99% of all malignant solid tumours diagnosed in Finland [133] and that false positive diagnoses are not registered as cancers [146]. The registration of some haematological malignancies is slow, and many of them might never be registered without extra efforts by the Cancer Registry staff. According to a comparison of codes of diagnoses from the Hospital Discharge Register including all hospitalizations in Finland, there were 9% of multiple myelomas and over 20% of non-acute leukaemias treated in hospitals during 1985-88 but still missing in the Cancer Registry in October 1993 [133]. The completeness of the registration of skin basaliomas is not known. There are problems in the registration of benign brain tumours (undercoverage almost 20%).

Out of the primary sites studied in the present study, only for chronic lymphocytic leukaemia, multiple myeloma, benign brain tumours and possibly basal cell carcinomas is there such an incompleteness in registration that it could theoretically cause a discernible bias in social class and occupational SIR patterns. Furthermore, the undercoverage is not likely to be strongly associated with social class or occupation, and the possible bias is thus minimal.

Comparison to other types of study

Most of the known occupational causes of cancer have been identified through epidemiological observations with subsequent confirmation by laboratory studies [147]. In some cases (vinyl chloride, mustard gas, 4-aminobiphenyl), the risks were detected in humans after the substances had been shown to induce tumours in laboratory animals, but little attention was given to the experimental studies when first reported. Thus epidemiological studies among human beings are important.

In the case of rare types of cancer in communities with a high prevalence of a specific risk factor, occupational carcinogens can be first identified from clinical observations. The mesothelioma risk of shipyard workers (which later was found to be associated with the use of asbestos) is a typical example of this approach. If the disease is more common or the causal factor more evenly spread throughout the population, a systematic surveillance system may be the only way to generate clues for causal risk associations.

Ecological vs. individual level

The association between the way of life and cancer incidence has been evaluated in ecological analyses both on the international level and within countries. In Finland municipalities (mean population 5,000) were classified according to various determinants of the way of life and welfare, and incidence rates of different cancers were calculated in these categories [148]. Growing trends with an increasing standard of living were obtained for many cancers, the steepest ones for cancers of the kidney, colon, breast and all female genitals as well as for skin melanoma and lung cancer among women. The only clearly opposite trend was that for male lip cancer.

Most of the risk patterns measured in ecological studies are in a parallel direction with the social class trends seen in individual-based studies. However, there are exceptions, the most striking in the above example being that of cervical cancer. The incidence in the wealthiest category of Finnish municipalities was — depending on the categorizing variable — 1.5 to 2.0-fold that of the poorest category, but still the incidence of cervical cancer was higher the lower the woman's own social status was [149]. Unskilled workers and women with only primary school education had a more than three times higher SIR for cervical cancer than managerial workers or women with college or university education respectively. The explanation given for this discrepancy was that in well-to-do municipalities there is a small minority of poor women with an exceptionally high risk.

In figure 43 the cancer incidence pattern in Finland in 1971-85 is given by social class from the present study series, and by municipality categories classified by the average social status of its population aged 35-69 years. The social status of a municipality was operationalised by the percentage of persons belonging to social

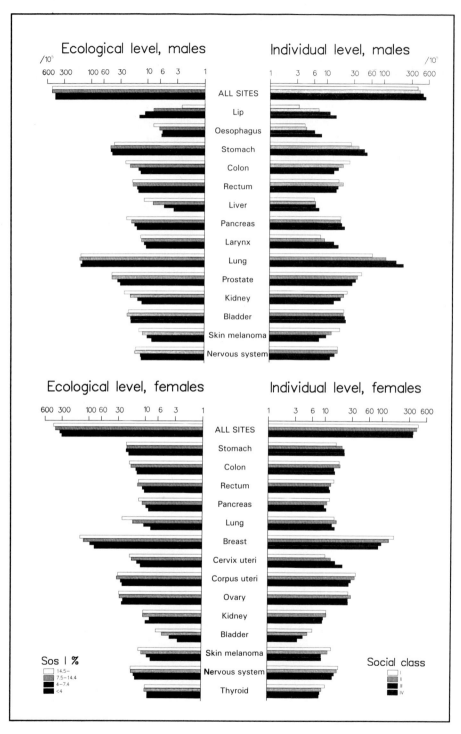

Fig. 43. Social class variation of age-adjusted incidence of selected cancers among men and women in Finland in 1971-85 as measured on ecological and on individual level. *Ecological level*: incidence among men in ages 35-69 in municipalities classified by the percentage of persons belonging to the social class I. *Individual level*: social class division and age limits of the present study series.

class I in that municipality. Other possible operationalisations would have given essentially similar results [148]. In this example one can see the opposite slopes for cervical cancer on individual and ecological levels but also for oesophageal cancer and laryngeal cancers among males. Liver cancer in men and lung cancer in women were much more common in well-to-do areas than in poor ones, although there was almost no variation on the individual level. The opposite was true for lung cancer among men, maybe due to migration. Men who move from rural areas to cities represent lower social classes, and they have a significantly higher risk of lung cancer than both rural and native urban men when adjusted for smoking and occupational exposures [150]. More generally, the well-being of individuals is relative to the standards which are common or customary in the place or society, i.e., some factors may affect differently in different ecological environments [151, 152].

For most sites ecological analyses give parallel results with studies based on individual data if the risk factors concern relatively large fraction of population. Only in exceptional cases are ecological analyses able to reveal risk associations of small population fractions like single occupational categories. One such exception is vinyl chloride exposure, since its target disease, hemangiosarcoma of the liver, virtually does not exist in people other than vinyl chloride workers. Anyhow, the example in fig. 43 proves that any observation obtained in an ecological study has to be confirmed on the individual level. Only few exposures — mainly environmental ones — are affecting all individuals of the area so similarly that the exposure can be generalised to apply the whole population [153].

Mortality vs. incidence

Most of the studies on social and occupational variation in cancer risk are based on mortality, and often these results are thought to be almost equal to those based on incidence. However, there are some problems which may bias the mortality pattern. First, the principles in definition of the underlying cause of death may vary by time, by period, and even by social class or occupation. Secondly, the mortality from competing causes of death may vary in these subgroups. For example in Finland mortality from all main disease categories and also from violent causes of death in 1971-85 was greatest in the lowest social classes, and the social class difference was increasing with time [46]. Finally, the survival of cancer patients in different social classes varies, both because of stage distribution — the well-to-do get their cancers diagnosed on average at an earlier stage — and because of better treatment. In Finland, where health care should be similarly available to everybody, not depending on wealth, breast cancer patients in social class IV had a 28% higher risk of dying from breast cancer than those in social class I, even when corrected for competing causes of death and for stage [154], and similar differences were seen for most other common cancer types [155].

In Finland the reliability of official causes of death is high [146], and thus the error caused by misclassification of cancer deaths is minimal. Still the social class

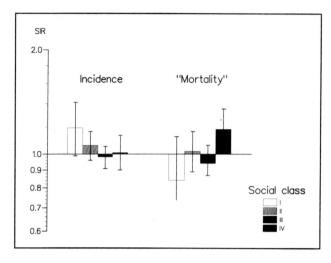

Fig. 44. Standardized incidence ratios with 95% confidence interval of rectal cancer among working-aged Finnish women in 1971-75 (incidence) and the corresponding pattern for those patients who died from rectal cancer by the end of 1992 ("mortality"), by social class.

patterns of non-fatal cancers can be rather different when based on incidence or on mortality. Figure 44 demonstrates the social class pattern of rectal cancer in women in the present study series in two ways: 1) SIRs based on all incident cases in 1971-85 and 2) the corresponding pattern of those incident cases from 1971-85 who, by the end of 1992, died from rectal cancer ("mortality"). The positive social class gradient in the incidence is changed to a negative one in "mortality" due to the better survival in upper social classes. Rectal cancer is one of those sites where the present Finnish results (slightly positive gradient with high social class) differ from those published in many other countries. Besides possible differences in the prevalence and distribution of aetiological factors in difference countries, one of the reasons for the different conclusions may be that many of the results abroad are based on mortality and not on incidence rates.

In the case of most fatal cancers (pancreas, liver, gallbladder and oesophagus, all with a relative five-year survival rate below 10% [156]) there is almost no difference between incidence and mortality patterns, whereas mortality-based studies of the cancers with a five-year survival exceeding 90% (lip, non-melanoma skin) are seldom valid to demonstrate differences in a etiology.

Proportionate analyses

Proportionate analysis has been used in occupational studies if the sizes of occupational categories are not known. In proportionate analysis the risk ratio for a given cancer is defined as the ratio of the proportion of cases of the cancer in question out of all cancer cases in that occupational category, relative to the proportion of that cancer out of all cancer cases in the reference population. In a proportionate analysis it is impossible to calculate risk ratios for total cancer and the risk ratios are biased if there is occupational variation also in the risk of total cancer [157, 158].

In table 51 some of the standardised proportional incidence ratios (SPIRs) reported by a large Danish study [18] are compared with the SIRs of the present study. There are not many common occupational categories in these two studies, since the Danish study did not separate white-collar and blue-collar workers within each industrial branch. The SPIRs among Danish male farmers for cancer of the buccal cavity and pharynx, cancer of the stomach, and for leukaemia were significantly elevated. However, when corrected with the SIR of total cancer among male farmers in Denmark (0.69) [10], the risk estimates of these cancers were close to 1.0 and also very close to the corresponding Finnish SIRs (table 51). An opposite bias is seen among seamen, whose SIR for total cancer in Denmark is above unity (1.34) and the SPIRs thus too low. When multiplied by the SIR for total cancer, the Danish risk estimates again resemble the SIRs achieved by the present Finnish study, indicating increased risk of alcohol-related cancers among seamen in both countries.

The present study showed that there are manyfold differences in the incidence of total cancer by occupation (tables 46-47). Therefore the feasibility of proportionate analysis in occupational cancer studies is sometimes questionable and one has to be careful in the interpretation of the proportional risk ratios.

General case-control vs. general cohort study

In most countries large cohort studies such as the present one are impossible to run because of a lack of linkable population-based registries. Therefore, e.g., in the Metropolitan Montreal area in Canada (population 2.7 million) a study with a similar goal was designed as a large case-control study [159]. The occupational histories and data about some potential confounder (mean census tract income, ethnic group, marital status, smoking and alcohol consumption) of male cancer patients aged 35 to 70 were recorded immediately after the diagnosis of cancer. Certain cancer patients and cancer types (e.g., leukaemia and cancers of the brain, buccal cavity and larynx) had to be excluded for practical reasons, but still the researchers were able to catch a data set of 4,576 patients representing 24 a priori selected primary sites. Similar occupational and confounder data were also collected for 375 population controls (69% of eligible subjects selected from electoral lists). The number of control patients remained small due to high expenses, and for most comparisons the control group was formed from cancer patients or noncancer patients from the same institutions believed to be unrelated to occupational exposures [159]. Using diseased patients as controls is problematic, if it is not quite sure the diseases of control patients are not associated with study factors.

In the Canadian case control study it was possible to identify the occupational exposures more precisely than in the present study based on a single occupational title. Moreover, the data on confounding factors were gathered in detail, and the adjustment for these factors could be made better than in the present study in which social class was used as a proxy for all lifestyle associated confounders. In table 52

Table 51. Standardized proportional incidence ratios (SPIR) reported from the Danish Pension Fund cohort study 1970-79 [18], and standardized incidence ratios (SIR_c) of the present cohort study among male farmers and seamen in selected primary sites

Occupation / Cancer site	Denmark				Finland		
	n	SPIR	95% CI	$SPIR_{corr}$[1]	n	SIR_c	95% CI
Farmers; $SIR_{DK}=0.69$							
Danish industry code 111[2], Finnish occupational code 300[3]							
Buccal cavity and pharynx	51	1.5	1.1-1.9	1.0	419	1.2	1.1-1.3
Oesophagus	10	0.8	0.4-1.5	0.6	91	0.9	0.7-1.1
Stomach	69	1.3	1.0-1.6	0.9	881	1.0	1.0-1.1
Small intestine, colon, rectum	141	1.1	0.9-1.2	0.7	555	0.8	0.8-0.9
Pancreas	36	1.0	0.7-1.3	0.7	294	0.8	0.7-0.9
Larynx	17	0.8	0.5-1.2	0.5	172	0.7	0.6-0.9
Lung	197	0.8	0.7-0.9	0.6	2355	0.8	0.8-0.8
Prostate	97	1.1	0.9-1.4	0.8	656	0.9	0.9-1.0
Kidney	17	0.6	0.4-1.0	0.4	241	0.7	0.6-0.8
Skin melanoma	16	0.7	0.4-1.1	0.5	179	0.9	0.8-1.1
Non-Hodgkin's lymphoma	28	1.2	0.8-1.8	0.8	249	1.0	0.9-1.2
Leukaemia	50	1.6	1.2-2.1	1.1	213	1.0	0.8-1.1
Seamen; $SIR_{DK}=1.34$							
Danish industry code 712[2], Finnish occupational codes 50-51[3]							
Buccal cavity and pharynx	31	1.0	0.7-1.5	1.4	13	1.3	0.7-2.2
Oesophagus	18	1.7	1.1-2.6	2.2	7	2.5	1.0-5.1
Stomach	39	0.8	0.6-1.1	1.1	22	0.9	0.6-1.5
Small intestine, colon, rectum	110	1.0	0.8-1.2	1.3	16	0.8	0.4-1.3
Liver	16	1.7	1.0-2.7	2.2	3	3.3	0.2-2.7
Pancreas	25	0.8	0.5-1.1	1.0	9	0.9	0.4-1.6
Larynx	24	1.3	0.9-1.9	1.7	9	1.4	0.6-2.6
Lung	251	1.2	1.1-1.4	1.6	86	1.1	0.9-1.4
Prostate	72	1.0	0.8-1.3	1.4	20	1.2	0.7-1.8
Testis	27	0.9	0.6-1.3	1.2	2	1.5	0.2-5.4
Kidney	23	0.9	0.6-1.4	1.2	17	1.5	0.9-2.5
Skin melanoma	12	0.6	0.3-1.0	0.8	10	1.3	0.6-2.4
Non-Hodgkin's lymphoma	12	0.6	0.4-1.1	0.8	6	0.8	0.3-1.6
Leukaemia	22	0.9	0.6-1.3	1.2	7	1.0	0.4-2.1

[1] SPIR multiplied by the SIR_{DK} = SIR for overall cancer in the respective occupational category in Denmark [32].
[2] Corresponds closely to the International Standard Industrial classification of all Economic Activities [161].
[3] Occupational codes of the Finnish study: cf. appendix table A.

some of the ORs reported from the Canadian study [160] are compared with the SIRs of the present study.

There are great similarities suggesting that these two approaches in many instances give similar results, but there are also differences. It is hard to evaluate

Table 52. Odds ratios (OR) reported from a Canadian case-control [160], and social class adjusted standardized incidence ratios (SIR_a) of the present cohort study among male workers in comparable occupations and primary sites

Occupation Cancer site	T[1]	C[2]	Canada			Finland		
			n	OR	90% CI[3]	n	SIR_a	95% CI
Forestry workers (34[4])								
Stomach	A	C	22	2.7	1.8-4.1	169	1.2	1.0-1.4
Rectum	A	C	14	1.8	1.0-3.0	38	0.9	0.7-1.2
Lung	F	C	47	1.2	0.8-1.8	602	1.1	1.0-1.2
Lung, small cell[5]	A	C	13	1.7	0.9-3.0	119	1.2	1.0-1.4
Sheet metal workers (653[4])								
Lung, squamous cell	A	C	29	1.4	0.9-2.0	47	1.7	1.2-2.2
Bladder	A	C	39	1.5	1.1-2.1	16	1.4	0.8-2.2
Plumbers and pipefitters (654[4])								
Stomach	F	C	8	2.4	1.2-4.6	39	1.1	0.8-1.5
Lung, adenocarcinoma	A	P	4	1.4	0.5-4.2	27	1.9	1.2-2.7
Lung, small cell[5]	A	C	9	2.0	1.0-4.2	26	1.3	0.8-1.8
Kidney	F	C	5	2.1	0.9-4.6	15	0.9	0.5-1.5
Welders and flame cutters (655[4])								
Lung	A	C	36	1.6	1.1-2.4	101	1.2	1.0-1.4
Lung, squamous cell	A	C	19	2.0	1.2-3.2	43	1.4	1.0-1.9
Prostate	F	C	11	1.2	0.6-2.2	23	1.5	1.0-2.2
Bladder	A	C	16	1.5	0.9-2.6	18	1.4	0.9-2.3
Printers (701[4])								
Rectum	A	P	6	2.6	0.9-7.3	4	2.0	0.6-5.2
Pancreas	A	C	6	2.1	0.8-5.2	4	1.7	0.8-5.2
Lung	A	C	26	2.1	1.2-3.7	19	1.1	0.7-1.7
Kidney	F	C	5	3.4	1.4-7.9	5	2.0	0.6-4.6
Bladder	A	P	10	2.3	0.9-6.0	6	2.4	0.9-5.1

[1] Canadian target population (A: All, F: French).
[2] Control group (P: Population, C: Cancer).
[3] 90% confidence interval.
[4] Occupational code of the Finnish study: cf. appendix table A.
[5] In Canadian study called *oat cell* carcinoma.

whether these differences are due to the incomplete control for confounders or the misclassification of occupational histories, or whether different risk estimates are due to differences in the exposure levels or other aetiological factors associated with work between Canada and Finland. Even when the Canadian study is one of the largest case-control occupational studies ever made, numbers of cases are usually only one-tenth of those in the Finnish study and the confidence intervals are thus wider. In the

Canadian study, comparisons were always made with two different reference groups (cancer controls, population controls), and separately for the French population and the total population, and even these comparisons often gave inconsistent results. (It should be noted that the comparison between the Canadian and the Finnish study is one-sided, i.e., there are many associations showing elevated risks in Finland but not reported among the high-light results of the Canadian study and thus missing from table 52.)

It can be concluded that in cancer surveys based on linkable high-quality population-based registers the occupational exposure and confounder data might be somewhat less exact than the large-scale case-control studies which, however, were compensated by the larger amount and better coverage of cancers, and by a cheaper price. The data collection for the present study from existing registers, including all the computer-work and human-power, cost at least ten times less than the data collection of the twenty times smaller series of the Canadian study [159].

Specific studies vs. general surveillance system

In table 53 there are results from traditional occupational cohort studies in Finland in which as detailed as possible occupational histories have been collected from payrolls of the companies or other similar sources. Since the present survey is restricted to the years 1971-85 and the age limitation excludes 30% of cases, the numbers of series in specific cohort studies in branches where all workers in the country can be caught into the cohort, e.g., through trade union membership registers (teachers [162], locomotive drivers [100], hairdressers [93]) can be even larger than in the present study series. When the specific cohorts have to be collected basicly from single plants (e.g., workers of sawmills [164] and machine shops [163]), the general surveillance system provides a larger study base.

In general, the general surveillance system seems to give very similar risk estimates for various cancers as the specific cohort studies (table 53). Non-melanoma skin cancer among sawmill workers and hairdressers seem to be an exception. This is possibly due to the age distribution of non-melanoma skin cancer: a large proportion of the cases are diagnosed in ages above 70 and have therefore been excluded from the present study, but not necessarily from the specific studies.

In the case of rubber industry workers the SIRs seem to have decreased from those published from the period 1953-76 [166]. The earlier observations were based on very small numbers and were thus possibly subject to chance variation, but the change in the risk pattern may also be true and indicate the decrease of hazardous agents in working conditions in rubber industry.

It is difficult to find case-referent studies in Finland in which cancer risks would have been analysed in occupations comparable to the classification of the present study. A recent questionnaire study [167] on risk factors of pancreatic cancer (using deceased stomach cancer and colorectal cancer patients as controls) also reported odd ratios by occupational branch. These rates — adjusted for age, gender, smoking, alcohol consumption and diabetes — are very similar to the social class-adjusted SIRs

Table 53. Standardized incidence ratios reported from specific control studies (SIR) and of the present general survey (SIR_c; not adjusted for social class) among workers in comparable occupations and primary sites

Occupation / Cancer site	Specific cohort study			General survey		
	n	SIR	95% CI	n	SIR_c	95% CI
051[1] Teachers of physical education and languages, women 1967-91 [162]						
Stomach	24	0.8	0.5-1.1	5	0.4	0.1-0.9
Colon	35	1.3	0.9-1.8	10	0.9	0.4-1.6
Rectum	16	0.9	0.5-1.5	4	0.5	0.1-1.3
Lung	12	0.7	0.3-1.2	3	0.3	0.1-1.0
Breast	228	1.5	1.3-1.7	154	1.6	1.4-1.9
Cervix uteri	3	0.2	0.0-0.5	4	0.4	0.1-1.0
Corpus uteri	49	1.5	1.1-2.0	28	1.4	0.9-2.0
Ovary	51	1.6	1.2-2.1	26	1.2	0.8-1.8
Kidney	15	1.1	0.6-1.9	7	1.2	0.5-2.4
All sites	621	1.2	1.1-1.3	304	1.1	1.0-1.2
530[1] Locomotive drivers, men 1953-91 [100]						
Oral cavity and pharynx	17	1.8	1.0-2.8	3	1.7	0.3-4.9
Stomach	86	0.8	0.6-0.9	8	0.5	0.2-1.1
Colon and rectum	65	0.9	0.7-1.2	13	1.0	0.5-1.7
Lung	236	0.9	0.8-1.0	34	0.7	0.5-0.9
Mesothelioma	8	4.1	1.8-8.0	2	3.6	0.4-13
Prostate	112	1.1	0.9-1.3	11	1.1	0.6-2.0
Kidney	38	1.2	0.9-1.7	10	1.4	0.7-2.5
Bladder	48	1.1	0.8-1.4	8	1.0	0.4-2.1
Skin, non-melanoma	32	1.5	1.0-2.1	4	1.6	0.4-4.0
Non-Hodgkin's lymphoma	19	0.8	0.5-1.2	5	1.0	0.3-2.3
All sites	915	1.0	0.9-1.0	146	0.9	0.8-1.0
65[1] Machine shop/steelworkers, men 1953-81 [163]						
Stomach	105	0.8	0.7-1.0	280	1.1	1.0-1.2
Colon and rectum	63	0.9	0.7-1.1	214	1.0	0.9-1.1
Nose	3	0.8	0.2-2.2	7	0.7	0.3-1.5
Larynx	32	1.0	0.7-1.4	92	1.3	1.0-1.6
Lung	337	1.1	1.0-1.2	1060	1.2	1.2-1.3
Prostate	87	1.1	0.9-1.3	171	1.0	0.8-1.1
Bladder	40	1.1	0.8-1.5	145	1.1	1.0-1.3
Skin, non-melanoma	21	1.1	0.7-1.7	58	1.3	1.0-1.6
Lymphoma (incl. Hodgkin's disease)	24	0.8	0.5-1.2	122	1.0	0.9-1.2
Leukaemia	28	1.1	0.7-1.5	72	1.0	0.8-1.2
All sites	987	1.0	0.9-1.0	3095	1.1	1.1-1.1
671[1] Sawmill workers 1961-80 [164]						
Lip, mouth and pharynx	7	1.6	0.7-3.4	23	1.6	1.0-2.5
Stomach	16	0.9	0.5-1.5	38	1.0	0.7-1.4
Colon and rectum	15	1.5	0.8-2.4	35	1.0	0.7-1.4
Lung	28	1.1	0.7-1.5	94	0.8	0.6-1.0
Bladder	3	0.9	0.2-2.7	16	0.9	0.5-1.5
Skin, non-melanoma	8	2.7	1.2-5.3	4	0.6	0.2-1.5
Lymphoma (incl. Hodgkin's disease)	4	1.4	0.4-3.5	16	1.0	0.6-1.6
Leukaemia	7	2.3	0.9-4.8	6	0.5	0.2-1.2
All sites	145	1.1	0.9-1.3	409	0.9	0.8-1.0

Table 53 (continued)

Occupation Cancer site	Specific cohort study			General survey		
	n	SIR	95% CI	n	SIR$_c$	95% CI
710/712/713[1] Glass factory workers 1953-86 [165]						
Stomach	34	0.9	0.6-1.3	12	1.8	0.9-3.2
Colon and rectum	21	0.8	0.5-1.2	5	0.8	0.3-1.8
Lung	69	1.3	1.0-1.6	22	1.3	0.8-1.9
Breast	39	0.9	0.7-1.2	5	0.5	0.2-1.1
Bladder	9	1.0	0.4-1.8	4	1.5	0.4-3.8
All sites	303	0.9	0.8-1.0	91	1.1	0.9-1.3
751[1] Rubber industry workers 1953-76 [166]						
Digestive organs	7	1.4	0.5-2.8	26	1.2	0.8-1.8
Respiratory organs	3	1.5	0.3-4.4	17	0.9	0.5-1.5
Lymphatic and hematopoietic tissue	2	1.3	0.2-4.5	6	0.9	0.3-1.9
Bladder	2	6.7	0.8-24	1	0.4	0.1-2.0
All sites	21	1.1	0.7-1.7	100	1.0	0.8-1.2
840[1] Hairdressers, women 1970-87 [93]						
Stomach	14	1.2	0.6-1.9	10	0.9	0.4-1.7
Colon and rectum	21	1.3	0.8-2.0	18	1.1	0.6-1.1
Pancreas	9	1.5	0.7-2.8	11	2.0	1.0-3.6
Lung	13	1.7	0.9-2.9	10	1.2	0.6-2.2
Breast	70	1.2	1.0-1.6	77	1.1	0.9-1.4
Cervix uteri	11	1.5	0.8-2.8	10	1.2	0.6-2.1
Corpus uteri	18	1.3	0.8-2.1	21	1.1	0.8-1.8
Ovary	21	1.6	1.0-2.5	27	1.6	1.1-2.4
Skin, non-melanoma	6	2.0	0.7-4.3	-	exp 2.4	0-1.6
Leukaemia	4	1.0	0.3-2.5	5	1.2	0.4-2.8
All sites	247	1.3	1.1-1.4	262	1.2	1.1-1.4

[1] Occupational code in the present survey: cf. appendix table A.

of the present study, showing an elevated risk of pancreatic cancer, e.g., among hairdressers (table 54).

Criticisms against the surveillance systems based on death certificates and disease registers have been raised, because the inconsistencies, e.g., in occupational classifications tend to diminish the real risk differences. However, the risk estimates given by specific studies and by the present survey are in most instances almost identical (tables 53-54). The diluting effect in the general surveillance approach thus seems not to be essentially more disturbing than in specific studies on occupational cancer risks.

Table 54. Odds ratios (OR) reported from a case-referent study on *pancreatic cancer* in Finland 1984-87 [167] and social class adjusted standardized incidence ratios (SIR_a) of the present general cohort survey in comparable occupational branches

Branch[1]	Case-referent study			General survey		
	n	OR[2]	95% CI	n	SIR_a	95% CI
Agriculture, forestry, fishing (3)	169	0.8	0.7-1.0	555	0.9	0.8-0.9
Mining and quarrying (4)	6	1.5	0.6-4.2	14	1.5	0.8-2.6
Transport and communication (5)	54	1.0	0.7-1.5	204	1.2	1.0-1.3
Textiles and clothes (60,61)	12	0.7	0.4-1.4	42	0.8	0.6-1.1
Sawmilling (671)	10	1.3	0.6-2.9	17	1.0	0.6-1.6
Printing (70)	9	1.7	0.7-4.1	14	1.2	0.6-1.9
Paper and board (735)	17	1.4	0.8-2.5	15	1.6	0.9-2.6
Restautants, cafés, snack bars (82)	7	1.8	0.3-1.9	21	1.3	0.8-2.1
Hairdressing, manicure (840,841)	4	1.8	0.5-6.4	14	2.1	1.2-2.3

[1] The occupational categories of the present survey corresponding as precisely as possible to the industrial branch titles of the case-referent study are given in parentheses.
[2] Odds ratios adjusted for age, gender, smoking, alcohol consumption and diabetes.

Limits of the present study

Classification of social class and occupation

Social class can be defined as a segment of the population widely sharing similar types and levels of resources with broadly similar styles of living and some shared perception of their collective condition [44]. Traditionally, inequalities have been portrayed through a characterization of class by ranking occupations according to their social status and prestige. A variety of other factors may be said to play a part in determining class: income, wealth, type of housing tenure, education, style of consumption, mode of behaviour, social origins and family and local connections. They are interrelated, and none of them should be regarded sufficient in itself [44]. There are studies indicating that different determinants of social class tend to give parallel results, e.g., in patterns of general mortality [168] or cancer incidence [105].

Historically, occupation has been selected as a principal indicator of social class. Occupation does not simply designate the type of work and occupation-related hazardous agents but also tends to broadly show how strenuous or unhealthy it is in general, what the likely working conditions are — for example whether it is indoors or outdoors — and what amenities and facilities are available. Pay and fringe benefits will determine the family living standard, and family members may be indirectly affected by some features of the working conditions, like the risk of intermittent employment or the stress of disablement and of shift work.

Occupation-based classifications of social class most often have two main problems [169]: classifications are too rigid and do not take into account the changes in society and the occupational groups are too heterogenous in income and education. The classification used in the 1970 Population Census of Finland was not a mechanical one but used results from sociological studies on social class and occupation in Finland. The occupational status of a patient was assessed before the cancer had been diagnosed, i.e., the bias caused by a downward drift in the social hierarchy as a result of disease [170] should have been avoided.

Defining the social class of women includes more problems than that for men. Using the woman's own occupation as a determinant of her social class has been criticised because it may be an insufficient measure of deprivation and poor life circumstances. A measure combining a woman's own and her relatives' occupations and education might prove useful [171]. Different indicators of social class may give different results, e.g., in regard to subjective health or the use of gynaecological services, but in the case of most cancer types all social class indicators discriminate women similarly [172, 173].

The accuracy of the occupational codes in Finnish population censuses has been evaluated and was proven to be high: the net error in the 3-digit level occupational codes in the 1980 Census was less than 2% [174]. The occupational stability between Censuses of 1975 and 1980 and between Censuses of 1980 and 1985 was 85-86% in both sexes [174]. The stability in 1980-85 was highest (96-97%) among dentists, policemen and physicians. Low stability was characteristic, e.g., for messengers (56%), labourers (61%), housekeepers (62%) and building hands (66%). It can be assumed that in occupations with a professional or vocational training, the occupational category of the 1970 Population Census usually represents relatively well the life-long occupational history, whereas in less specialised occupations there is more heterogeneity. E.g., many of the persons who moved from farming occupations to towns belong to unskilled workers.

In future analyses the occupational stability can be taken into account by combining subsequent censuses. The occupational risks should be best visible among those who did not change their occupation (unless the changes were due to exposure). In some occupational categories the exposures could be better pointed out when persons with a similar occupation title would be divided into groups by the industry of their employer. This will be done in the next update of the Finnish cancer surveillance system.

Job exposure matrices

When precise occupational titles are used as such, many of the single categories are small and therefore usually fail to show convincing risk estimates. One effective way to gather the scattered data is to classify occupational categories by exposure to the risk factors to be studied and then add up the observed and expected numbers of

Table 55. Incidence of leukaemia and tumours of the nervous system among male industrial workers aged 25 to 64 years in Finland in 1971-80, by category of occupational exposure to ELF magnetic fields [136]

Cancer type	Exposure	Obs[1]	Exp[2]	RR[3]	95% CI	p for trend[4]
Leukaemia	Probable	10	6.4	1.85	1.0-3.5	
	Possible	94	77.7	1.42	1.1-1.8	*0.005*
	No exposure	117	136.9	1.0	ref.	
Nervous system	Probable	13	11.1	1.31	0.7-2.3	
	Possible	149	128.1	1.29	1.0-1.6	*0.02*
	No exposure	204	226.8	1.0	ref.	

[1] Observed number of cases.
[2] Expected number of cases based on age and period-specific incidence rates in all industrial occupations.
[3] Relative risk adjusted for age and period by a log-linear model, with 95% confidence interval (CI).
[4] p-value for testing the existence of linear trend effect of exposure.

cases for categories with similar exposure levels. This type of combining was done in an earlier set of Finnish occupational cancer incidence data by exposure to the extremely low frequency (ELF) magnetic fields [136]. The blue collar occupational titles of the 1970 Population Census were *a priori* classified by the likelihood of ELF magnetic field exposure, and then the occupation-specific observed and expected numbers of leukaemia and central nervous system tumours were added up according to these exposure categories. Although none of the single occupational categories with ELF magnetic field exposure showed any apparent excess when studied one by one, the combined SIRs for both leukaemia and nervous system tumours increased significantly by increasing exposure probability (table 55).

Construction of an extensive Finnish job exposure matrix (FINJEM) which systematically classifies all occupational categories of the Finnish population censuses by the likelihood and level of exposure to numerous known or suspected agents such as solvents and organic dusts is already in its final straight. This matrix will be done mainly by work environmental hygienists of the Institute of Occupational Health in Finland and will then be linked with the occupational cancer surveillance system of the Finnish Cancer Registry. FINJEM also includes historical data about the change of exposure levels from the 1920s to the 1980s and thus allows the monitoring of cancer risk trends following varying exposure levels. While the classical work place exposures have been reduced after getting to know their health hazards, some new potential work-related factors come up. Therefore FINJEM will be supplemented by variables such as physical strain, work stress, monotony and irregulatory, which in the future are likely to affect the occupational risk pattern much more than chemical agents.

The present study did not focus on single agents in working environments. This may be considered as a weakness. On the other hand, there are numerous examples showing that even after most careful examinations it has proved better to define the whole industrial process as hazardous rather than single agents included in the process [39]. Exposure to chemical mixtures may be considerably more hazardous than to individual chemicals [5]. Precise occupational titles, perhaps further specified by industrial codes, thus provide in many instances a rather good basis for searching occupational hazards.

Social class in controlling for confounding

Social class is a satisfactory proxy only for such confounding factors, the prevalence of which strongly correlates with it. Smoking, and many dietary factors are known to correlate with social class in Finland [48, 49]. Consumption of fruit and vegetables is clearly highest among highly educated well-to-do people. Consumption of meat and fat used to be highest among the richest Finns, but nowadays the low-fat products are most popular in the highest social classes. A similar shift has been seen in smoking among women, which first was a habit of highly educated urban women but has since the 1970s increased especially among women with only basic education.

Physical exertion used to be hardest in blue-collar occupations, but it has decreased with automatization. Leisure-time physical activity is most popular among white-collar professions. Some reproductive factors are known to vary by social class: the age at menarche is lowest and at menopause and first birth highest among women of higher social classes. There is only a slight variation between socioeconomic classes in the average number of children (from 2.7 among 40-49-year-old blue-collar workers to 2.4 among upper-level clerical workers), although the variation between occupational categories is relatively large [57]. Alcohol consumption is not systematically associated with social class, but there are population subgroups with higher-than-average alcohol consumption in each social class [56]. Therefore the occupations with a low average number of children tend to have high SIRs of cancers associated with high fertility, and those with high alcohol consumption high SIRs of alcohol-related cancers even after adjustment for social class.

Controlling of confounding using social class information is even at its best incomplete because of the intermixing of confounding factors throughout the social strata. Thus the social class adjusted rates (SIR_a) in comparison to unadjusted rates (SIR_c) rather indicate the direction of correction, but there always remains some residual confounding in the SIR_as. On the other hand, in many studies social class has been considered as a risk determinant of cancer even when no specific aetiological factors can be pointed out. Social class adjustment may control for factors or interactions which today are not yet known to be involved in cancer causation. Socioeconomic differences in health necessarily belong to any society with a hierarchial structure, and it has been suggested that one should perhaps study social status as a whole as a causal factor of health instead of searching for single factors associated with different ways of life [152].

Social class is mostly based on occupation. Especially in large occupational categories of social class IV (forestry workers, building hands, labourers) the possibility of overadjustment should be taken into account when interpreting the occupation-specific SIR_as, because each category has a great impact on the reference incidence in social class IV. Therefore, the SIR_c should also always be studied in the case of these occupations. E.g., the SIR_a of small cell lung carcinoma among Finnish forestry workers (1.2) shown in table 52 is much smaller than the odds ratio among the Canadian ones but the SIR_c in Finland is exactly the same as the OR in Canada (1.7).

Data on risk factors, neither those associated with occupational categories nor those associated with social class, are seldom systematically available in numerical form for comparable classifications, especially not for older time periods relevant in the causation of cancers of the study period, 1971-85. Thus, no numerical parameters for associations were calculated, and no multivariate analyses for studying the independent roles or various factors were done in the present study. These can be done in further studies restricted to associations of specific occupations, social classes and cancer sites.

Multiple tests

This study produced over 30,000 occupation, cancer site and sex specific crude SIRs and 30,000 social class adjusted SIRs. It is difficult to conclude which of the numerous excess risks are just chance findings and which are true. The number of observed statistically significant SIRs compared with the corresponding expected number may tell whether or not the occupational variation for a certain cancer site is larger than just by chance. There should be about 2.5% of the occupation-specific SIRs significantly both below and above 1.0 on the 95% significance level. In practice, when some of the expected numbers are small and the number of observed cases is a discrete variable, the expected number of significant SIRs is smaller, especially in the case of SIRs below 1.0.

Out of a total of about 70 occupational branches (two-digit level of occupational code) and over 320 specific occupational categories (three-digit codes) the average number of men working in that occupation was less than 100 in 2 occupational branches and 56 specific categories among men and in 11 branches and 117 specific categories among women. In a category of 100 workers the expected number of cases (all sites) is 5-6. This means that the SIR has to be below 0.2 or very high above 2.0 to reach statistical significance ($p<0.05$). For specific cancer sites the respective limits are even more extreme: e.g., for colon cancer the expected number in a category of 100 workers is around 0.25 in each sex and only an SIR exceeding 8.3 would be statistically significant. If the expected number of cases is less than 3.69 the SIR can never be significantly below 1.0.

General discussion

Table 56 gives the numbers of significantly low and high SIR_as in the present study on 95%, 99% and 99.9% significence levels among three-digit occupational categories. On 95% significance level only total cancer and cancers of the lung (small cell carcinoma and squamous cell carcinoma) and the breast exceeded the theoretical expected number of significantly elevated SIR_as (2.5% of the observations), thus confirming the larger than chance occupational variation of these cancers. Numbers of significant excesses on higher significance levels indicate that at least cancers of the cervix uteri, lip and kidney may belong to the occupation-related ones, too.

The justification whether or not an observed association is likely to be true should not be based on statistical significance only. Other knowledge about the meaningfulness of the association such as similar earlier observations and theories of possible causal mechanisms should be taken into account. If this evaluation is done properly, it should actually not make any difference whether the risk estimate stems from a multiple test system or from a specific study designed to investigate just that association [175, 176].

Age, period, latency

The age range of this study, 35-64 years at the beginning of each five-year period is close to what has been considered optimal in occupational cancer studies [177]. Cancers — particularly solid tumours — diagnosed before 35 years of age are not likely to be associated with occupational exposures, since the minimum latency between the first exposure and the onset of cancer is at least five years, with a large proportion of cases appearing between 10 and 30 years after exposure [5, 147]. In the older ages other factors than occupational ones become so dominant that the possible occupational component may be nonidentifiable. To date, no agent has been solely identified through study of retired persons [5].

There are, however, some carcinogenic agents with such long inducing times that the upper age limit of this study series, 64-69 years is too low. E.g., the risk pattern of mesothelioma remained relatively uninformative, because asbestos-related mesotheliomas may appear more than 40 years after the first exposure [102, 178]. The upper age limit of the present study also seems to be too low, e.g., when estimating the long-term cumulative effects of UV-radiation on the risk of non-melanoma skin cancer.

Most of the major occupational hazards known today had been recognised by the early 1970s [5, 179]. In the last 30 years production and use of carcinogens has been regulated, and exposure to carcinogens in many industrialised countries has been decreasing. Exposure levels, especially in large plants of industrialised countries, are now sometimes several orders of magnitude lower than in the past, whereas industrial hygiene may not be adequate in small plants with only a few workers in many countries [5]. Industrial processes which have been discontinued or strictly regulated in industrialised countries may continue or be exported elsewhere. Therefore, it would also be important to include in the cancer surveillance systems older periods both for cancer follow-up and especially for occupational exposure.

Table 56. Number of occupation-specific (three-digit occupational code level) social class adjusted SIRs significantly above 1.0 in 1971-85, by sex and significance level

Primary site	Males			Females		
	95%	99%	99.9%	95%	99%	99.9%
Expected significant excesses[1]	8.3	1.7	0.2	8.1	1.6	0.2
All sites	**28**	**15**	**10**	**17**	**8**	**3**
Lip	5	4	2	3	-	-
Tongue	3	-	-	3	1	-
Salivary glands	2	-	-	-	-	-
Oral cavity	1	-	-	2	1	-
Nasopharynx	2	1	-	1	-	-
Pharynx excl. nasopharynx	5	-	-	1	-	-
Oesophagus	5	-	-	2	-	-
Stomach	5	-	-	1	1	-
Small intestine	1	1	-	6	1	1
Colon	3	1	-	2	1	-
Rectum	3	1	-	2	-	-
Liver	8	2	-	5	-	-
Gallbladder, biliary tract	2	-	-	3	-	-
Pancreas	8	2	2	4	-	-
Nose, nasal sinuses	5	1	-	-	-	-
Larynx	7	2	-	5	1	-
Lung, trachea	32	19	9	14	4	3
adenocarcinoma	*9*	*3*	-	*3*	*1*	-
small cell carcinoma	*14*	*5*	*1*	*6*	*1*	-
squamous cell carcinoma	*22*	*12*	*3*	*9*	*4*	*2*
Mesothelioma	5	2	-	1	-	-
Breast	-	-	-	20	6	3
Cervix uteri	.	.	.	5	1	1
Corpus uteri	.	.	.	5	1	-
Ovary	.	.	.	8	2	-
Vulva	.	.	.	2	-	-
Vagina	.	.	.	2	-	-
Prostate	5	-	-	.	.	.
Testis	3	-	-	.	.	.
Penis	1	-	-	.	.	.
Kidney	7	4	2	3	1	1
renal pelvis	*4*	*1*	-	*5*	*1*	-
Bladder, ureter, urethra	3	-	-	6	2	-
Skin melanoma	2	-	-	2	-	-
head and neck	-	-	-	*3*	-	-
trunk	*3*	*1*	-	*4*	-	-
limbs	*3*	*1*	-	*6*	*1*	-
Other skin	3	1	-	2	1	-
Eye	4	-	-	3	-	-
Brain, nervous system	4	1	-	6	1	-
Thyroid	5	1	-	3	2	1
Other endocrine glands	3	-	-	2	1	-
Bone	3	-	-	3	1	-
Soft tissue	3	-	-	2	-	-
Unspecified	5	-	-	2	1	-
Non-Hodgkin's lymphoma	6	-	-	1	1	-
Hodgkin's disease	4	1	-	2	-	-
Multiple myeloma	2	-	-	4	-	-
Leukaemia	5	1	-	5	-	-
Not included above:						
Skin, basal cell carcinoma	9	4	-	11	6	3

Reference: economically active population.

[1] Due to the small numbers of expected cases in many occupational categories and the discrete nature of the observed number of cases, the actual expected number of significantly high SIR_ss is always smaller than the theoretical one, the difference being the larger the less common the disease.

Unfortunately, the oldest computerised population census in Finland is relatively recent, dating only from 1970. Occupational data from the 1960 Population Census would have added to the knowledge of occupational histories and occupational stability, thereby strengthening the results. Because occupational stability in Finland before 1970, especially among specialised workers, was relatively high, the observation period of the present study, i.e., 1971-85, should anyway sufficiently reflect the occupational circumstances in the 1940s to 1960s. Since cancer usually cannot be diagnosed in a preclinical phase, the healthy worker effect related to selection at recruitment in a study based on incident cancer cases is minimal [5]. Thus, starting the follow-up immediately after the date of the 1970 Population Census should theoretically not cause any major bias in this study. The relative risks observed during the first five-year follow-up period were not systematically lower than in the latter ones.

Although the occupational cancer risks caused by work place exposures tend to strongly decrease some decades after the cancerogenecity of the exposures becomes known, new occupation-related risk factors come up. In the modern work environment non-chemical factors may become important. Such factors are included, e.g., in sedentary jobs and jobs with work stress. Therefore, repeatable surveillance systemsare of great value. If Finland, the basic work for an update of the present occupational cancer data base up to the early 1990s has already been done.

Upper social classes as predictors of future cancer incidence

The living standard in Finland rose constantly until very recent years, and by the end of the 1980s Finland's gross national product per inhabitant was among the ten highest countries in the world, more evenly distributed between all citizens than in many other industrial countries. This has meant that it has been possible for people of low social classes to come close to the living standard of higher classes, learning features of their way of life relatively soon after them. E.g., the adopting of new and healthier dietary habits typically happens about ten years later in the lowest social class than in the highest one [51, 180]. There is also a shift towards higher social classes among people, i.e., the proportions of different social classes in the population change with time.

If the way of life for the high social classes later becomes common for the rest of the population, the cancer incidence of lifestyle-associated cancers should also follow that of the high social classes with a certain delay. The present data set provides an opportunity to study this delay with real observations. Figure 45 shows the incidence trends of the most common and selected other cancer sites among Finnish men and women aged 35-69 years as recorded by the Finnish Cancer Registry. The total population seemed to reach the overall cancer incidence level of social classes I-II in 1971-75 some 10-15 years later and for many cancer sites even sooner.

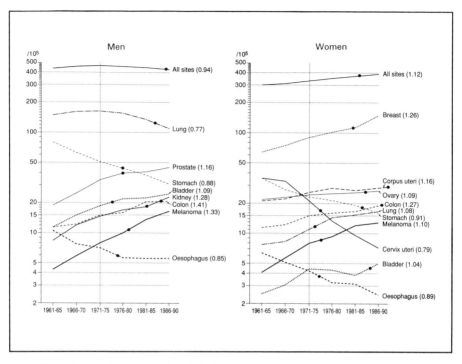

Fig. 45. Trends of age-adjusted incidence of most common and selected other sites cancer sites among Finnish men and women aged 35-69, with dots (●) indicating when the incidence among the total population reached the combined incidence level of social classes I and II as it was in 1971-75.

For cancers of the corpus uteri and colon among women, the delay was more than 15 years, and for cancers of the rectum and pancreas there was no consistent change in incidence over time, i.e., this exercise was irrelevant for these sites.

It can to be concluded that for cancers with a clearly decreasing or increasing incidence trend the incidence of upper social classes serves as a predictor of future incidence for the whole population with a delay from some years to almost 20 years, depending on the cancer site.

Preventability

Social class variation

All of the three most important risk factors of cancer, i.e., diet, smoking and reproductive factors [1], vary by social class in Finland, and much of the observed social class variation seen for different cancer types can be explained by general lifestyle factors. In tables 57 and 58 it has been calculated how much less the number

Table 57. Numbers of cancer cases in 1971-85 (Obs.) and difference to the expected number of cases assuming that the incidence in all social classes would be same as in the social class with the lowest SIR (⋈), given as absolute number of cases (Diff.) and as percentage of the site-specific total (%) for selected primary sites, by social class (I-IV); age 35-64 at the beginning of each 5-year follow-up period, males

Primary site	I			II			III			IV			Total			%/Total[1]
	Obs.	Diff.	%	Obs.	Diff.	%	Obs.	Diff.	%	Obs.	Diff.	%	Obs.	Diff.	%	
ALL SITES	3,195	⋈	⋈	9,533	1,013	10.6	25,873	5,703	22.0	8,577	2,579	30.1	47,178	9,344	19.8	19.8
Lip	26	⋈	⋈	166	92	55.5	620	446	72.0	234	181	77.5	1,046	719	68.8	1.5
Oral cavity	21	10	47.7	31	⋈	⋈	100	39	39.4	37	21	57.5	189	75	39.5	0.2
Pharynx excl. nasopharynx	22	7	31.7	50	10	19.4	117	⋈	⋈	42	14	33.8	231	53	23.0	0.1
Oesophagus	34	⋈	⋈	101	18	17.8	332	140	42.0	132	76	57.2	599	237	39.5	0.5
Stomach	226	⋈	⋈	834	228	27.4	2,485	1,031	41.5	819	379	46.2	4,364	1,642	37.6	3.5
Colon	213	93	43.8	444	131	29.6	875	153	17.5	212	⋈	⋈	1,744	386	22.1	0.8
Rectum	143	19	13.4	439	103	23.5	857	65	7.5	239	⋈	⋈	1,678	191	11.4	0.4
Liver	49	⋈	⋈	144	12	8.1	346	36	10.3	119	27	22.8	658	75	11.4	0.2
Gallbladder, biliary tract	22	⋈	⋈	84	26	31.0	175	37	21.4	60	19	30.9	341	83	24.3	0.2
Pancreas	148	6	3.9	400	⋈	⋈	1,006	90	9.0	337	65	19.1	1,891	173	9.2	0.4
Larynx	65	⋈	⋈	213	44	20.7	733	326	44.5	258	133	51.6	1,269	507	40.0	1.1
Lung, trachea	526	⋈	⋈	2,514	1,087	43.2	8,964	5,555	62.0	3,609	2,571	71.2	15,613	9,224	59.1	19.6
adenocarcinoma	77	⋈	⋈	306	92	30.2	977	465	47.6	327	172	52.5	1,687	728	43.1	1.5
small cell carcinoma	95	⋈	⋈	425	162	38.1	1,440	817	56.7	552	364	66.0	2,512	1,343	53.4	2.8
squamous cell carcinoma	160	⋈	⋈	847	417	49.3	3,129	2,113	67.5	1,237	931	75.3	5,373	3,466	64.5	7.3
Prostate	316	96	30.5	760	136	17.8	1,721	201	11.7	473	⋈	⋈	3,270	425	13.0	0.9
Testis	38	26	68.2	48	20	42.4	82	20	24.7	16	⋈	⋈	184	67	36.7	0.1
Kidney	200	80	39.8	474	156	33.0	975	232	23.8	215	⋈	⋈	1,864	469	25.1	1.0
Bladder, ureter, urethra	171	7	4.2	452	⋈	⋈	1,141	75	6.6	357	37	10.3	2,121	123	5.8	0.3
Skin melanoma	164	91	55.5	306	120	39.3	562	137	24.4	116	⋈	⋈	1,148	348	30.4	0.7
Other skin	67	9	13.7	154	⋈	⋈	406	37	9.2	118	9	7.3	745	54	7.2	0.1
Brain, nervous system	150	34	22.6	383	90	23.6	791	119	15.0	180	⋈	⋈	1,504	241	16.0	0.5
Thyroid	28	12	41.9	84	43	50.7	165	71	42.9	25	⋈	⋈	302	125	41.3	0.3
Soft tissue	27	2	7.0	67	⋈	⋈	164	15	9.4	50	9	17.5	308	28	9.2	0.1
Unspecified	46	⋈	⋈	167	60	35.8	461	215	46.7	183	114	62.2	857	394	46.0	0.8
Non-Hodgkin's lymphoma	123	17	14.0	315	40	12.8	704	72	10.3	186	⋈	⋈	1,328	140	10.5	0.3
Hodgkin's disease	43	1	2.9	96	-	-	231	-	-	58	⋈	⋈	428	1	0.2	0.0
Multiple myeloma	37	⋈	⋈	146	36	24.6	288	17	5.8	92	6	6.9	563	56	10.0	0.1
Leukaemia	111	21	19.2	264	28	10.5	635	86	13.5	153	⋈	⋈	1,163	131	11.3	0.3
Sum of above sites	3,016	531	17.6	9,134	2,480	27.1	24,936	9,215	37.0	8,320	3,661	44.0	45,408	15,967	35.2	33.8

[1] Excess number of cases as percentage of all cancer cases of men in the present study population.

Table 58. Numbers of cancer cases in 1971-85 (Obs.) and difference to the expected number of cases assuming that the incidence in all social classes would be same as in the social class with the lowest SIR (⋈), given as absolute number of cases (Diff.) and as percentage of the site-specific total (%) for selected primary sites, by social class (I-IV); age 35-64 at the beginning of each 5-year follow-up period, females

Primary site	I			II			III			IV			Total			%/Total[1]
	Obs.	Diff.	%	Obs.	Diff.	%	Obs.	Diff.	%	Obs.	Diff.	%	Obs.	Diff.	%	
ALL SITES	3,769	685	18.2	13,596	1,848	13.6	21,438	317	1.5	8,050	⋈	⋈	46,853	2,938	6.3	6.3
Oesophagus	10	⋈	⋈	78	34	44.0	253	159	63.0	121	80	66.4	462	273	59.2	0.6
Stomach	134	⋈	⋈	661	166	25.1	1,360	369	27.1	543	148	27.3	2,698	689	25.5	1.5
Colon	156	29	18.5	618	127	20.5	906	⋈	⋈	351	-	-	2,031	121	6.0	0.3
Rectum	123	24	19.3	421	39	9.4	744	⋈	⋈	300	19	6.4	1,588	104	6.5	0.2
Liver	19	⋈	⋈	104	48	46.0	182	85	46.6	70	33	46.7	375	170	45.4	0.4
Gallbladder, biliary tract	48	6	12.4	184	⋈	⋈	356	40	11.2	164	37	22.7	752	103	13.7	0.2
Pancreas	102	27	26.1	354	60	17.0	621	⋈	⋈	273	46	17.0	1,350	185	13.7	0.4
Lung, trachea	123	11	8.6	528	94	17.7	838	⋈	⋈	379	60	15.8	1,868	187	10.0	0.4
Breast	1,466	622	42.4	4,524	1,349	29.8	5,867	411	7.0	1,925	⋈	⋈	13,782	2,325	16.9	5.0
Cervix uteri	91	⋈	⋈	432	174	40.4	936	446	47.7	458	265	58.0	1,917	909	47.4	1.9
Corpus uteri	299	66	22.2	1,125	239	21.2	1,797	203	11.3	621	-	-	3,842	526	13.7	1.1
Ovary	232	-	-	989	64	6.5	1,557	⋈	⋈	588	⋈	⋈	3,366	64	1.9	0.1
Vulva and vagina	20	⋈	⋈	107	41	43.5	168	42	25.0	85	37	43.5	380	123	32.4	0.3
Kidney	91	12	13.3	358	55	15.3	596	44	7.4	224	⋈	⋈	1269	123	9.7	0.3
Bladder, ureter, urethra	51	23	46.0	163	55	33.8	263	53	20.3	87	⋈	⋈	564	135	23.9	0.3
Skin melanoma	121	39	32.0	398	87	21.8	523	⋈	⋈	192	10	5.3	1,234	145	11.7	0.3
Other skin	46	15	31.9	132	12	9.5	288	56	19.4	82	⋈	⋈	548	75	13.6	0.2
Brain, nervous system	160	37	23.2	575	120	20.8	897	129	14.4	311	⋈	⋈	1,943	323	16.6	0.7
Thyroid	95	20	21.1	315	32	10.1	497	18	3.7	174	⋈	⋈	1,081	72	6.6	0.2
Soft tissue	29	8	28.3	87	7	7.8	157	16	10.3	48	⋈	⋈	321	27	8.3	0.1
Unspecified	46	⋈	⋈	216	36	16.7	423	87	20.6	181	52	28.8	866	175	20.2	0.4
Non-Hodgkin's lymphoma	74	13	17.6	287	52	18.3	516	72	14.0	172	⋈	⋈	1,049	136	12.9	0.3
Hodgkin's disease	22	1	6.3	77	-	-	117	⋈	⋈	45	-	-	261	1	0.4	0.0
Multiple myeloma	25	⋈	⋈	127	42	32.9	268	107	39.9	112	48	43.1	532	200	37.6	0.4
Leukaemia	55	⋈	⋈	255	34	13.3	473	47	9.9	184	13	7.0	967	93	9.6	0.2
Sum of above sites	3638	9,53	26.2	13,115	2,967	22.6	20,603	2,384	11.6	7,690	848	11.0	45,046	7,284	16.2	15.6

[1] Excess number of cases as percentage of all cancer cases of women in the present study population.

of cases of each cancer site would be if the total population would have in each age-group an incidence rate as low as the social class with the lowest age-adjusted rate.

Men of social class IV showed the lowest SIRs for more than every second primary site analysed in this study (table 57). Still, the total cancer incidence among men in social class IV was the highest of all social classes due to the high incidence of some of the most common cancers (lung, stomach, bladder, pancreas). Over 2,500 cancer cases (30%) of working-aged Finnish men of social class IV would have been prevented if men in social class IV had had the same total cancer incidence as men in social class I. All this difference would actually have been gained in lung cancer alone. Adding up the theoretical numbers of preventable cases of all social classes gives a total of 9,300, i.e., 20% of all cases. Great relative site-specific gains would have been achieved in cancers of the lip (69%), lung (59%), thyroid (41%), larynx (40%), oesophagus (40%), oral cavity (40%), stomach (38%) and testis (36%). The absolute importance of these gains is relative to the frequency of each cancer type: the theoretical number of preventable lung cancer cases comprises almost 20% of all cancer cases, stomach cancer 3.5%, lip cancer 1.5% and laryngeal cancer 1.1%.

The above sites also form the most important potential of cancer prevention among men in social classes III and IV. In social class II lung cancer is the greatest absolute problem, but the preventable number of colorectal cancers exceeds that of stomach cancer. In the highest social class the largest gains would be achieved if the incidence of cancers of prostate, colon, kidney and skin melanoma would be reduced down to the level of social class IV. The absolute importance of each of these gains would, however, be less than 3% of the total number of cancer cases in men in social class I.

Due to a smaller social class variation in the total cancer incidence among women than among men, the proportion of theoretically preventable cancers estimated on the basis of total cancer incidence among women is only 6% (table 58). In most leading cancer sites in women the incidence was lowest in lower social classes, and therefore the theoretical proportion of preventable cancer cases of total cancer is largest (18%) in social class I. However, the largest site-specific relative proportions of preventable cases are found among sites with the lowest incidence in social class I, i.e., in oesophageal cancer (59%), cancer of the cervix uteri (47%), liver cancer (45%) and multiple myeloma (38%). Taking into account the absolute incidence of each cancer, the largest gains can be achieved in cancers of the breast (5.0% of all cases of working-aged women), cervix uteri (1.9%), stomach (1.5%) and corpus uteri (1.1%).

Almost all of the potential for prevention among women of social class I is attributable to breast cancer, with endometrial cancer and colorectal cancer taking the next positions in absolute importance (table 58). The same sites are also most important in social class II. In social classes III and IV cancer of the cervix uteri becomes most important, and cancers of the stomach and oesophagus also serve a relatively large target for prevention.

Since the risk factors of different cancers can be opposite, it is not realistic to believe that the "preventability" of the total cancer incidence would be the sum of the potentially prevented proportions of individual cancer types. This sum for all cancer sites analysed in the present study is 35% for males and 16% for females, i.e., much larger than the "preventability" based on the real social class-specific SIRs for total cancer (20% and 6%, respectively).

Earlier estimates of preventable proportions of colorectal and stomach cancers [181] assuming arbitrary shifts in dietary factors towards the most favourable category (as indicated by various case-control studies) are similar to those obtained here, i.e., some 30% for stomach cancer and 10-20% for colorectal cancer. The target incidence levels of the above calculations are a reality in a large proportion of the Finnish population, and the prevalence of many of the factors contributing to these differences — primarily, smoking — could really be changed. Thus, in many instances, primary prevention of cancer among working-aged Finnish men and women could set itself an optimistic goal based on the above proportions of avoidable cancer cases.

Occupational variation

Part of the residual occupational variation behind the social class variation may in principle be accounted for by real occupational exposures. Various methods for evaluating the magnitude of this excess have been used, e.g., all the cases above the upper limit of the statistical confidence interval may have been defined as occupation-related excess cases [182]. Although all such estimates are more or less artificial — for instance they usually do not pay any attention to the rates below the average — the size and shape of the upper end of the distribution of occupation-specific risk ratios gives some indication of possible occupation-related component in causation of each cancer form.

One may believe that part of the excess cases included in the highest relative risk ratios are likely to be attributable to occupation-related factors. In tables 59 and 60 excesses going beyond the expected number of cases (Exp_a) by more than 20% and 100% have been summed up over all three-digit occupational categories with at least 4 observed cases for selected cancer sites of the present study. The proportions of these sums — hereafter referred to as occupation-related excesses — out of the site-specific total number of cases among men were largest for cancers of the nasopharynx and renal pelvis, but the absolute numbers of these excess cases were very small (table 59). Among more common cancer sites high occupation-related excess proportions were seen, e.g., for cancers of the lip, oesophagus and liver. The highest absolute number of excess cases was still in lung cancer. The 466 excess cases on the 20% excess level constituted 3.8% of all lung cancer cases and 1.2% of all cancer cases of the men in the study series. The second largest proportions of occupation-related excess out of all cancer cases were those for the kidney and lip (0.3% each).

The sum of site-specific excess cases among men over all primary sites analysed in this study on a 20% excess level was 5.5% and on a 100% excess level 0.8% out

Table 59. Number of all cancer cases (Obs.) in 1971-85 and numbers of sums of occupation-specific fractions of observed cases exceeding the social class-adjusted expected numbers of cases by ≥20% and by ≥100%, given both as absolute number of excess cases (n) and as percentage of site-specific total (%). For the 20% excess level also given the percentage out of all cancer cases among economically active men (%/Total). Reference: Economically active men. Ages 35-69, males. Only three-digit occupational categories with ≥4 cases are included.

Primary site	Obs.	Excess ≥20%			Excess ≥100%	
		n	%	%/Total	n	%
All sites	39175	308	0.8	0.8	4	0.0
Lip	737	98	13.3	0.3	9	1.3
Tongue	83	16	19.8	0.0	2	1.9
Salivary glands	52	5	10.1	0.0	3	5.2
Oral cavity	55	10	17.9	0.0	2	4.0
Nasopharynx	12	5	38.5	0.0	4	30.8
Pharynx excl. nasopharynx	81	17	20.9	0.0	5	5.7
Oesophagus	317	34	10.7	0.1	10	3.1
Stomach	3483	74	2.1	0.2	1	0.0
Small intestine	62	6	9.8	0.0	0	0.8
Colon	1314	95	7.2	0.2	13	1.0
Rectum	1282	76	5.9	0.2	11	0.8
Liver	353	55	15.6	0.1	11	3.2
Gallbladder, biliary tract	172	19	11.0	0.0	2	0.9
Pancreas	1404	89	6.3	0.2	11	0.8
Nose, nasal sinuses	55	9	15.7	0.0	1	1.8
Larynx	838	70	8.3	0.2	6	0.7
Lung, trachea	12153	466	3.8	1.2	61	0.5
adenocarcinoma	*1219*	*80*	*6.6*	*0.2*	*19*	*1.5*
small cell carcinoma	*1926*	*130*	*6.8*	*0.3*	*25*	*1.3*
squamous cell carcinoma	*4114*	*247*	*6.0*	*0.6*	*28*	*0.7*
Mesothelioma	27	4	15.1	0.0	3	10.4
Prostate	2540	93	3.7	0.2	11	0.4
Testis	64	9	14.4	0.0	4	5.9
Penis	33	2	7.0	0.0	0	0.0
Kidney	1470	125	8.5	0.3	18	1.2
renal pelvis	*32*	*10*	*30.4*	*0.0*	*6*	*17.9*
Bladder, ureter, urethra	1585	91	5.8	0.2	9	0.6
Skin melanoma	865	56	6.5	0.1	3	0.3
Other skin	473	35	7.3	0.1	5	1.1
Eye	72	14	18.9	0.0	7	9.2
Brain, nervous system	1152	62	5.3	0.2	3	0.3
Thyroid	148	25	17.0	0.1	8	5.6
Other endocrine glands	45	6	13.7	0.0	4	9.5
Bone	44	7	16.4	0.0	3	7.7
Soft tissue	173	24	13.8	0.1	5	3.2
Unspecified	556	36	6.5	0.1	6	1.0
Non-Hodgkin's lymphoma	978	56	5.7	0.1	4	0.4
Hodgkin's disease	240	20	8.4	0.1	5	2.0
Multiple myeloma	359	23	6.3	0.1	3	0.8
Leukaemia	827	45	5.4	0.1	12	1.4
chronic lymphocytic	*230*	*24*	*10.4*	*0.1*	*4*	*1.8*
acute myelocytic	*197*	*19*	*9.4*	*0.0*	*4*	*2.1*
other	*219*	*22*	*10.2*	*0.1*	*8*	*3.8*
Sum of all analysed sites	**34112**	**1877**	**5.5**	**4.8**	**264**	**0.8**
Not included above:						
Skin, basal cell carcinoma	5428	159	2.9	.	13	0.2

Table 60. Number of all cancer cases (Obs.) in 1971-85 and numbers of sums of occupation-specific fractions of observed cases exceeding the social class-adjusted expected numbers of cases by $\geq 20\%$ and by $\geq 100\%$, given both as absolute number of excess cases (n) and as percentage of site-specific total (%). For the 20% excess level also given the percentage out of all cancer cases among economically active women (%/Total). Reference: Economically active women. Ages 35-69, females. Only three-digit occupational categories with ≥ 4 cases are included.

Primary site	Obs.	Excess $\geq 20\%$			Excess $\geq 100\%$	
		n	%	%/Total	n	%
All sites	**27829**	**206**	**0.7**	**0.7**	**9**	**0.0**
Lip	22	6	27.9	0.0	3	13.2
Tongue	33	2	5.4	0.0	0	0.0
Salivary glands	42	7	15.9	0.0	2	4.1
Oral cavity	29	4	12.3	0.0	1	4.3
Pharynx excl. nasopharynx	21	2	10.9	0.0	0	0.0
Oesophagus	169	16	9.6	0.1	3	1.9
Stomach	1332	56	4.2	0.2	12	0.9
Small intestine	29	2	6.6	0.0	0	0.0
Colon	1064	43	4.0	0.2	5	0.5
Rectum	751	38	5.1	0.1	3	0.4
Liver	109	10	8.9	0.0	1	1.3
Gallbladder, biliary tract	264	20	7.5	0.1	3	1.1
Pancreas	606	41	6.7	0.1	5	0.8
Nose, nasal sinuses	23	3	14.7	0.0	0	0.0
Lung, trachea	966	129	13.4	0.5	40	4.2
adenocarcinoma	*237*	*20*	*8.6*	*0.1*	*4*	*1.9*
small cell carcinoma	*91*	*21*	*23.5*	*0.1*	*5*	*5.4*
squamous cell carcinoma	*109*	*20*	*18.1*	*0.1*	*12*	*11.2*
Breast	8576	214	2.5	0.8	11	0.1
Cervix uteri	973	73	7.5	0.3	11	1.2
Corpus uteri	2140	68	3.2	0.2	4	0.2
Ovary	1965	84	4.3	0.3	10	0.5
Vulva	68	7	9.8	0.0	3	3.9
Vagina	26	5	19.0	0.0	2	8.6
Kidney	578	21	3.6	0.1	7	1.2
Bladder, ureter, urethra	225	22	9.9	0.1	5	2.4
Skin melanoma	643	24	3.7	0.1	1	0.1
Other skin	209	15	7.2	0.1	1	0.6
Eye	48	8	17.6	0.0	2	4.0
Brain, nervous system	1008	58	5.8	0.2	10	1.0
Thyroid	528	35	6.6	0.1	10	1.9
Other endocrine glands	16	2	13.6	0.0	0	0.0
Bone	16	2	10.9	0.0	0	0.0
Soft tissue	101	16	15.6	0.1	1	0.7
Unspecified	351	26	7.3	0.1	1	0.4
Non-Hodgkin's lymphoma	475	26	5.5	0.1	5	1.1
Hodgkin's disease	67	3	4.7	0.0	0	0.0
Multiple myeloma	203	22	11.0	0.1	5	2.4
Leukaemia	416	33	8.0	0.1	5	1.2
chronic lymphocytic	*66*	*7*	*10.2*	*0.0*	*1*	*2.1*
acute myelocytic	*128*	*13*	*10.5*	*0.0*	*3*	*2.5*
other	*123*	*17*	*13.6*	*0.1*	*5*	*4.0*
Sum of all analysed sites	**24105**	**1143**	**4.7**	**4.1**	**172**	**0.7**
Not included above:						
Cervix uteri, carcinoma in situ	767	100	13.0	.	23	3.0
Skin, basal cell carcinoma	3972	82	2.1	.	9	0.2

of all cases. Among women the corresponding proportions were 4.7% and 0.7%, respectively (table 60). High site-specific proportions of occupation-related excesses among women were obtained, e.g., for cancers of the lip, vagina and soft tissue, as well as for small cell carcinoma of the lung. The absolute numbers of excess cases were largest for cancers of the breast, lung and female genital organs.

This very rough approach gives an estimate that some 5% of all cancer cases would be occupation-related, if the a priori selected threshold of SIR_a 1.2 is used. If the threshold is put to 2.0, the proportion is less than 1%. Most estimates of the risk attributable to occupational factors fall within these margins [1-5]. Cancer types generally considered as mostly occupation-related showed large excess proportions. Hence, this mechanistic exercise seems to reveal similar aspects as specialist evaluations based on extensive reviews of published studies.

VII. Summary and Conclusions

Method

The present surveillance system systematically produced standardised incidence ratios (SIRs) among working-aged Finnish men and women for all main cancer sites by social class and occupation. It was based on the computerised record linkage of the nationwide population-based Finnish Cancer Registry and the 1970 Population Census including social class and occupational data from a time-point 0-15 years prior to the cancer diagnosis. Because of the high coverage and accuracy of the linked files, the cancer risk estimates, both by occupation and social class, can be considered very reliable, and the large numbers of cases downplay the role of chance variation even in the case of relatively rare cancer forms. Still, for the many small occupational categories only international collaborative studies can give meaningful risk evaluations.

The occupation at one point in time may not always correspond to the lifelong occupational history of a person. However, comparison with results of special occupational cancer studies indicates that the risk diluting effect of misclassification is small. The system was able to find known occupational risks such as a high lip cancer incidence in farmers and a high risk of nasal cancer among woodworkers. Even the numerical relative risk estimates were similar to those obtained in many other studies.

The non-occupational component included in occupation-specific cancer risk estimates was controlled by using social class as a proxy for all these factors, which is likely to leave residual confounding particularly caused by factors which are not associated with social class or would be better separated by using some other classification of socio-economic status. In practice the importance of such known factors is relatively small, and social class may actually control to a certain extent also unknown lifestyle factors. Comparison with specific studies with precise adjustment for many known confounding factors showed that the present social class adjustment usually gave almost identical results.

Because the present survey was based on incidence rates and exact person-year calculations, there was no bias caused by social class and occupational variation in cancer survival and in mortality from competing causes of death. Comparative examples of results of the present study and of surveillance systems using alternative, less reliable methodologies, i.e., proportionate analysis or an ecological analyses, concretisised how different the risk estimates can be.

Findings

There was a some 30% higher overall cancer incidence among men in the lowest social class (IV) than in the highest one (I). In women the trend was opposite. Cancers of the lip, oesophagus, stomach, larynx and nose, and multiple myeloma were associated with low social class in both sexes, cancers of cervix uteri and vagina in women and lung cancer in men. Cancers of the colon, breast, testis and soft tissue, and skin melanoma in the trunk and limbs were most common in high social classes throughout the whole observation period 1971-85, whereas for cancers of the corpus uteri, kidney and nervous system as well for non-Hodgkin's lymphoma the positive social class association disappeared by the early 1980s. In lung cancer among women there was a rapid change from a disease of a high social class to a disease of a low one in about five years.

Much of the largest social class differences, i.e., of those in cancers of the lung and larynx, can be accounted for by smoking. More than one-fifth of all cancer cases among men would be prevented if the incidence of these two cancers in the whole population would be reduced to the level of social class I. Other important factors behind social class variation are dietary factors (colon, stomach, oesophagus) and reproductive factors (breast, uterus).

Social class explained a lot of the occupational variation of many cancers, but there were many occupations with a total cancer incidence of more than 50% above the incidence of the whole economically active population of their own social class, such as asphalt roofers, insulators, tobacco industry workers, glass and ceramics decorators, miners and hairdressers. The risk was low, e.g., among sport coaches, priests and male medical workers. Farmers had relatively low risks of most cancer types.

From the numerous site and occupation-specific risk ratios one can pick up known or suspected associations such as a high risk of nasal cancer among woodworkers, lung cancer among asbestos and silica dust exposed workers, pancreatic cancer among painters and hairdressers, and cancers of the upper gastrointestine tract possibly associated with a dusty working environment. Viruses and infectious diseases possibly transmit cancers of the bone and soft tissue, multiple myeloma and leukaemia, which were found in excess in workers treating people or animals. Sedentary workers tend to have increased risk of cancers of the colon and breast, and indoor workers have relatively more skin melanoma in those parts of their bodies which are not used to sun radiation and thus easily burn due to intensive sunbathing during the holidays. Cumulative UV radiation seems to cause excess risk of non-melanoma skin cancer among outdoor workers.

Several new associations came up, and these should be confirmed in other studies before they can be believed to be true causal associations. Cooks who are likely to burn their lips in work had a high risk of lip cancer. Sauna attendants, cooks, flame cutters and some other workers in very warm working conditions experienced a high risk of pancreatic cancer.

Cancers of the lung, pancreas, liver, kidney and lip showed features of clear occupation-dependance. Unexpectedly, bladder cancer did not seem to be so much occupation-related, whereas, e.g., in ovarian cancer there was a cluster of chemical-exposed occupations with a high risk. Even cancers of the colon, prostate and cervix uteri gave some clues about possible chemical or dust exposure association. Persons in occupations with work stress (e.g., managers) seemed to have high risk of colon cancer even when compared to their own social class.

Occupation-related social factors seem to be more important determinants of some cancer risks than the real occupational ones. There were high risks of alcohol-related cancers (pharynx, oesophagus, liver, larynx) among workers having easy access to alcoholic beverages in their work, and women in occupations with an obvious seduction to frequent sexual contacts were at the highest risk of cervical cancer. However, data about such delicate life habits like drinking or sexual behaviour are very poorly known and any conclusions on the role of these factors are thus more or less speculative. Occupations can also create a protective environment against cancer: it is not suitable for a primary school teacher, dentist or priest to smoke at work (or elsewhere), which is reflected in a low incidence of smoking-related cancers.

The sum of cases exceeding the expected number of cases by more than 20% over the 335 occupations and 46 primary sites of this study is some 5% of all cancer cases both in males and in females. This is close to most international estimates of the proportion of cancers attributable to occupational factors. The sum of social class-specific cases exceeding the lowest social class-specific incidence is 35% in males and 16% in females. Thus, if it would have been possible for all social classes to maintain a way of life similar to that of the social class with the lowest incidence, some 24,000 malignant cancer cases of the total of 94,000 among working-aged Finns would have been avoided during 1971-85.

VIII. References

1. Doll R, Peto J: The causes of cancer: Quantitative estimates of avoidable risks of cancer in the United States today. Oxford, Oxford University Press, 1981.
2. Wynder EL, Gori GB: Contribution of the environment to cancer incidence: an epidemiologic exercise. J Natl Cancer Inst 1977;58:825-832.
3. Higginson J, Muir CS: Environmental carcinogenesis: Misconceptions and limitations to cancer control. J Natl Cancer Inst 1979;63:1290-1298.
4. Hemminki K, Vainio H: Human exposure to potentially carcinogenic compounds, in Berlin A, Draper K, Hemminki K, Vainio H (Eds): Monitoring Human Exposure to Carcinogenic and Mutagenic Agents. IARC Scientific Publications No. 59. Lyon, International Agency for Research on Cancer, 1984.
5. Simonato L: Occupational factors, in Higginson J, Muir CS, Muñoz N: Human Cancer: Epidemiology and Environmental Causes. Cambridge, Cambridge University Press, 1992, pp 97-113.
6. Registrar General. Fourteenth annual report of the Registrar General of births, deaths and marriages in England. London, Her Majesty's Stationery Office, 1855, pp 15-8.
7. Office of Population Censuses and Surveys: Occupational mortality: The Registrar General's decennial supplement for Great Britain, 1979-80, 1982-83. London, Her Majesty's Stationary Office, 1986.
8. Pott P: Chirurgical Observations Relative to the Cataract, the Polypos of the nose, the Cancer of the Scrotum, the Different Kinds of Ruptures, and the Mortification of the Mortification of the Toes and Feet. London, Hawse, Clark and Collins, 1775, pp 63-68.
9. Fox AJ, Adelstein AM: Occupational mortality: Work or way of life? J Epidemiol Community Health 1978;32:73-78.
10. Lynge E, Thygesen L: Occupational cancer in Denmark. Cancer incidence in the 1970 census population. Scand J Work Environ Health 1990;16:Suppl 2.
11. Pearce NE, Howard JK: Occupation, social class and male cancer mortality in New Zealand 1974-78. Int J Epidemiol 1986;15:456-462.
12. Milham S: Occupational mortality in Washington State 1950-1979. Cincinnati (OH), National Institute for Occupational Safety and Health, 1983.
13. Kelley BC, Gute DM: Surveillance cooperative agreement between NIOSH and States (Scans) Program: Rhode Island 1980-82. Cincinnati (OH), US Department of Health and Human Services, 1986.
14. Petersen GR, Milham S: Occupational mortality in the State of California, 1959-61. DHEW (NIOSH) Publication No 80-104. Cincinnati (OH), National Institute for Occupational Safety and Health, 1980.
15. Dubrow R, Wegman DH: Occupational characteristics of white male cancer victims in Massachusets 1971-1973. Cincinnati (OH), National Institute for Occupational Safety and Health, 1982.
16. Mack TM: Cancer surveillance program in Los Angeles county. Natl Cancer Inst Monogr 1977;99-101.
17. Pearce NE, Sheppard RA, Howard JK, Fraser J, Lilley BM: Leukaemia among New Zealand agricultural workers. Am J Epidemiol 1986;124:402-409.
18. Olsen JH, Jensen OM: Occupation and risk of cancer in Denmark. An analysis of 93810 cancer cases, 1970-1979. Scand J Work Environ Health 1987;13:Suppl 1.
19. Decouflé P, Stanislawczyk K: A retrospective survey of cancer in relation to occupation. DHEW (NIOSH) publication no 77-178. Cincinnati (OH), National Institute for Occupational Safety and Health, 1977.
20. Williams R, Stegens NL, Goldsmith JR: Associations of cancer site and type with occupation and industry from the Third National Survey Interview. J Natl Cancer Inst 1977;59:1147-1185.

21 Siemiatycki J, Wacholder S, Richardson L, Dewar R, Gérin M: Discovering carcinogens in the occupational environment: Methods of data collection and analysis of a large case-referent monitoring system. Scand J Work Environ Health 1987;13:486-492.
22 Borgan J-K, Kristofersen LB: Mortality by occupation and socio-economic group in Norway 1970-1980. Statistiske analyser 56. Oslo, Central Bureau of Statistics in Norway, 1986.
23 Statistiska Centralbyrån: Dödsfall-register 1961-70 [Death register 1961-70]. Promemorior från SBC 1981:5. Stockholm, Socialstyrelsen, 1982 (in Swedish).
24 Marin R: Occupational mortality in 1971-1980. Study No 129. Helsinki, Central Statistical Office of Finland, 1986.
25 Andersen O: Dødelighet og ehrverv 1970-80 [Occupational mortality 1970-80]. Statistiske undersøgelser nr 41. Copenhagen, Danmarks Statistik, 1985 (in Danish).
26 Occupational mortality in the Nordic countries 1971-1980. Statistical Reports of the Nordic Countries 49. Copenhagen, Nordic Statistical Secretariat, 1988.
27 Howe GR, Lindsay JP: A follow-up study of a ten-percent sample of the Canadian Labour Force: I. Cancer mortality in males 1965-73. J Natl Cancer Inst 1983;37-44.
28 Fox AJ, Goldblatt PO: Longitudial study: socio-demographic mortality differentials. A first report on mortality in 1971-1975 according to 1971 Census characteristics, based on data collected in the OPCS Longitudial study. Office of Population Censuses and Surveys, Series LS no. 1. London, Her Majesty's Stationery Office, 1982.
29 Andersen Aa, Bjelke E, Langmark F: Cancer in waiters. Br J Cancer 1989;60:112-115.
30 Cancer-Miljöregisternämnden: Cancer-Miljöregistret uppdaterat: Omfattar nu över 600,000 cancerfall [Cancer-environment-register updated: Now includes more than 600,000 cancer cases]. Läkartidningen 1983;80:123-124 (in Swedish).
31 Pukkala E: Occupation, socioeconomic status and education as risk determinants of cancer. Cancer Detect Prev 1989;14:87.
32 Lynge E, Thygesen L: Use of surveillance systems for occupational cancer: Illustrated with data from a nationwide system in Denmark. Int J Epidemiol 1988;17:493-500.
33 Leon DA: Longitudial study: Social distribution of cancer. Office of Population Censuses and Surveys, Series LS no. 3. London, Her Majesty's Stationary Office, 1988.
34 Tüchsen F, Bach E: Ehrverv og hospitalization 1981-84 [Occupation and hospitalization 1981-84]. Copenhagen, Arbejdtilsynet, 1989 (in Danish).
35 Hirayama T: Life-style and mortality. A large-scale census-based cohort study in Japan. Contributions to Epidemiology. Basel, Karger, 1990, vol 7.
36 Dubrow R, Sestito JP, Lalich NR, Burnett CA, Salg JA: Death certificate-based occupational mortality surveillance in the United States. Am J Ind Med 1987;11:329-342.
37 CANCER-CD™ June 1992-November 1993. Comprehensive database of cancer-related records from CANCERLITR and EMBASE. National Cancer Institute/National Library of Medicine. Norwood, SilverPlatter Information, 1994.
38 IARC Monographs on the evaluation of the carcinogenic risks to humans. List of IARC evaluations. Lyon, International Agency for Research on Cancer, October 1994.
39 Overall evaluations of carcinogenicity: an updating of of IARC Monographs 1 to 42. IARC Monographs on the evaluation of the carcinogenic risk of chemicals to humans, Suppl 7. Lyon, International Agency for Research on Cancer, 1987.
40 Occupational cancer: prevention and control, in Occupational Safety and Health Series No 39. Geneva, International Labor Office, 1988, pp 1-122.
41 Heikkilä P, Kauppinen T: Occupational exposure to carcinogens in Finland. Am J Ind Med 1992;21:467-480.
42 Valkonen T: Socio-economic differences in male mortality in selected countries in Europe. Sosiaalilääket Aikak 1988;25:13-22 (in Finnish, with an English summary).
43 Vågerö D, Norrell SE: Mortality and social class in Sweden - Exploring a new epidemiological tool. Scand J Soc Med 1989;17:49-58.
44 Black D, Morris JN, Smith C, Townsend P: The Black report, in Townsend P, Davidson N (eds): Inequalities in health. Harmondsworth, Penguin Books, 1982, pp 33-213.

45 Valkonen T, Martelin T, Rimpelä A, Notkola V, Savela S: Socio-economic mortality differences in Finland in 1981-90. Population 1993:1. Helsinki, Statistics Finland, 1993.
46 Valkonen T, Martelin T, Rimpelä A: Inequality in the face of death. Socio-economic mortality differences in Finland in 1971-85. Studies 176. Helsinki, Central Statistical Office of Finland, 1990 (in Finnish).
47 Household survey for 1966. Statistical Report No. 51. Helsinki, Central Statistical Office of Finland, 1972.
48 Rimpelä M: Adult use of tobacco in Finland in the 1950s to 1970s. The state of smoking in autumn 1976, changes in cigarette smoking in 1968-1976 and conclusions of development of smoking habits. Publications on Public Health M 40/78. Tampere, University of Tampere, Dept of Public Health, 1978 (in Finnish).
49 Prättälä R, Berg M-A, Leino P, Puska P: Lifestyles in different occupational groups among Finnish men in 1978-1990. Publication No 20. Helsinki, LEL Työeläkekassa, 1992 (in Finnish with an English summary).
50 Seppänen R, Karinpää A: The quality of the Finnish diet. Results of the dietary questionnaire of the Mini-Finland Health Survey. Publications of the Social Incurance Institution ML:58. Helsinki, Social Incurance Institution, Finland 1986 (in Finnish, with an English summary).
51 Aro S, Räsänen L, Telama R: Social class and changes in health-related habits in Finland in 1973-83. Scand J Soc Med 1986;14:39-47.
52 Martelin T: The development of smoking habits according to survey data in Finland. Publications of the National Board of Health. Health Education. Series Original Reports 1/1984. Helsinki, National Board of Health, Finland 1984 (in Finnish, with an English summary).
53 Fougstedt G: Trends and factors of fertility in Finland. Commentationes Scientiarum Socialium No. 7. Helsinki, Societas Scientiarum Fennica, 1977.
54 Rimpelä A, Rimpelä M: Biological growth and maturation, in Health Habits Among Finnish Youth. Health Education. Series Original Reports 4/1984. Helsinki, National Board of Health, 1983.
55 Simpura J: Finnish drinking habits and work. Alkoholipolitiikka 1979;44:63-70 (in Finnish, with an English summary).
56 Salaspuro A: Alcohol-related utilization of health services in Finland 1972. Studies No 29. Helsinki, Alcohol Research Foundation, 1978 (in Finnish).
57 Pukkala E: Number of children among 40-49 year-old women by occupation, 1985. A study based on a record linkage data of Statistics Finland. Helsinki, Finnish Cancer Registry 1995 (unpublished).
58 Jensen OM, Carstensen B, Glattre R, Malker B, Pukkala E, Tulinius H: Atlas of cancer incidence in the Nordic countries. A collaborative study of the five Nordic Cancer Registries. Helsinki, Nordic Cancer Union, 1988.
59 Vital statistics 1991. Population 1994:2. Helsinki, Statistics Finland, 1994.
60 Karjalainen S: Geographical variation in cancer patient survival in Finland: change, confounding or effect of treatment? J Epidemiol Community Health 1990;44:210-214.
61 Purola T, Kalimo E, Nyman K: Health services use and health status under national sickness insurance. An evaluation resurvey of Finland. Publications of the Social Insurance Institution, Finland A:11. Helsinki, Research Institute for Social Security, 1974.
62 Kalimo E, Nyman K, Klaukka T, Tuomikoski H, Savolainen E: Need, use and expences of health services in Finland 1964-1976. Publications of the Social Insurance Institution, Finland A:18. Helsinki, Social Insurance Institution, 1982 (in Finnish, with an English summary).
63 Härö S: Health expenditure by area in Finland - an indicator of equity. Health Policy 1987;7:299-315.
64 Salmela R: General hospital inpatient care in Finland in 1980-85. Studies 10. Helsinki, National Agency for Welfare and Health, 1991 (in Finnish, with an English summary).
65 Häkkinen U: Health care utilization, health and socioeconomic equality in Finland. Studies 20, Helsinki, National Agency for Welfare and Health, 1992 (in Finnish, with an English summary).

66 Population census 1970: Occupation and social position. Official Statistics of Finland VI C:104, vol IX. Helsinki, Central Statistical Office of Finland, 1974.
67 Sauli H: Occupational mortality in 1971-75. Studies No. 54. Helsinki, Central Statistical Office of Finland, 1979.
68 Rauhala U: Suomalaisen yhteiskunnan sosiaalisten kerrostumien määrälliset vahvuudet. [Social structures of the Finnish society]. Social Review No 6. Helsinki, Ministry of Social Affairs and Health 1966 (in Finnish).
69 Manual of tumor nomenclature coding. Atlanta, American Cancer Society, 1951.
70 Lindqvist C: Risk factors in lip cancer: A questionnaire survey. Amer J Epidemiol 1979;109:521-530.
71 Kolstad H, Lynge E, Olsen J, Sabroe S: Occupational causes of some rare cancers. A literature review. Scand J Soc Med 1992;Suppl 48:1-148.
72 Mabuchi K, Bross DS, Kessler II: Cigarette smoking and nasopharyngeal carcinoma. Cancer 1985;55:2874-2876.
73 Higginson J, Muir CS, Muñoz N: Human cancer: Epidemiology and environmental causes. Cambridge, Cambridge University Press, 1992.
74 Decouflé P: Cancer risks associated with employment in the leather and leather product industry. Arch Environ Health 1979;34:33-37.
75 Winn DM, Blot WJ, Shy CM, Fraumeni JF Jr: Occupation and oral cancer among women in the South. Am J Ind Med 1982;3:161-167.
76 Muir C, Waterhouse J, Mack T, Powell J, Whelan S (eds): Cancer incidence in five continents, volume V. IARC Scientific Publication No 88. Lyon, International Agency for Research on Cancer, 1987.
77 Yu MC, Garabrandt DH, Peters JM, Mack TM: Tobacco, alcohol, diet, occupation and carcinoma of the oesophagus. Cancer Res 1988;48:3843-3848.
78 Norell S, Lipping H, Ahlbom A, Österblom L: Oesophageal cancer and vulcanization work. Lancet 1983;i:462-623.
79 Cocco P, Palli D, Buiatti E, Cipriani F, DeCarli A, Manca P, Ward MH, Blot WJ, Fraumeni JF Jr: Occupational exposures as risk factors for gastric cancer in Italy. CCC 1994;5:241-248.
80 Lightdale CJ, Koepsell TD, Sherlock P: Small intestine, in Schottenfed D, Fraumeni J Jr. (eds): Cancer epidemiology and prevention. Philadelphia, Saunders, 1982, pp 692-702.
81 Chow W-H, Linet MS, McLaughlin JK, Hsing AW, Co Chieng HT, Blot WJ: Risk factors for small intestine cancer. CCC 1993;4:163-169.
82 Pukkala E, Teppo L: Socioeconomic status and education as risk determinants of gastrointestinal cancer. Prev Med 1986;15:127-138.
83 Demers RY, Demers P, Hoar SK, Deighton K: Prevalence of colorectal cancer polyps among Michigan pattern and model makers. J Occup Med 1985;27:809-812.
84 Gerhardsson M, Norell SE, Kiviranta H, Pedersen NL, Ahlbom A: Sedentary jobs and colon cancer. Am J Epidemiol 1986;128:490-503.
85 Berg M-A, Niemensivu H, Piha T, Puska P: Health behaviour among Finnish adult population, Spring 1989. Publications B1/1990. Helsinki, National Public Health Institute, 1990.
86 Aro S: Stress, morbidity, and health-related behaviour. A five-year follow-up study among metal industry employees. Scand J Soc Med 1981;Suppl 25.
87 Alcohol drinking. IARC Monographs on the evaluation of the carcinogenic risk of chemicals to humans, Vol. 44. Lyon, International Agency for Research on Cancer, 1988.
88 Goldbohm RA, Van den Brandt PA, Van't Veer P, Dorant E, Sturmans F, Hermus RJJ: Prospective study on alcohol consumption and the risk of cancer of the colon and rectum in the Netherlands. CCC 1994;5:95-104.
89 Hernberg S, Kauppinen T, Riala R, Korkala M-L, Asikainen U: Increased risk for primary liver cancer among women exposed to solvents. Scand J Work Environ Health 1988;14:356-365.
90 Skov T, Weiner J, Pukkala E, Malker H, Andersen A, Lynge E: Risk for cancer of the pharynx and oral cavity among male painters in the Nordic countries. Arch Environ Health 1993;48:178-180.

91 Lowenfels AB, Lindstrom CG, Conway MJ, Hastings PR: Gallstones and risk of gallbladder cancer. J Natl Cancer Inst 1985;75:77-80.
92 Malker HS, McLaughlin JK, Malker BK, Stone BJ, Weiner JA, Ericsson JL, Blot WJ: Biliary tract cancer and occupation in Sweden. Brit J Ind Med 1986;43:257-262.
93 Pukkala E, Nokso-Koivisto P, Roponen P: Changing cancer risk pattern among Finnish hairdressers. Int Arch Occup Environ Health 1992;64:39-42.
94 Mohtashamipur E, Norpoth K, Lühmann F: Cancer epidemiology of woodworking. J Cancer Res Clin Oncol 1989;115:503-515.
95 Nylander LA, Dement JM: Carcinogenic effects of wood dust: Review and discussion. Am J Ind Med 1993;24:619-647.
96 Brinton LA, Blot WJ, Becker JA, Winn DM, Browder JP, Farmer JC Jr, Fraumeni JF Jr: A case-control study of cancers of the nasal cavity and paranasal sinuses. Am J Epidemiol 1984;119:896-906.
97 Hirayama T: Cancer mortality in non-smoking women with smoking husbands based on a large-scale cohort study in Japan. Prev Med 1984;6:680-690.
98 Hayes RB, Kardaun JW, Bruyn A: Tobacco use and sinonasal cancer: A case-control study. Br J Cancer 1987;56:843-846.
99 Partanen T, Pukkala E, Vainio H, Hannunkari I, Kurppa K, Koskinen H: Increased incidence of lung and skin cancer in Finnish silicotics. J Occup Med 1994;36:616-22.
100 Nokso-Koivisto P, Pukkala E: Past exposure to asbestos and combustion products and incidence of cancer among Finnish locomotive drivers. Occup Environ Med 1994;51:330-334.
101 Meurman LO, Kiviluoto R, Hakama M: Mortality and morbidity among the working population of anthophyllite asbestos miners in Finaland. Brit J Industr Med 1974;31:105-112.
102 Meurman LO, Pukkala E, Hakama M: Incidence of cancer among anthophyllite asbestos miners in Finland. Occup Environ Med 1994;51:421-425.
103 Parkin DM, Muir CS, Whelan SL, Gao YT, Ferlay J, Powell J (eds): Cancer incidence in five continents. Volume VI. IARC Scientific Publications No 120. Lyon, International Agency for Research on Cancer, 1992.
104 Tuomi T: Fibrous minerals in the lungs of mesothelioma patients. Comparison data on SEM, TEM and personal interview information. Am J Ind Med 1992;21:155-162.
105 Rimpelä A, Pukkala E: Cancers of affluence: positive social class gradient and rising incidence trend in some cancer forms. Soc Sci Med 1987;24:601-606.
106 Knekt P, Albanes D, Seppänen R, Aromaa A, Järvinen R, Hyvönen L, Teppo L, Pukkala E: Dietary fat and risk of breast cancer. Am J Clin Nutr 1991;52:903-908.
107 Frisch RE, Wyshak G, Albright NL, Albright TE, Schiff I, Jones KP, Witschi J, Shiang E, Koff EA, Marguaglio M: Lower prevalence of breast cancer and cancers of the reproductive system among former college athletes compared to non-athletes. Br J Cancer 1985;52:885-891.
108 Vihko VJ, Apter DL, Pukkala E, Oinonen MT, Hakulinen TR, Vihko RK: Risk of breast cancer among female teachers of physical education and languages. Acta Oncol 1992;31:201-204.
109 Baverstock KF, Papworth D, Vennart J: Risks of radiation at low dose rates. Lancet 1981;i:430-433.
110 Wang J-X, Boice JD Jr, Li B-X, Zhang J-Y, Fraumeni JF Jr: Cancer among medical diagnostic X-ray workers in China. J Natl Cancer Inst 1988;80:344-50.
111 Hakama M: To screen or not to screen for cervical cancer. Eur J Cancer 1993;29A:2218-2220.
112 Fortelius P, Haapoja H, Hakulinen T: Reasons for non-participation in mass-screening of vaginal cytology. Duodecim 1974;90:597-601 (in Finnish, with an English summary).
113 Kallio M, Kauraniemi T, Nousiainen A-R, Hanstén S, Rytsölä J, Heikkilä M, Hakama M: Naisten osallistuminen kohdunkaulan syövän seulontoihin [Participation of women in mass screening for cervical cancer]. Duodecim 1994;110:1061-1067 (in Finnish).
114 Schiffman MH, Bauer HM, Hoover RN, Glass AG, Cadell DM, Rush BB, Scott DR, Sherman ME, Kurman RJ, Wacholder S, Stanton CK, Manos MM: Epidemiologic evidence showing that human paillomavirus infection causes most cervical intraepithelial neoplasia. JNCI 1993;85:958-964.

115 Shapiro S, Kelly JP, Rosenberg L, Kaufman DW, Helmrich SP, Rosenheim NB, Lewis JL Jr, Knapp RC, Stolley PD, Schottenfeld D: Risk of localized and widespread endometrial cance in relation to recent and discontinued use of cojugated estrogens. N Engl J Men 1985;313:969-972.
116 Hunt K, Vessey M, McPherson K, Coleman M: Long-term surveillance of mortality and cancer incidence in women receiving hormone replacement therapy. Br J Obstet Gynaecol 1987;94:620-635.
117 Luoto R, Hemminki E, Topo P, Uutela A, Kangas I: Hysterectomy among Finnish women: Prevalence and women's own opinions. Scand J Soc Med 1992;20:209-212.
118 Beryllium, cadmium and mercury and exposures in the glass manufacturing industry. IARC Monographs on the evaluation of the carcinogenic risk of chemicals to humans, Vol. 58. Lyon, International Agency for Research on Cancer, 1993.
119 Teppo L: Testicular cancer in Finland. Acta Path Microbiol Scand Sect A 1973;Suppl 238.
120 Baird DD, Wilcox AJ: Future fertility after prenatal exposure to cigarette smoke. Fertil Steril 1986;46:368-372.
121 Tuohimaa P, Wichmann L: Sperm count of men working under heavy-metal or organic solvent exposure, in Hemminki K, Sorsa M, Vainio H (eds): Occupational Hazards and Reproduction. Washington, Hemisphere, 1982, pp 73-79.
122 Asal NR, Lee ET, Geyer JR, Kadamani S, Risser DR, Cherng N: Risk factors in renal cell carcinoma. II. Medical history, occupation, multivariate analysis, and conclusions. Cancer Detect Prev 1988;13:263-279.
123 Kitchen DN: Neoplastic renal effects of unleaded gasoline in Fischer 344 rats, in Mehlman MA, Hemsteet GP, Thorpe JJ, Weaver NK (eds): Renal Effects of Petroleum Hydrocarbons, Advances in Modern Environmental Toxicology. Princeton, Princeton Scientific Publishers, 1984, vol VII, pp 65-71.
124 Partanen T, Heikkilä P, Hernberg S, Kauppinen T, Moneta G, Ojajärvi A: Renal cell cancer and occupational exposure to chemical agents. Scand J Work Environ Health 1991;17:231-239.
125 McLaughlin JK: Renal cell cancer and exposure to gasoline: A review. Environmental Health Perspectives Suppl 1993;101:111-114.
126 Mellemgaard A, Engholm G, McLaughlin JK, Olsen JH: Occupational risk factors for renal-cell carcinoma in Denmark. Scand J Work Environ Health 1994;20:160-165.
127 Ross RK, Paganini-Hill A, Landolph J, Gerkins V, Henderson BE: Analgesics, cigarette smoking, and other risk factors for cancer of the renal pelvis and ureter. Cancer Res 1989;49:1045-1048.
128 Tobacco smoking. IARC Monographs on the evaluation of the carcinogenic risk of chemicals to humans, Vol. 38. Lyon, International Agency for Research on Cancer, 1986.
129 Smith EM, Miller ER, Woolson RF, Brown CK: Bladder cancer risk among auto and truck mechanics and chemically related occupations. Am J Pub Health 1985;75:881- 883.
130 Claude JF, Frenzel-Beyme RR, Kunze E: Occupation and risk of cancer of the lower urinary tract among men. A case-control study. Int J Cancer 1988;41:371-379.
131 Whiteman D, Green A: Melanoma and sunburn. CCC 1994;5:564-72.
132 Østerlind A, Tucker MA, Stone BJ, Jensen OM: The Danish case-control study of cutaneous malignant melanoma. II. Importance of UV-light exposure. Int J Cancer 1988;42:319-324.
133 Teppo L, Pukkala E, Lehtonen M: Data quality and quality control of a population- based cancer registry. Experience in Finland. Acta Oncol 1994;33:365-369.
134 Polednak AP, Stehney AF, Rowland RE: Mortality among women first employed before 1930 in the U.S. radium dial painting industry. Am J Epidemiol 1978;107:179- 195.
135 Floderus B, Persson T, Stenlund C, Wennberg A, Öst Å, Knave B: Occupational exposure to electromagnetic fields in relation to leukemia and brain tumors: A case- control study in Sweden. CCC 1993;4:465-476.
136 Juutilainen J, Läärä E, Pukkala E: Incidence of leukaemia and brain tumours in Finnish workers exposed to ELF magnetic fields. Int Arch Occup Environ Health 1990;62:289-293.
137 Franssila KO: Is the differentiation between papillary and follicular thyroid carcinoma valid? Cancer 1973;32:853-864.

138 Hardell L, Sandström A: A case-control study: Soft-tissue sarcomas and exposure to phenoxyacetic acids or chlorophenols. Br J Cancer 1979;39:711-717.
139 Asp S, Riihimäki V, Hernberg S, Pukkala E: Mortality and cancer morbidity of Finnish chlorophenoxy herbicide applicators - an 18-year prospective follow-up. Am J Ind Med 1994;26:243-253.
140 Shore RE: Occupational radiation studies: Status, problems, and prospects. Health Physics 1990;59:63-68.
141 BEIR V: Health effects of exposure to low levels of ionizing radiation. Washington DC, National Academy Press, 1990.
142 Kokko S, Vuori H, Rimpelä M: Lääkärien tupakointitavat Suomessa 1973. [Smoking habits of Finnish physicians in 1973]. Suomen Lääkärilehti 1974;29:1451-1454 (in Finnish).
143 Labour force statistics 1992. Labour market 1993:17. Helsinki, Statistics Finland, 1993.
144 Pukkala E, Teppo L, Hakulinen T, Rimpelä M: Occupation and smoking as risk determinants of lung cancer. Int J Epidemiol 1983;12:290-6.
145 Pukkala E: Use of record linkage in small-area studies, in Elliott P, Cuzick J, English D, Stern R (eds): Geographical & Environmental Epidemiology: Methods for Small- Area Studies. Oxford, Oxford University Press, 1992, pp 125-131.
146 Saxén E: Cancer registry: Aims, functions and quality control. Arch Geschwulstforsch 1980;50:588-597.
147 Decouflé P: Occupation, in Schottenfed D, Fraumeni J Jr (eds): Cancer Epidemiology and Prevention. Philadelphia, Saunders, 1982.
148 Teppo L, Pukkala E, Hakama M, Hakulinen T, Herva A, Saxén E: Way of life and cancer incidence in Finland. A municipality-based ecological analysis. Scand J Soc Med 1980;Suppl 19.
149 Hakama M, Hakulinen T, Pukkala E, Saxén E, Teppo L: Risk indicators of breast and cervical cancer on ecologic and individual levels. Amer J Epidemiol 1982;116:990- 1000.
150 Tenkanen L: Migration to towns, occupation, smoking and lung cancer: Experience from the Finnish-Norwegian lung cancer study. CCC 1993;4:133-141.
151 Townsend P: Poverty in the United Kingdom. Harmondsworth, Penguin Books, 1979.
152 Hasan J: Social class, disease and death. An essay in social medicine. Proc Soc Hornphysiol No 6. Tampere, University of Tampere, 1988.
153 Schwartz S: The fallacy of the ecological fallacy: the potential misuse of a concept and the consequences. Am J Public Health 1994;84:819-824.
154 Karjalainen S, Pukkala E: Social class as a prognostic factors in breast cancer survival. Cancer 1990;66:819-826.
155 Auvinen A, Karjalainen S, Pukkala E: Social class as prognostic factor in cancer. Am J Epidemiol (submitted for publication 1994).
156 Hakulinen T, Pukkala E, Hakama M, Lehtonen M, Saxén E, Teppo L: Survival of cancer patients in Finland in 1953-1974. Ann Clin Res 1981;13:Suppl 31.
157 Wong O, Decouflé P: Methodological issues involving the standardized mortality ratio and proportionate mortality ratio in occupational studies. J Occup Med 1982;24:299- 304.
158 Alderson M: Occupational cancer. London, Butterworths, 1986.
159 Siemiatycki J, Richardson L: Case-control design and fielwork methods, in Siemiatycki J (ed): Risk Factors for Cancer in the Workplace. Boca Raton, CRC Press, 1991, pp 29-44.
160 Siemiatycki J, Gérin M, Dewar R, Nadon L, Lakhani RZ, Bégin D, Richardson L: Associations between occupational circumstances and cancer, in Siemiatycki J (ed): Risk Factors for Cancer in the Workplace. Boca Raton, CRC Press, 1991, pp 141- 196.
161 United Nations: Indexes to the international standard industrial classification of all economic activities. New York, Statistical Office of United Nations, 1968.
162 Pukkala E, Poskiparta M, Apter D, Vihko V: Life-long physical activity and cancer risk among Finnish female teachers. Eur J Cancer Prev 1993;2:369-376.
163 Tola S, Kalliomäki P-L, Pukkala E, Asp S, Korkala M-L: Cancer incidence among welders, platers, machinists and pipe fitters in shipyards and machine shops. Brit J Ind Med 1988;45:209-218.

164 Jäppinen P, Pukkala E, Tola S: Cancer incidence of workers in a Finnish sawmill. Scand J Work Environ Health 1989;15:18-23.
165 Sankila R, Karjalainen S, Pukkala E, Oksanen H, Hakulinen T, Teppo L, Hakama M: Cancer risk among glass factory workers: An excess of lung cancer? Brit J Ind Med 1990;47:815-818.
166 Kilpikari I, Pukkala E, Lehtonen M, Hakama M: Cancer incidence among Finnish rubber workers. Int Arch Occup Environ Health 1982;51:65-71.
167 Partanen T, Kauppinen T, Degerth R, Moneta G, Mearelli I, Ojajärvi A, Hernberg S, Koskinen H, Pukkala E: Pancreatic cancer in industrial branches and occupations in Finland. Am J Ind Med 1994;36:616-622.
168 Whitehead M: The health divide, in Townsend P, Davidson N (eds): Inequalities in health. Harmondsworth, Penguin Books, 1988, pp 221-381.
169 Liberatos P, Link BG, Kelsey JL: The measurement of social class in epidemiology. Epidemiol Rev 1988;10:87-121.
170 Wilkinson RG: Class and health: Research and longitudinal data. London, Tavistock, 1986.
171 Hemminki E, Malin M, Rahkonen O: Mother's social class and perinatal problems in a low-problem area. Int J Epid 1990;19:983-990.
172 Luoto R: Measurement of women's socioeconomic position in the Finnish Journal of Social Medicine - a review. J Soc Med 1991;28:159-165 (in Finnish, with an English summary).
173 Malin M, Topo P, Hemminki E: The indicators of women's social class and their connection on health differences and the use of health services. J Soc Med 1993;30:369-378 (in Finnish, with an English summary).
174 Kolari R: Occupational mobility in Finland 1975/1980/1985. Studies 160. Helsinki, Central Statistical Office of Finland, 1989.
175 Miettinen O: Theoretical epidemiology. Principles of occurrence research in medicine. New York, Wiley, 1985.
176 Rothman KJ: No adjustments are needed for multiple comparisons. Epidemiology 1990;1:43-46.
177 Siemiatycki J: Epidemiological approaches to discovering occupational carcinogens, in Siemiatycki J (ed): Risk Factors for Cancer in the Workplace. Boca Raton, CRC Press, 1991, pp 17-28.
178 Karjalainen A, Meurman LO, Pukkala E: Four cases of mesothelioma among Finnish anthophyllite miners. OEM 1994;51:212-215.
179 McClure KM, MacMahon B: An epidemiologic perspective of environmental carcinogenesis. Epidemiol Rev 1980;2:19-48.
180 Prättälä R, Berg M-A, Puska P: Diminishing or increasing contrasts? Social class variation in Finnish food consumption patterns, 1979-1990. Eur J Clin Nutr 1992;46:279-287.
181 Wahrendorf J: An estimate of the proportion of colo-rectal and stomach cancers which might be prevented by certain changes in dietary habits. Int J Cancer 1987;40:625- 628.
182 Siemiatycki J, Dewar R: Statistical methods, in Siemiatycki J (ed): Risk Factors for Cancer in the Workplace. Boca Raton, CRC Press, 1991, pp 115-140.

Appendix tables

A. Average number of persons under follow-up, by occupation, social class and sex.

B. Numbers of cancer cases and standardised incidence ratios, by primary site, sex, social class and period.

C. Numbers of cancer cases and crude and social class adjusted standardised incidence ratios for all main occupational branches and selected specific occupational categories, by primary site and sex.

Appendix table A

Average number of persons under follow-up in 1971-1985, by occupation, social class and sex. Included are those 35-64 years of age at the beginning of each five-year follow-up period. Persons with unknown social status (1.0% of the economically active population) are included in social class III. Full-length "official" headers are given *in Italics* for occupational categories with shorter headers used in text and tables.

Occupation	Sex	Social class				
		Total	I	II	III	IV
WHOLE POPULATION	M	725,868	69,540	170,167	385,567	100,595
	F	825,528	63,354	236,451	389,528	136,195
ECONOMICALLY ACTIVE PERSONS	M	667,121	67,649	160,306	352,823	86,342
	F	513,110	32,455	163,746	223,772	93,137
0 Technical, humanistic, etc. work	M	75,036	37,579	36,879	546	32
Technical, physical and social science, humanistic and artistic work	F	76,752	28,423	32,616	15,709	5
00 Technical professions	M	9,846	9,844	2	-	-
	F	412	412	-	-	-
000 Architects	M	612	612	-	-	-
	F	204	204	-	-	-
001 Civil engineers	M	2,504	2,504	-	-	-
	F	45	45	-	-	-
002 Electrical engineers	M	1,290	1,290	-	-	-
	F	5	5	-	-	-
003 Teletechnical engineers	M	622	622	-	-	-
	F	4	4	-	-	-
004 Mechanical engineers	M	2,848	2,846	2	-	-
	F	16	16	-	-	-
005 Chemotechnical engineers	M	830	830	-	-	-
	F	63	63	-	-	-
006 Mining engineers *Engineers in mining and metallurgy*	M	215	215	-	-	-
	F	2	2	-	-	-
007 Engineers NOS *Engineers in other technical fields*	M	523	523	-	-	-
	F	70	70	-	-	-
008 Surveyors	M	404	404	-	-	-
	F	4	4	-	-	-
01 Technical work	M	26,640	-	26,639	1	-
	F	4,025	4	4,021	-	-
010 Civil engineering technicians	M	8,940	-	8,940	-	-
	F	81	-	81	-	-
011 Power technicians	M	2,321	-	2,321	-	-
	F	12	-	12	-	-
012 Teletechnicians	M	1,281	-	1,281	-	-
	F	8	-	8	-	-
013 Mechanical technicians	M	7,107	-	7,107	-	-
	F	35	-	35	-	-

Occupation	Sex	Social class				
		Total	I	II	III	IV
014 Chemotechnicians	M	756	-	756	-	-
	F	34	-	34	-	-
015 Mining technicians *Technicians in mining and metallurgy*	M	303	-	303	-	-
	F	1	-	1	-	-
016 Technicians NOS *Technicians in other technical fields*	M	2,664	-	2,664	-	-
	F	109	-	109	-	-
017 Cartographers *Surveyor technicians and cartographers*	M	766	-	766	-	-
	F	31	-	31	-	-
018 Draughtsmen, survey assistants	M	1,543	-	1,542	1	-
	F	1,177	4	1,173	-	-
019 Laboratory assistants	M	958	-	958	-	-
	F	2,538	-	2,538	-	-
02 Chemical/physical/biological work	M	4,137	2,195	1,942	-	-
	F	1,389	439	950	-	-
020 Chemists	M	439	439	-	-	-
	F	220	220	-	-	-
021 Physicists	M	125	125	-	-	-
	F	6	6	-	-	-
022 Geologists	M	147	147	-	-	-
	F	12	12	-	-	-
023 Meteorologists, hydrologists	M	91	52	39	-	-
	F	60	8	52	-	-
024 Chemical/physical workers NOS *Other chemical and physical occupations*	M	3	3	-	-	-
	F	1	1	-	-	-
025 Veterinary surgeons	M	294	294	-	-	-
	F	26	26	-	-	-
026 Biologists	M	93	93	-	-	-
	F	41	41	-	-	-
027 Consultancy, agriculture *Research and consultancy (agriculture, horticulture, fishing)*	M	1,268	284	984	-	-
	F	1,009	111	897	-	-
028 Consultancy, forestry *Research and consultancy (forestry)*	M	1,678	759	919	-	-
	F	15	14	1	-	-
03 Medical work and nursing	M	3,947	2,582	823	510	32
	F	34,494	2,363	16,479	15,648	5
030 Medical doctors	M	2,148	2,148	-	-	-
	F	805	805	-	-	-
031 Dentists	M	433	433	-	-	-
	F	1,093	1,093	-	-	-
032 Nurses	M	58	1	57	-	-
	F	10,666	406	10,260	-	-
033 Doctor's/dentist's receptionists	M	1	-	-	1	-
	F	750	59	4	687	-
034 Midwives	F	1,480	-	1,480	-	-

Cancer Risk by Social Class and Occupation

Occupation	Sex	Social class				
		Total	I	II	III	IV
035 Psychiatric nurses	M	755	-	755	-	-
	F	2,265	-	2,265	-	-
036 Auxiliary nurses	M	67	-	-	67	-
	F	14,526	-	0	14,526	-
037 Technical nursing assistants	M	36	-	-	36	-
	F	371	-	-	371	-
038 Institutional children's nurses	M	4	-	4	-	-
	F	2,424	-	2,424	-	-
039 Medical workers NOS	M	446	-	7	407	32
Other medical occupations	F	115	-	46	64	5
04 Health-care related work	M	812	274	503	35	-
Other medical professions	F	4,321	2,620	1,641	60	-
040 Pharmacists	M	272	272	-	-	-
Pharmacists, owner-directors of pharmacies	F	2,620	2,608	12	-	-
041 Physiotherapists	M	149	-	149	-	-
Physiotherapists, occupational therapists	F	598	-	598	-	-
042 Health inspectors	M	223	-	223	-	-
	F	88	-	88	-	-
043 Masseurs, etc.	M	153	-	117	35	-
	F	308	-	247	60	-
044 Pharmaceutical assistants	M	7	1	6	-	-
	F	658	10	648	-	-
049 Health-care workers NOS	M	9	1	8	-	-
Other health-care occupations	F	48	1	46	-	-
05 Teaching	M	16,894	14,160	2,734	-	-
	F	22,276	17,893	4,383	-	-
050 University teachers	M	1,479	1,479	-	-	-
University/tertiary level teachers	F	400	400	-	-	-
051 Subject teachers	M	3,523	3,523	-	-	-
Specialist-subject teachers (especially in secondary school)	F	6,206	6,206	-	-	-
052 Primary school teachers	M	6,784	6,784	-	-	-
	F	9,661	9,661	-	-	-
053 Teachers of practical subjects	M	940	635	306	-	-
	F	2,851	1,114	1,737	-	-
054 Vocational teachers	M	3,555	1,418	2,137	-	-
	F	1,831	383	1,448	-	-
055 Preschool teachers	M	1	-	1	-	-
	F	1,010	-	1,010	-	-
056 Education officers	M	526	284	242	-	-
	F	120	29	91	-	-
059 Teaching workers NOS	M	85	38	47	-	-
Other teaching occupations	F	197	99	98	-	-
06 Religious professions	M	1,478	983	495	-	-
	F	1,181	115	1,066	-	-
060 Clergy and lay preachers	M	1,266	951	315	-	-
Ministers, priests and lay preachers	F	396	100	296	-	-

Appendix Table A

Occupation	Sex	Social class				
		Total	I	II	III	IV
061 Deacons and social workers	M	210	32	178	-	-
	F	775	16	759	-	-
069 Religious workers NOS *Other religious occupations*	M	2	-	2	-	-
	F	10	-	10	-	-
07 Legal professions	M	1,681	1,523	158	-	-
	F	329	318	11	-	-
070 Barristers and judges	M	411	411	-	-	-
	F	59	59	-	-	-
071 Senior police officials *Prosecutors and senior police officials*	M	282	282	-	-	-
	F	1	1	-	-	-
072 Lawyers	M	325	325	-	-	-
	F	21	21	-	-	-
073 Solicitors	M	464	464	-	-	-
	F	224	224	-	-	-
079 Juridical workers NOS *Other juridical occupations*	M	200	43	158	-	-
	F	25	14	11	-	-
08 Artistic and literary professions	M	4,829	3,139	1,690	-	-
	F	2,703	1,659	1,044	-	-
080 Sculptors, painters, etc.	M	495	490	5	-	-
	F	182	175	7	-	-
081 Commercial artists	M	397	-	397	-	-
	F	105	-	105	-	-
082 Window dressers, etc. *Window dressers and lettering artists*	M	189	-	189	-	-
	F	163	-	163	-	-
083 Authors	M	109	109	-	-	-
	F	76	76	-	-	-
084 Journalists *Journalists, editors, copywriters*	M	1,540	1,310	230	-	-
	F	1,128	691	437	-	-
085 Industrial designers	M	214	156	58	-	-
	F	349	269	79	-	-
086 Performing artists	M	366	318	48	-	-
	F	297	226	70	-	-
087 Musicians	M	1,159	512	648	-	-
	F	177	101	77	-	-
088 Film and radio producers *Radio, television and film producers*	M	241	241	-	-	-
	F	117	116	1	-	-
089 Art-related workers NOS *Other art-related professions*	M	117	3	114	-	-
	F	109	5	104	-	-
09 Humanistic and social work etc. *Other occupations in group 0*	M	4,772	2,878	1,894	-	-
	F	5,623	2,600	3,022	-	-
090 Auditors	M	284	271	13	-	-
	F	121	85	36	-	-
091 Social workers	M	968	301	667	-	-
	F	2,524	791	1,733	-	-
092 Librarians, museum officials *Librarians, archivists, museum officials*	M	342	228	114	-	-
	F	1,615	893	722	-	-

Occupation	Sex	Social class				
		Total	I	II	III	IV
093 Community planning professions *Community research and planning professions*	M F	381 117	381 117	- -	- -	- -
094 Systems analysts, programmers	M F	938 178	771 83	167 96	- -	- -
095 Psychologists	M F	117 223	117 223	- -	- -	- -
096 PR officers *Personnel and public relations officers*	M F	1,450 540	590 194	860 346	- -	- -
099 Humanistic/scientific workers NOS *Other occupations in group 09*	M F	293 305	220 215	74 90	- -	- -
1 Administrative and clerical work *Administrative, managerial and clerical professions*	M F	39,883 73,828	23,894 3,261	15,988 70,564	- 3	- -
10 Public administration 100 Public sector managers *Senior officials in public administration*	M F	3,592 1,178	3,592 1,178	- -	- -	- -
11 Corporate administration *Administrators in companies and organizations*	M F	19,137 1,577	19,137 1,577	- -	- -	- -
110 Corporate managers	M F	7,769 548	7,769 548	- -	- -	- -
111 Technical managers	M F	1,813 49	1,813 49	- -	- -	- -
112 Commercial managers	M F	5,439 221	5,439 221	- -	- -	- -
113 Administrative managers *Administrative managers, budgeting and accounting*	M F	1,146 159	1,146 159	- -	- -	- -
114 Managers of ideal organizations *Senior officials in commercial and non-profit associations*	M F	713 112	713 112	- -	- -	- -
119 Private sector managers NOS *Other private sector managers*	M F	2,257 488	2,257 488	- -	- -	- -
12 Clerical work	M F	1,519 15,632	372 166	1,147 15,464	- 2	- -
120 Book-keepers, accountants	M F	1,299 7,105	372 162	927 6,941	- 2	- -
121 Office cashiers	M F	135 2,927	- 4	135 2,922	- -	- -
122 Bank and post office cashiers	M F	8 1,235	- -	8 1,235	- -	- -
123 Shop and restaurant cashiers	M F	35 4,279	- -	35 4,279	- -	- -
129 Book-keeping workers/cashiers NOS *Other book-keeping/cashier occupations*	M F	42 86	- -	42 86	- -	- -

Appendix Table A

Occupation	Sex	Social class				
		Total	I	II	III	IV
13 Stenographers and typists	M	328	0	327	-	-
	F	7,352	5	7,346	-	-
130 Private secretaries	M	214	0	214	-	-
Private secretaries, correspondents, stenographers	F	4,192	5	4,186	-	-
131 Typists	M	113	-	113	-	-
	F	3,160	-	3,160	-	-
14/15 Clerical work NOS	M	15,307	793	14,514	-	-
Other clerical work	F	48,089	335	47,754	1	-
140 Computer book-keepers	M	11	-	11	-	-
	F	178	-	178	-	-
141 Computer operators	M	248	-	248	-	-
	F	181	-	181	-	-
142 Data storage assistants	M	9	-	9	-	-
	F	769	-	769	-	-
143 Photocopier operators etc.	M	278	-	278	-	-
Computing assistants, photocopier operators, etc.	F	1,168	-	1,167	1	-
144 Office clerks	M	2,485	2	2,483	-	-
	F	31,190	106	31,084	-	-
145 Bank clerks	M	1,297	579	719	-	-
	F	6,798	201	6,596	-	-
146 Insurance clerks	M	482	174	308	-	-
	F	1,646	18	1,628	-	-
147 Social insurance clerks	M	200	-	200	-	-
Health social insurance clerks	F	699	-	699	-	-
148 Travel agents	M	51	-	51	-	-
	F	343	-	343	-	-
149 Shipping agents	M	936	-	936	-	-
	F	190	-	190	-	-
150 Property managers, warehousemen	M	6,902	-	6,902	-	-
	F	975	-	975	-	-
151 Bid calculators, orders clerks	M	623	37	585	-	-
	F	270	2	268	-	-
159 Clerical workers NOS	M	1,785	1	1,784	-	-
Other clerical occupations	F	3,683	8	3,676	-	-
2 Sales professions	M	37,022	1,126	23,898	11,998	-
	F	53,775	106	13,830	39,839	0
20 Wholesale and retail dealers	M	7,964	136	7,828	-	-
	F	6,325	15	6,310	-	-
200 Wholesalers	M	363	136	228	-	-
	F	33	15	18	-	-
201 Retailers	M	7,601	-	7,601	-	-
	F	6,292	-	6,292	-	-
21 Real estate, services, securities	M	2,581	460	2,120	-	-
	F	325	82	242	-	-
210 Insurance salesmen	M	1,381	39	1,341	-	-
	F	44	1	43	-	-

Occupation	Sex	Social class				
		Total	I	II	III	IV
211 Real estate/stockbrokers	M	295	-	295	-	-
	F	48	-	48	-	-
212 Advertising sales	M	823	421	402	-	-
	F	208	81	127	-	-
219 Real estate etc. workers NOS *Other occupations related to group 21*	M	82	-	82	-	-
	F	24	-	24	-	-
22 Sales representatives	M	8,994	0	8,993	-	-
	F	903	1	902	-	-
220 Commercial travellers, etc. *Sales staff, commercial travellers*	M	8,472	0	8,472	-	-
	F	833	1	832	-	-
221 Sales agents	M	521	-	521	-	-
	F	70	-	70	-	-
23 Sales work *Other sales work*	M	17,484	530	4,956	11,998	-
	F	46,222	7	6,375	39,839	0
230 Buyers, office sales staff	M	3,060	529	2,531	-	-
	F	1,091	5	1,086	1	-
231 Shop personnel	M	11,463	-	257	11,205	-
	F	43,620	1	4,642	38,976	0
232 Door-to-door salesmen	M	760	1	702	57	-
	F	505	1	413	91	-
233 Service station attendants	M	1,387	-	1,387	-	-
	F	165	-	165	-	-
239 Sales staff NOS *Other sales staff*	M	815	-	78	736	-
	F	842	-	70	772	-
3 Farming, forestry and fishing	M	158,090	1,414	34,091	79,351	43,235
	F	100,640	620	17,315	57,742	24,963
30 Agricultural/forestry management *Managerial professions in agriculture, forestry and horticulture*	M	120,755	1,304	31,863	73,356	14,232
	F	22,095	143	2,446	11,766	7,740
300 Farmers, silviculturists *Farmers, silviculturists, horticulturists*	M	113,105	1,269	25,527	72,103	14,205
	F	21,388	141	2,230	11,409	7,608
301 Agricultural managers	M	612	-	612	-	-
	F	9	-	9	-	-
302 Forestry managers	M	5,003	-	5,003	-	-
303 Horticultural managers	M	657	33	624	-	-
	F	167	2	165	-	-
304 Livestock breeders	M	256	1	36	199	19
	F	428	-	35	261	132
305 Fur-bearing animal breeders	M	801	-	61	735	5
	F	97	-	8	90	-
306 Reindeer breeders	M	321	1	1	318	2
	F	6	-	-	6	-
31 Farming, animal husbandry *Agriculture and horticulture, animal husbandry*	M	12,157	103	2,180	3,897	5,977
	F	78,239	476	14,867	45,835	17,061
310 Agricultural workers	M	9,632	94	2,020	3,433	4,086
	F	7,668	120	1,858	4,374	1,317

Appendix Table A

Occupation	Sex	Social class				
		Total	I	II	III	IV
311 Gardeners	M	1,053	-	1	30	1,022
	F	2,713	1	12	523	2,178
312 Livestock workers	M	1,097	8	159	417	513
	F	67,451	355	12,996	40,705	13,395
313 Fur-farm workers	M	222	-	-	9	213
Fur-bearing animal farm workers	F	324	-	2	222	101
314 Reindeer herders	M	125	-	-	7	118
	F	11	-	-	9	2
319 Agricultural workers NOS	M	28	-	-	1	27
Other agricultural occupations	F	70	-	-	3	68
32 Game protection and hunting						
320 Gamekeepers and hunters	M	23	-	17	6	-
	F	3	-	-	2	1
33 Fishing	M	1,371	7	24	1,202	138
	F	142	1	1	125	15
330 Fishermen	M	1,310	1	-	1,193	116
	F	127	1	-	120	6
331 Fish farmers	M	61	7	24	9	22
	F	15	-	1	5	9
34 Forestry work						
340 Forestry and log floating	M	23,785	-	7	891	22,887
	F	162	-	1	15	146
4 Mining and quarrying	M	3,954	-	306	3,576	72
	F	138	-	7	125	5
40 Mining and quarrying						
400 Miners, blasters, etc.	M	2,303	-	176	2,113	14
	F	9	-	3	6	-
41 Deep drilling						
410 Drilling-machine operators	M	494	-	73	419	2
	F	1	-	-	1	-
42 Concentration plant work						
420 Concentration plant staff	M	286	-	-	286	-
	F	58	-	-	58	-
49 Mining and quarrying NOS						
490 Mining workers NOS	M	870	-	56	758	56
Other workers in mining and quarrying	F	70	-	4	61	5
5 Transport and communications	M	70,447	1,698	22,970	45,465	315
	F	17,330	18	10,916	4,654	1,742
50 Ship's officers	M	2,666	637	2,029	-	-
	F	2	-	2	-	-
500 Ship's masters and mates	M	1,196	637	560	-	-
	F	2	-	2	-	-
501 Ship pilots	M	532	-	532	-	-
502 Chief engineers in ships	M	938	-	938	-	-
51 Deck and engine-room crew	M	2,309	-	54	2,167	87
	F	15	-	1	11	3
510 Deck crew	M	1,573	-	53	1,433	87
	F	15	-	1	11	3

Occupation	Sex	Social class				
		Total	I	II	III	IV
511 Engine-room crew	M	735	-	1	734	0
52 Air traffic						
520 Pilots, flight engineers, etc.	M	195	164	19	12	-
53 Engine drivers						
530 Engine-drivers, driver's assistants	M	2,902	-	-	2,901	0
54 Road transport	M	46,290	4	15,522	30,696	69
	F	700	-	499	177	24
540 Motor-vehicle and tram drivers	M	46,193	4	15,493	30,696	-
	F	676	-	499	177	-
541 Draymen	M	57	-	29	-	28
	F	1	-	-	-	1
542 Messengers, etc.	M	41	-	-	-	41
	F	23	-	-	-	23
55 Transport services	M	5,501	-	1,167	4,298	37
	F	1,546	-	108	1,434	3
550 Railway staff	M	5,328	-	1,047	4,280	1
	F	167	-	25	141	1
551 Flight operations officers	M	155	-	120	-	35
	F	83	-	81	-	2
552 Bus/tram services	M	18	-	-	18	-
	F	1,296	-	2	1,293	-
56 Traffic supervisors	M	3,162	893	2,270	-	-
	F	625	18	608	-	-
560 Port traffic supervisors	M	395	76	320	-	-
	F	7	1	6	-	-
561 Air traffic supervisors	M	129	101	28	-	-
	F	2	1	1	-	-
562 Railway traffic supervisors	M	1,451	174	1,277	-	-
	F	543	5	538	-	-
563 Road transport supervisors	M	1,175	532	644	-	-
	F	73	10	63	-	-
569 Traffic managers NOS	M	11	10	2	-	-
Other traffic managers	F	1	1	-	-	-
57 Post and telecommunications	M	1,714	-	1,714	-	-
	F	9,691	-	9,691	-	-
570 Post/telecommunications officials	M	1,304	-	1,304	-	-
	F	4,184	-	4,184	-	-
571 Telephone operators	M	62	-	62	-	-
Telephone operators long-distance and local calls)	F	3,328	-	3,328	-	-
572 Switchboard operators	M	7	-	7	-	-
Telephone switchboard operators	F	1,613	-	1,613	-	-
573 Telegraphists	M	342	-	342	-	-
Telegraphists, radio-communication operators etc.	F	565	-	565	-	-
58 Postal services/couriers	M	4,262	-	178	3,964	119
	F	4,668	-	4	2,952	1,711
580 Postmen	M	3,071	-	-	2,993	79
Postmen and sorters	F	4,132	-	-	2,563	1,569

Appendix Table A

Occupation	Sex	Social class				
		Total	I	II	III	IV
581 Caretakers/messengers	M	1,190	-	178	971	41
	F	536	-	4	389	143
59 Communication work NOS *Other transport and communications work*	M	1,446	-	17	1,427	2
	F	83	-	4	79	1
590 Lighthouse keepers	M	67	-	7	60	-
	F	1	-	-	1	-
591 Canal/harbour guards, ferrymen	M	241	-	1	239	1
	F	36	-	-	35	1
599 Communication workers NOS *Other occupations in communications*	M	1,138	-	9	1,129	1
	F	47	-	4	43	-
6/7 Industrial and construction work *Industrial, mechanical and construction work*	M	251,297	3	14,462	195,394	41,439
	F	90,800	3	4,511	77,758	8,528
60 Textiles	M	2,372	-	87	2,274	12
	F	9,929	-	570	9,307	52
600 Pre-process yarnworker	M	103	-	1	102	0
	F	491	-	-	489	2
601 Spinners etc.	M	206	-	12	194	0
	F	2,186	-	5	2,172	9
602 Weavers	M	240	-	52	187	1
	F	3,253	-	410	2,820	22
603 Textile machine setters/operators	M	835	-	-	834	2
	F	24	-	-	24	-
604 Knitters	M	79	-	7	72	1
	F	1,274	-	37	1,235	1
605 Textile finishers/dyers	M	710	-	2	700	8
	F	1,247	-	1	1,230	16
606 Textile quality controllers	M	34	-	-	34	-
	F	778	-	-	778	-
609 Textile workers NOS *Other occupations in textiles*	M	165	-	14	151	-
	F	677	-	117	559	1
61 Cutting/sewing etc. *Cutting, sewing and upholstering etc.*	M	2,000	-	558	1,440	2
	F	18,878	2	2,671	16,170	36
610 Tailors	M	423	-	166	256	-
	F	346	-	87	255	5
611 Dressmakers	M	27	-	17	10	-
	F	3,362	-	2,125	1,235	2
612 Furriers	M	157	-	55	102	-
	F	338	-	60	277	2
613 Milliners	M	41	-	10	31	-
	F	697	-	136	560	0
614 Upholsterers	M	742	-	243	499	1
	F	414	-	38	374	2
615 Patternmakers and cutters *Patternmakers and cutters (incl. leather and gloves)*	M	269	-	1	268	-
	F	1,758	-	16	1,731	11
616 Garment workers *Garment workers (incl. leather and gloves)*	M	253	-	50	202	1
	F	11,124	2	152	10,958	12

Occupation	Sex	Social class				
		Total	I	II	III	IV
619 Cutting/sewing workers NOS	M	88	-	17	71	-
Other occupations in group 61	F	838	-	57	779	2
62 Shoes and leather	M	1,714	-	500	1,210	4
	F	3,451	-	224	3,208	18
620 Shoemakers and cobblers	M	434	-	311	121	1
	F	73	-	53	20	-
621 Shoe cutters etc.	M	234	-	-	234	-
	F	264	-	-	264	-
622 Shoe sewers	M	49	-	-	49	-
	F	1,350	-	10	1,334	5
623 Lasters	M	168	-	-	168	-
	F	90	-	-	90	-
624 Sole fitters etc.	M	166	-	-	166	-
	F	135	-	-	134	1
625 Shoemakers NOS	M	230	-	-	229	1
Other shoemakers	F	827	-	0	816	10
626 Saddlers, leather sewers etc.	M	433	-	189	243	1
	F	712	-	160	550	2
63 Smelting, metal and foundry work	M	6,632	-	471	6,115	46
	F	805	-	4	799	2
630 Smelter furnacemen	M	1,290	-	0	1,281	10
	F	45	-	-	45	-
631 Hardeners, temperers, etc.	M	140	-	-	140	-
Heat treaters, hardeners, temperers etc.	F	14	-	-	13	2
632 Hot-rollers	M	322	-	-	319	2
	F	17	-	-	17	-
633 Cold-rollers	M	128	-	-	128	-
	F	8	-	-	8	0
634 Blacksmiths	M	1,289	-	442	840	8
	F	36	-	-	36	-
635 Founders	M	1,965	-	3	1,942	20
	F	250	-	2	248	-
636 Wire and tube drawers	M	279	-	-	279	-
	F	34	-	-	34	-
639 Metalworkers NOS	M	1,218	-	26	1,186	7
Other occupations related to group 63	F	400	-	2	398	-
64 Precision mechanical work	M	2,920	1	932	1,986	1
	F	310	-	60	247	3
640 Precision mechanics	M	1,007	-	44	962	0
	F	73	-	0	72	-
641 Watchmakers	M	628	-	364	263	-
	F	14	-	7	7	-
642 Opticians	M	202	-	85	118	-
	F	37	-	13	23	-
643 Dental technicians	M	358	1	200	156	1
	F	41	-	23	17	1
644 Goldsmiths, silversmiths etc.	M	640	-	217	423	-
	F	96	-	13	82	2

Appendix Table A

Occupation	Sex	Social class				
		Total	I	II	III	IV
645 Jewellery engravers	M	86	-	22	64	-
	F	49	-	4	45	-
65 Machine shop/steelworkers	M	55,978	-	3,487	52,325	165
	F	3,511	-	78	3,414	19
650 Turners, machinists	M	10,647	-	319	10,310	18
	F	696	-	10	681	5
651 Fitter-assemblers etc.	M	5,585	-	126	5,436	23
	F	49	-	2	47	-
652 Machine and motor repairers	M	13,468	-	1,546	11,888	35
	F	84	-	24	57	3
653 Sheetmetalworkers	M	5,376	-	427	4,937	12
	F	76	-	10	66	-
654 Plumbers	M	7,485	-	587	6,877	21
	F	1	-	-	1	-
655 Welders and flame cutters	M	6,985	-	143	6,839	3
	F	185	-	1	182	2
656 Plate/constructional steel workers *Metal-plate workers and constructional steel erectors*	M	1,608	-	12	1,592	3
	F	1	-	-	1	-
657 Metal platers and coaters	M	316	-	21	290	5
	F	254	-	1	252	1
659 Machine shop/steelworkers NOS *Other occupations in group 65*	M	4,508	-	305	4,158	44
	F	2,165	-	31	2,126	8
66 Electrical work	M	17,482	-	725	16,720	36
	F	2,109	-	53	2,052	3
660 Electricians (indoors) *Electricians (indoor installation)*	M	9,557	-	362	9,185	11
	F	93	-	3	88	1
661 Electric machine operators	M	1,065	-	2	1,054	10
	F	4	-	-	4	-
662 Electric fitters *Electric fitters (high intensity)*	M	377	-	-	377	1
	F	11	-	-	11	-
663 Electronics and telefitters *Electronics fitters and repairmen (not telephone)*	M	1,132	-	226	906	0
	F	36	-	4	31	-
664 Telephone installers and repairmen	M	2,767	-	-	2,766	1
	F	56	-	-	56	-
665 Linemen	M	1,621	-	-	1,609	12
666 Electronic equipment assemblers *Electrical and electronic equipment assemblers*	M	517	-	-	517	0
	F	1,755	-	-	1,754	1
669 Electrical workers NOS *Other electrical occupations*	M	445	-	136	308	1
	F	155	-	46	108	1
67 Woodwork	M	42,838	-	2,325	40,339	173
	F	7,590	-	96	7,369	125
670 Round-timber workers	M	1,102	-	60	1,034	8
	F	196	-	3	193	-
671 Timber workers	M	5,876	-	366	5,460	50
	F	1,469	-	8	1,435	26

Occupation	Sex	Social class				
		Total	I	II	III	IV
672 Plywood makers	M	1,853	-	-	1,845	8
	F	3,605	-	-	3,583	22
673 Construction carpenters	M	25,143	-	483	24,630	30
	F	9	-	1	8	-
674 Boatbuilders etc.	M	989	-	219	766	4
Wooden boatbuilders, coach-body builders	F	19	-	3	16	-
675 Bench carpenters	M	2,510	-	748	1,759	3
	F	78	-	33	44	1
676 Cabinetmakers etc.	M	1,748	-	243	1,501	5
Cabinetmakers, joiners, etc.	F	214	-	16	190	9
677 Woodworking machine operators etc.	M	2,734	-	137	2,589	8
	F	911	-	14	874	24
678 Wooden surface finishers	M	291	-	16	255	21
	F	425	-	3	419	3
679 Woodworkers NOS	M	592	-	55	499	37
Other woodwork	F	662	-	15	607	40
68 Painting and lacquering	M	9,665	-	1,211	8,446	8
	F	1,032	-	32	900	100
680 Painters	M	8,745	-	1,087	7,652	6
Painters, decorators	F	712	-	16	605	91
681 Lacquerers	M	919	-	124	794	1
	F	320	-	16	295	9
69 Construction work NOS	M	36,338	-	768	11,765	23,805
Other construction work	F	3,332	-	16	163	3,153
690 Bricklayers and tile setters	M	4,369	-	166	4,186	17
Bricklayers, plasterers and tile setters	F	68	-	3	51	15
691 Reinforced concreters etc.	M	181	-	2	179	-
Reinforced concreters, stonemasons etc.						
692 Reinforcing iron workers	M	1,336	-	-	1,308	28
	F	7	-	-	5	1
693 Concrete/cement shutters	M	3,262	-	110	3,152	-
Concrete shutterers, cement finishers	F	10	-	1	9	-
694 Asphalt roofers	M	344	-	4	340	-
	F	2	-	-	2	-
695 Insulators	M	1,315	-	118	1,197	-
	F	64	-	5	59	-
696 Glaziers	M	283	-	47	236	-
	F	28	-	1	27	-
697 Building hands	M	15,332	-	-	-	15,332
	F	2,754	-	-	-	2,754
698 Roadbuilding hands	M	8,428	-	-	-	8,428
Other construction hands	F	383	-	-	-	383
699 Construction workers NOS	M	1,489	-	322	1,167	-
Other occupations related to group 69	F	16	-	6	9	-
70 Printing	M	4,415	0	94	4,303	17
	F	3,521		49	3,445	28

Appendix Table A

Occupation	Sex	Social class				
		Total	I	II	III	IV
700 Typographers etc.	M	1,706	0	-	1,704	2
	F	637	-	1	635	1
701 Printers	M	1,446	-	3	1,440	3
	F	645	-	-	631	15
702 Lithographers	M	478	-	1	470	8
	F	166	-	-	161	5
703 Bookbinders	M	455	-	2	453	-
	F	1,698	-	5	1,692	2
709 Printing workers NOS Other occupations related to printing	M	329	-	89	236	4
	F	374	-	43	327	4
71 Glass and ceramic work Glass, ceramic and pottery	M	1,562	-	40	1,509	13
	F	1,340	-	9	1,317	14
710 Glass formers	M	547	-	-	545	2
	F	295	-	-	292	3
711 Potters	M	447	-	23	417	7
	F	406	-	5	395	7
712 Kiln operators Kilnmen (glass and ceramics)	M	219	-	3	215	1
	F	59	-	1	57	1
713 Glass and ceramics decorators Glass and ceramics decorators, glaziers	M	136	-	1	135	-
	F	243	-	0	241	2
714 Glass and clay mixers	M	53	-	0	52	-
	F	14	-	-	14	-
719 Glass/ceramic workers NOS Other occupations related to this group	M	160	-	13	144	2
	F	323	-	3	318	2
72 Food industry	M	5,855	-	516	5,304	34
	F	10,858	1	376	10,253	229
720 Grain millers	M	723	-	141	577	5
	F	47	-	8	37	2
721 Bakers and pastry chiefs	M	1,474	-	312	1,154	8
	F	4,832	-	345	4,307	180
722 Chocolate and confectionery makers	M	168	-	7	160	1
	F	707	-	9	695	3
723 Brewers and beverage producers Brewers, beverage producers and distillers	M	277	-	1	274	2
	F	489	-	1	487	1
724 Food preservation	M	238	-	9	227	2
	F	504	-	4	500	-
725 Butchers and sausage makers	M	1,701	-	39	1,653	9
	F	983	-	2	971	11
726 Dairy workers	M	758	-	3	754	0
	F	2,443	1	4	2,421	17
727 Prepared foods	M	33	-	2	31	-
	F	495	-	1	484	10
728 Sugar processers	M	248	-	-	244	4
	F	89	-	-	87	2
729 Food-product workers NOS Other food-product occupations	M	236	-	3	229	4
	F	269	-	2	265	2

Occupation	Sex	Social class				
		Total	I	II	III	IV
73 Chemical process/paper making	M	9,191	-	10	9,096	86
	F	2,872	-	3	2,836	33
730 Distillers	M	99	-	-	99	0
	F	1	-	-	1	-
731 Cookers (chemical processes) *Cookers and furnacemen (chemical processes)*	M	520	-	-	516	4
	F	58	-	-	56	2
732 Crushers and calender operators *Crushers, grinders and calender operators (chemical processes)*	M	213	-	-	212	1
	F	54	-	-	50	4
733 Wood grinders	M	531	-	-	524	7
	F	31	-	-	31	-
734 Pulp mill workers	M	2,362	-	-	2,335	27
	F	225	-	-	223	2
735 Paper and board mill workers	M	3,754	-	0	3,724	30
	F	1,603	-	1	1,584	18
739 Chemical process workers NOS *Other chemical process work*	M	1,713	-	10	1,686	17
	F	899	-	2	890	7
74 Tobacco industry	M	78	-	-	76	1
	F	346	-	-	344	2
740 Preprocess tobacco treatment	M	40	-	-	38	1
	F	111	-	-	111	1
741 Cigar makers	M	5	-	-	5	-
	F	63	-	-	63	-
742 Cigarette makers	M	23	-	-	23	-
	F	119	-	-	118	1
749 Tobacco workers NOS *Other tobacco-making occupations*	M	10	-	-	10	-
	F	53	-	-	53	-
75 Industrial work NOS *Other industrial work*	M	5,899	1	628	5,234	36
	F	5,655	-	196	5,408	51
750 Basket and brush makers	M	228	-	187	41	0
	F	170	-	58	112	-
751 Industrial rubber products	M	971	-	10	957	4
	F	933	-	0	930	3
752 Plastics	M	1,319	-	76	1,239	4
	F	1,291	-	22	1,261	8
753 Tanners and pelt dressers	M	344	-	12	332	0
	F	393	-	6	387	-
754 Photolab. workers *Workers in photograph laboratories*	M	101	-	29	73	-
	F	437	-	55	380	3
755 Musical instrument makers etc.	M	122	-	29	94	-
	F	16	-	-	16	-
756 Stone cutters	M	504	-	126	376	2
	F	14	-	3	11	-
757 Paper products	M	669	-	1	661	7
	F	1,052	-	3	1,025	24
758 Cast concrete products *Concrete-mixer operators and cast concrete products*	M	854	1	59	783	11
	F	51	-	4	41	5

Appendix Table A

Occupation	Sex	Social class				
		Total	I	II	III	IV
759 Industrial workers NOS	M	787	-	101	679	7
Other industrial workers	F	1,297	-	45	1,244	8
76 Packing and labelling						
760 Packers and labellers	M	2,411	-	4	2,372	36
	F	8,861	-	24	8,778	59
77 Machinists	M	22,565	-	2,099	20,327	139
Machine and engine operators (stationary plants)	F	1,903	-	15	946	943
770 Crane and hoist operators	M	1,848	-	-	1,829	19
	F	606	-	-	606	-
771 Forklift operators	M	3,609	-	1	3,593	15
	F	145	-	-	144	1
772 Construction machinery operators etc.	M	8,199	-	1,940	6,226	33
	F	12	-	12	1	-
773 Operators of stationary engine	M	4,442	-	-	4,422	21
	F	94	-	-	91	3
774 Greasers	M	1,827	-	157	1,621	48
	F	1,046	-	3	104	939
775 Industrial personnel, riggers	M	2,640	-	0	2,637	3
Industrial personnel (not in textile industry) and riggers						
78 Dock and warehouse work	M	14,379	0	6	4,552	9,821
	F	3,838	-	34	802	3,002
780 Dockers	M	3,298	-	-	2,973	324
	F	365	-	-	328	38
781 Freight handlers	M	2,286	-	6	97	2,184
Other freight handlers	F	188	-	33	15	140
782 Warehousemen	M	8,778	0	0	1,482	7,296
	F	3,271	-	1	460	2,810
789 Dock/warehouse workers NOS	M	17	-	-	-	17
Other occupations in group 78	F	14	-	-	-	14
79 Labourers not classified elsewhere						
790 Labourers	M	7,003	-	-	-	7,003
	F	658	-	-	-	658
8 Services	M	25,303	241	9,060	14,753	1,250
	F	98,806	24	13,967	26,921	57,893
80 Watchmen, security guards	M	11,394	241	6,774	3,627	752
	F	313	-	104	145	64
800 Firemen	M	1,436	213	160	1,063	-
801 Policemen	M	4,500	-	4,500	-	-
	F	41	-	41	-	-
802 Customs/border control	M	1,974	27	1,947	-	-
	F	50	-	50	-	-
803 Prison guards	M	1,059	-	156	902	1
	F	66	-	8	58	-
804 Civilian guards	M	2,407	-	11	1,645	751
	F	146	-	3	78	64
809 Security workers NOS	M	17	-	-	17	-
Other occupations in group 80	F	10	-	2	8	-

Occupation	Sex	Social class				
		Total	I	II	III	IV
81 Housekeeping, domestic work, etc.	M	858	-	484	322	52
	F	33,765	11	6,266	10,108	17,380
810 Housekeepers	M	428	-	428	-	-
	F	3,290	-	3,290	-	-
811 Chefs, cooks etc.	M	208	-	4	205	-
	F	8,435	-	21	8,355	59
812 Kitchen assistants	M	48	-	2	-	45
	F	9,643	-	5	-	9,638
813 Domestic servants	M	12	-	0	5	6
	F	7,665	-	108	1,038	6,519
814 Communal home-help services	M	1	-	1	-	-
	F	2,785	-	1,611	20	1,154
815 Hotel reception clerks	M	104	-	-	104	-
	F	63	-	-	62	2
816 Pursers, stewardesses	M	31	-	31	-	-
	F	236	-	236	-	-
817 Guides	M	5	-	5	-	-
	F	27	-	27	-	-
818 Hotel/restaurant manageresses	M	10	-	10	-	-
	F	567	11	556	-	-
819 Housekeeping workers NOS	M	11	-	3	7	-
Other occupations in group 81	F	1,055	-	413	633	10
82 Waiters	M	616	-	452	164	1
	F	11,802	14	2,944	8,316	528
820 Waiters in restaurants	M	350	-	210	139	1
Head waiters, waiters	F	5,470	14	615	4,836	4
821 Waiters in cafés etc.	M	266	-	242	24	-
	F	6,332	-	2,329	3,479	524
83 Caretakers and cleaners	M	9,888	-	134	9,538	215
	F	43,027	-	195	5,703	37,129
830 Caretakers	M	8,773	-	10	8,727	36
	F	5,782	-	1	5,673	108
831 Cleaners	M	174	-	1	-	173
Cleaners, head cleaners	F	37,002	-	7	-	36,995
832 Chimney sweeps	M	787	-	1	779	6
	F	19	-	-	3	16
839 Caretakers/cleaners NOS	M	155	-	122	32	1
Other occupations in group 83	F	223	-	187	27	9
84 Hygiene and beauty services	M	194	-	137	55	2
	F	5,214	-	3,492	1,290	431
840 Hairdressers and barbers	M	139	-	110	28	1
	F	4,182	-	3,137	1,039	6
841 Beauticians	F	324	-	234	90	0
842 Pedicurists	F	93	-	62	30	1
843 Sauna attendants etc.	M	53	-	26	26	1
	F	603	-	58	121	424
849 Hygiene/beauty workers NOS	M	2	-	1	1	-
Other occupations in group 84	F	11	-	1	11	-

Appendix Table A

Occupation	Sex	Social class				
		Total	I	II	III	IV
85 Laundry and pressing	M	231	-	133	80	18
	F	3,845	-	512	1,253	2,079
850 Launderers	M	213	-	132	63	17
	F	3,213	-	508	639	2,067
851 Pressers	M	16	-	-	16	-
	F	620	-	3	607	9
859 Laundry workers NOS	M	2	-	1	0	1
Other occupations in group 85	F	11	-	1	7	3
86 Sports						
860 Sports coaches	M	169	-	169	-	-
Sports coaches, jockeys etc.	F	55	-	55	-	-
87 Photography						
870 Photographers and cameramen	M	651	-	651	-	-
	F	299	-	299	-	-
88 Undertakers						
880 Undertakers etc.	M	163	-	60	2	101
	F	62	-	60	2	-
89 Services NOS	M	1,138	-	64	965	109
Other services	F	425	-	40	104	281
890 Hotel porters	M	962	-	2	952	7
	F	94	-	-	86	8
891 Service workers NOS	M	177	-	62	13	102
Other service work	F	331	-	40	18	273
9 Work not classified elsewhere	M	6,091	1,696	2,653	1,741	-
	F	1,042	-	20	1,022	-
90 Military occupations	M	4,367	1,696	2,555	116	-
	F	47	-	1	46	-
900 Officers etc.	M	1,696	1,696	-	-	-
901 Non-commissioned officers	M	2,555	-	2,555	-	-
	F	1	-	1	-	-
902 Rank and file	M	116	-	-	116	-
	F	46	-	-	46	-
91 Occupation not specified						
910 Occupation not specified	M	1,723	-	98	1,625	-
	F	995	-	19	976	-
ECONOMICALLY INACTIVE PERSONS	M	58,747	1,890	9,861	32,744	14,252
	F	312,417	30,900	72,704	165,755	43,058

Total number of 1-digit categories (called in this publication as *main occupational branches*) 9.

Total number of 2-digit categories (*occupational branches*): men 70, women 88.

Total number of 3-digit categories (*specific occupations*): men 332, women 324. Out of them, 15 occupations among men and 13 among women were the only subcategories under the respective occupational branch and therefore were not used in tabulations as independent entities.

Appendix table B

Numbers of cancer cases (Obs.) and standardised incidence ratios (SIR) with 95% confidence intervals (95% CI) in 1971-85, by primary site, sex, social class and period. Ages 35-64 at the beginning of each five-year follow-up period. Reference: Economically active population.

Primary site Sex Social class	1971-75			1976-80			1981-85			1971-85		
	Obs.	SIR	95% CI	Obs.	SIR	95% CI	Obs.	SIR	95% CI	Obs.	SIR	95% CI
ALL SITES												
Males												
I	946	0.87	0.82-0.93	1057	0.85	0.80-0.90	1192	0.84	0.80-0.89	3195	0.85	0.82-0.88
II	3008	0.96	0.93-1.00	3193	0.93	0.90-0.97	3332	0.92	0.89-0.96	9533	0.94	0.92-0.96
III	8836	1.11	1.09-1.13	8572	1.07	1.05-1.09	8465	1.06	1.03-1.08	25873	1.08	1.07-1.09
IV	3175	1.21	1.17-1.25	2850	1.20	1.15-1.24	2552	1.21	1.16-1.26	8577	1.21	1.18-1.23
Total	15965	1.08	1.06-1.10	15672	1.04	1.02-1.06	15541	1.03	1.01-1.04	47178	1.05	1.04-1.06
Females												
I	1109	1.19	1.12-1.26	1245	1.14	1.08-1.20	1415	1.12	1.06-1.17	3769	1.14	1.11-1.18
II	3936	1.10	1.07-1.13	4531	1.08	1.05-1.11	5129	1.07	1.04-1.10	13596	1.08	1.06-1.10
III	7046	0.95	0.93-0.97	7166	0.94	0.92-0.96	7226	0.95	0.93-0.97	21438	0.95	0.93-0.96
IV	2824	0.95	0.92-0.99	2718	0.92	0.89-0.96	2508	0.95	0.91-0.99	8050	0.94	0.92-0.96
Total	14915	1.00	0.99-1.02	15660	0.99	0.97-1.00	16278	1.00	0.98-1.01	46853	1.00	0.99-1.00
Lip												
Males												
I	6	0.21	0.08-0.46	11	0.44	0.22-0.78	9	0.30	0.14-0.57	26	0.31	0.20-0.46
II	63	0.79	0.60-1.01	50	0.72	0.54-0.95	53	0.70	0.52-0.91	166	0.74	0.63-0.85
III	226	1.12	0.98-1.27	196	1.21	1.05-1.39	198	1.17	1.01-1.33	620	1.16	1.07-1.26
IV	94	1.43	1.16-1.75	72	1.50	1.17-1.89	68	1.52	1.18-1.93	234	1.48	1.30-1.67
Total	389	1.04	0.94-1.14	329	1.08	0.97-1.20	328	1.02	0.92-1.14	1046	1.05	0.98-1.11
Females												
I	2	1.95	0.24-7.06	2	1.21	0.15-4.38	-	-	0.00-1.72	4	0.83	0.23-2.12
II	4	1.03	0.28-2.63	5	0.77	0.25-1.80	2	0.24	0.03-0.86	11	0.58	0.29-1.05
III	7	0.82	0.33-1.70	21	1.72	1.06-2.63	12	0.80	0.41-1.39	40	1.12	0.80-1.52
IV	8	2.36	1.02-4.64	10	2.05	0.98-3.77	13	2.21	1.18-3.78	31	2.19	1.49-3.11
Total	21	1.25	0.77-1.91	38	1.51	1.07-2.07	27	0.86	0.56-1.25	86	1.17	0.93-1.44
Tongue												
Males												
I	4	1.12	0.31-2.87	3	0.61	0.12-1.77	10	1.36	0.65-2.51	17	1.07	0.62-1.72
II	10	1.01	0.48-1.85	20	1.55	0.95-2.39	19	1.05	0.63-1.64	49	1.20	0.88-1.58
III	33	1.37	0.94-1.93	33	1.11	0.77-1.56	33	0.83	0.57-1.16	99	1.06	0.86-1.29
IV	5	0.67	0.22-1.57	5	0.60	0.20-1.41	13	1.29	0.68-2.20	23	0.89	0.56-1.34
Total	52	1.16	0.86-1.52	61	1.09	0.84-1.40	75	0.99	0.78-1.24	188	1.07	0.92-1.22
Females												
I	3	1.06	0.22-3.11	2	0.54	0.07-1.96	3	1.03	0.21-3.02	8	0.85	0.37-1.67
II	15	1.39	0.78-2.30	16	1.12	0.64-1.82	11	1.02	0.51-1.82	42	1.17	0.84-1.58
III	19	0.80	0.48-1.24	24	0.91	0.59-1.36	17	0.98	0.57-1.56	60	0.89	0.68-1.14
IV	5	0.52	0.17-1.20	10	0.97	0.47-1.79	6	1.00	0.37-2.17	21	0.81	0.50-1.23
Total	42	0.89	0.64-1.20	52	0.95	0.71-1.25	37	1.00	0.70-1.37	131	0.94	0.79-1.11

Primary site Sex Social class	1971-75			1976-80			1981-85			1971-85		
	Obs.	SIR	95% CI	Obs.	SIR	95% CI	Obs.	SIR	95% CI	Obs.	SIR	95% CI

Salivary glands

Males												
I	5	1.74	0.57-4.07	6	1.61	0.59-3.52	3	0.51	0.10-1.48	14	1.12	0.61-1.88
II	11	1.39	0.69-2.48	14	1.38	0.75-2.31	13	0.88	0.47-1.51	38	1.16	0.82-1.59
III	18	0.91	0.54-1.44	17	0.71	0.42-1.14	37	1.13	0.80-1.56	72	0.94	0.74-1.19
IV	6	0.95	0.35-2.07	6	0.86	0.31-1.86	7	0.83	0.33-1.72	19	0.87	0.53-1.37
Total	40	1.08	0.77-1.48	43	0.96	0.70-1.30	60	0.97	0.74-1.25	143	1.00	0.84-1.17
Females												
I	3	1.12	0.23-3.27	2	0.64	0.08-2.32	3	0.98	0.20-2.87	8	0.90	0.39-1.78
II	12	1.18	0.61-2.05	13	1.12	0.60-1.92	15	1.28	0.72-2.11	40	1.19	0.85-1.63
III	20	1.06	0.65-1.64	21	1.07	0.66-1.63	12	0.63	0.33-1.11	53	0.92	0.69-1.21
IV	13	1.79	0.95-3.06	12	1.68	0.87-2.94	9	1.34	0.61-2.55	34	1.61	1.12-2.25
Total	48	1.23	0.91-1.63	48	1.16	0.85-1.53	39	0.97	0.69-1.32	135	1.12	0.94-1.31

Oral cavity

Males												
I	2	0.65	0.08-2.34	9	1.65	0.75-3.13	10	1.50	0.72-2.77	21	1.38	0.86-2.11
II	7	0.80	0.32-1.64	10	0.71	0.34-1.31	14	0.86	0.47-1.45	31	0.79	0.54-1.13
III	23	1.04	0.66-1.57	38	1.17	0.83-1.61	39	1.08	0.77-1.48	100	1.11	0.90-1.33
IV	18	2.51	1.49-3.97	9	1.01	0.46-1.91	10	1.10	0.53-2.03	37	1.47	1.03-2.02
Total	50	1.22	0.90-1.60	66	1.08	0.84-1.38	73	1.08	0.84-1.35	189	1.11	0.96-1.28
Females												
I	3	1.67	0.35-4.89	6	1.78	0.65-3.87	5	1.43	0.46-3.34	14	1.62	0.88-2.71
II	8	1.18	0.51-2.33	15	1.13	0.63-1.86	17	1.30	0.76-2.08	40	1.21	0.86-1.64
III	18	1.23	0.73-1.95	20	0.79	0.48-1.22	21	1.00	0.62-1.53	59	0.97	0.74-1.25
IV	4	0.68	0.19-1.75	6	0.59	0.22-1.28	6	0.83	0.30-1.81	16	0.69	0.39-1.12
Total	33	1.14	0.78-1.60	47	0.90	0.66-1.20	49	1.09	0.81-1.45	129	1.02	0.86-1.21

Nasopharynx

Males												
I	6	2.40	0.88-5.23	3	1.58	0.33-4.62	4	1.22	0.33-3.13	13	1.69	0.90-2.90
II	6	0.85	0.31-1.84	9	1.78	0.81-3.37	14	1.72	0.94-2.88	29	1.43	0.96-2.05
III	15	0.85	0.48-1.40	7	0.60	0.24-1.23	14	0.78	0.42-1.30	36	0.76	0.53-1.05
IV	2	0.35	0.04-1.28	3	0.90	0.19-2.64	1	0.22	0.01-1.22	6	0.44	0.16-0.96
Total	29	0.88	0.59-1.27	22	1.00	0.63-1.52	33	0.97	0.67-1.36	84	0.95	0.75-1.17
Females												
I	-	-	0.00-5.80	-	-	0.00-2.63	1	1.41	0.04-7.85	1	0.36	0.01-2.03
II	2	0.77	0.09-2.79	5	0.95	0.31-2.21	5	1.82	0.59-4.26	12	1.13	0.58-1.97
III	9	1.69	0.77-3.21	7	0.75	0.30-1.54	6	1.41	0.52-3.08	22	1.16	0.73-1.76
IV	1	0.44	0.01-2.44	5	1.42	0.46-3.32	-	-	0.00-2.52	6	0.83	0.30-1.80
Total	12	1.11	0.57-1.93	17	0.87	0.51-1.39	12	1.31	0.68-2.29	41	1.04	0.74-1.41

Primary site Sex	1971-75			1976-80			1981-85			1971-85		
Social class	Obs.	SIR	95% CI	Obs.	SIR	95% CI	Obs.	SIR	95% CI	Obs.	SIR	95% CI

Other pharynx

Males												
I	8	1.78	0.77-3.50	7	1.44	0.58-2.96	7	1.05	0.42-2.16	22	1.37	0.86-2.07
II	17	1.32	0.77-2.12	21	1.56	0.96-2.38	12	0.71	0.37-1.24	50	1.16	0.86-1.52
III	41	1.26	0.91-1.71	33	1.04	0.71-1.46	43	1.14	0.82-1.53	117	1.15	0.95-1.36
IV	15	1.41	0.79-2.32	15	1.57	0.88-2.59	12	1.22	0.63-2.13	42	1.40	1.01-1.89
Total	81	1.34	1.06-1.66	76	1.27	1.00-1.59	74	1.04	0.82-1.31	231	1.21	1.06-1.37
Females												
I	-	-	0.00-1.45	-	-	0.00-1.66	3	2.74	0.56-8.00	3	0.51	0.11-1.50
II	10	1.00	0.48-1.84	9	1.04	0.47-1.97	5	1.14	0.37-2.67	24	1.04	0.67-1.55
III	15	0.72	0.40-1.19	13	0.76	0.40-1.30	14	1.86	1.02-3.12	42	0.92	0.67-1.25
IV	12	1.40	0.72-2.44	10	1.42	0.68-2.61	10	3.50	1.68-6.44	32	1.73	1.18-2.44
Total	37	0.88	0.62-1.22	32	0.91	0.62-1.29	32	2.02	1.38-2.85	101	1.09	0.89-1.31

Oesophagus

Males												
I	10	0.77	0.37-1.41	10	0.77	0.37-1.41	14	0.88	0.48-1.47	34	0.81	0.56-1.13
II	33	0.87	0.60-1.22	36	1.00	0.70-1.38	32	0.78	0.53-1.09	101	0.88	0.71-1.06
III	128	1.33	1.11-1.57	100	1.18	0.96-1.42	104	1.13	0.92-1.36	332	1.22	1.09-1.35
IV	53	1.66	1.24-2.17	36	1.42	1.00-1.97	43	1.75	1.27-2.36	132	1.61	1.35-1.90
Total	224	1.25	1.09-1.42	182	1.14	0.98-1.32	193	1.11	0.96-1.27	599	1.17	1.08-1.27
Females												
I	3	0.31	0.06-0.90	4	0.50	0.14-1.28	3	0.32	0.07-0.94	10	0.37	0.18-0.68
II	36	0.94	0.66-1.30	22	0.68	0.43-1.04	20	0.54	0.33-0.84	78	0.73	0.57-0.91
III	99	1.16	0.94-1.41	85	1.29	1.03-1.60	69	1.06	0.82-1.34	253	1.17	1.03-1.32
IV	50	1.39	1.03-1.83	30	1.08	0.73-1.54	41	1.63	1.17-2.22	121	1.36	1.13-1.61
Total	188	1.11	0.95-1.27	141	1.06	0.89-1.24	133	0.98	0.82-1.15	462	1.05	0.96-1.15

Stomach

Males												
I	79	0.68	0.54-0.85	79	0.67	0.53-0.84	68	0.58	0.45-0.74	226	0.65	0.56-0.73
II	311	0.93	0.83-1.04	275	0.86	0.76-0.96	248	0.83	0.73-0.94	834	0.88	0.82-0.94
III	927	1.08	1.01-1.15	817	1.09	1.02-1.17	741	1.12	1.04-1.20	2485	1.10	1.05-1.14
IV	343	1.20	1.08-1.33	262	1.18	1.04-1.33	214	1.24	1.08-1.41	819	1.20	1.12-1.29
Total	1660	1.04	0.99-1.09	1433	1.02	0.97-1.07	1271	1.02	0.96-1.07	4364	1.03	1.00-1.06
Females												
I	45	0.79	0.57-1.05	50	0.87	0.64-1.14	39	0.69	0.49-0.94	134	0.78	0.65-0.92
II	206	0.94	0.82-1.08	214	0.96	0.83-1.09	241	1.11	0.98-1.26	661	1.00	0.93-1.08
III	517	1.11	1.02-1.21	456	1.09	0.99-1.19	387	1.08	0.97-1.19	1360	1.09	1.04-1.15
IV	231	1.24	1.08-1.40	187	1.12	0.97-1.29	125	0.96	0.80-1.14	543	1.12	1.03-1.22
Total	999	1.08	1.01-1.15	907	1.05	0.98-1.12	792	1.04	0.97-1.11	2698	1.06	1.02-1.10

Appendix Table B

Primary site Sex Social class	1971-75			1976-80			1981-85			1971-85		
	Obs.	SIR	95% CI	Obs.	SIR	95% CI	Obs.	SIR	95% CI	Obs.	SIR	95% CI

Small intestine

Males												
I	6	1.82	0.67-3.95	14	2.52	1.38-4.23	10	1.82	0.87-3.36	30	2.09	1.41-2.99
II	6	0.65	0.24-1.41	14	0.93	0.51-1.57	13	0.94	0.50-1.61	33	0.87	0.60-1.22
III	27	1.16	0.77-1.69	26	0.74	0.49-1.09	27	0.88	0.58-1.29	80	0.90	0.72-1.12
IV	6	0.80	0.30-1.75	9	0.89	0.41-1.68	8	1.02	0.44-2.01	23	0.90	0.57-1.35
Total	45	1.04	0.76-1.39	63	0.96	0.74-1.23	58	1.01	0.76-1.30	166	1.00	0.85-1.15
Females												
I	5	1.79	0.58-4.17	5	1.83	0.59-4.26	5	1.19	0.39-2.78	15	1.54	0.86-2.54
II	12	1.12	0.58-1.96	12	1.15	0.59-2.01	13	0.81	0.43-1.39	37	1.00	0.70-1.37
III	23	1.04	0.66-1.55	22	1.16	0.73-1.75	29	1.15	0.77-1.65	74	1.11	0.87-1.40
IV	4	0.45	0.12-1.15	5	0.68	0.22-1.59	8	0.92	0.40-1.81	17	0.68	0.40-1.09
Total	44	0.99	0.72-1.32	44	1.11	0.81-1.50	55	1.02	0.76-1.32	143	1.03	0.87-1.21

Colon

Males												
I	61	1.72	1.31-2.21	67	1.49	1.16-1.90	85	1.29	1.03-1.59	213	1.45	1.27-1.66
II	128	1.26	1.05-1.49	151	1.24	1.05-1.45	165	0.98	0.84-1.14	444	1.14	1.03-1.24
III	239	0.94	0.82-1.06	261	0.92	0.81-1.03	375	1.01	0.91-1.11	875	0.96	0.90-1.02
IV	66	0.79	0.61-1.01	69	0.82	0.64-1.04	77	0.79	0.62-0.99	212	0.80	0.70-0.91
Total	494	1.04	0.95-1.13	548	1.02	0.94-1.11	702	1.00	0.93-1.07	1744	1.02	0.97-1.07
Females												
I	60	1.48	1.13-1.90	49	1.02	0.76-1.35	47	0.87	0.64-1.16	156	1.09	0.93-1.27
II	186	1.20	1.03-1.38	222	1.20	1.04-1.36	210	1.02	0.89-1.16	618	1.13	1.04-1.22
III	283	0.86	0.76-0.96	301	0.87	0.77-0.97	322	0.95	0.85-1.05	906	0.89	0.83-0.95
IV	116	0.87	0.72-1.04	112	0.82	0.67-0.98	123	1.00	0.83-1.19	351	0.89	0.80-0.99
Total	645	0.98	0.91-1.06	684	0.96	0.89-1.03	702	0.97	0.90-1.04	2031	0.97	0.93-1.01

Rectum

Males												
I	39	1.05	0.75-1.44	46	0.94	0.69-1.26	58	1.09	0.82-1.40	143	1.03	0.87-1.20
II	125	1.17	0.97-1.38	166	1.23	1.05-1.43	148	1.09	0.92-1.27	439	1.16	1.06-1.27
III	268	0.98	0.87-1.10	291	0.92	0.81-1.02	298	0.98	0.87-1.10	857	0.96	0.90-1.02
IV	84	0.93	0.74-1.15	87	0.91	0.73-1.13	68	0.85	0.66-1.08	239	0.90	0.79-1.02
Total	516	1.02	0.93-1.11	590	0.99	0.91-1.07	572	1.00	0.92-1.08	1678	1.00	0.95-1.05
Females												
I	41	1.43	1.02-1.93	41	1.12	0.80-1.52	41	1.08	0.78-1.47	123	1.19	0.99-1.41
II	116	1.05	0.87-1.25	151	1.05	0.89-1.23	154	1.06	0.90-1.23	421	1.06	0.96-1.16
III	258	1.07	0.95-1.21	256	0.94	0.83-1.06	230	0.94	0.82-1.06	744	0.98	0.91-1.05
IV	111	1.14	0.94-1.36	96	0.88	0.71-1.07	93	1.04	0.84-1.27	300	1.01	0.90-1.13
Total	526	1.10	1.01-1.20	544	0.97	0.89-1.05	518	1.00	0.92-1.09	1588	1.02	0.97-1.07

Primary site Sex Social class	1971-75			1976-80			1981-85			1971-85		
	Obs.	SIR	95% CI	Obs.	SIR	95% CI	Obs.	SIR	95% CI	Obs.	SIR	95% CI

Liver

Males												
I	11	0.81	0.41-1.45	15	1.00	0.56-1.65	23	1.18	0.75-1.78	49	1.02	0.76-1.35
II	48	1.22	0.90-1.62	46	1.09	0.80-1.46	50	0.99	0.74-1.31	144	1.09	0.92-1.28
III	118	1.18	0.98-1.41	108	1.08	0.89-1.30	120	1.07	0.88-1.27	346	1.11	1.00-1.23
IV	39	1.18	0.84-1.61	39	1.28	0.91-1.75	41	1.36	0.97-1.84	119	1.27	1.05-1.51
Total	216	1.16	1.01-1.32	208	1.11	0.96-1.27	234	1.10	0.96-1.25	658	1.12	1.04-1.21
Females												
I	6	0.99	0.36-2.16	6	0.97	0.36-2.12	7	0.70	0.28-1.44	19	0.86	0.52-1.34
II	34	1.44	1.00-2.02	27	1.10	0.73-1.61	43	1.11	0.80-1.49	104	1.20	0.98-1.44
III	63	1.26	0.97-1.61	58	1.21	0.92-1.57	61	0.91	0.70-1.17	182	1.11	0.95-1.27
IV	19	0.92	0.56-1.44	23	1.16	0.74-1.74	28	1.12	0.74-1.61	70	1.07	0.83-1.35
Total	122	1.22	1.01-1.44	114	1.16	0.96-1.38	139	0.99	0.83-1.16	375	1.11	1.00-1.22

Gallbladder, biliary tract

Males												
I	7	1.10	0.44-2.27	7	0.75	0.30-1.55	8	0.69	0.30-1.36	22	0.81	0.51-1.22
II	21	1.16	0.72-1.77	29	1.13	0.75-1.62	34	1.15	0.80-1.61	84	1.14	0.91-1.42
III	43	0.94	0.68-1.27	59	0.97	0.74-1.25	73	1.11	0.87-1.40	175	1.02	0.87-1.17
IV	21	1.40	0.87-2.14	16	0.88	0.50-1.43	23	1.34	0.85-2.00	60	1.19	0.91-1.53
Total	92	1.08	0.87-1.32	111	0.97	0.80-1.16	138	1.11	0.94-1.31	341	1.05	0.95-1.17
Females												
I	15	1.39	0.78-2.29	10	0.68	0.32-1.24	23	1.44	0.91-2.15	48	1.15	0.85-1.53
II	49	1.18	0.88-1.56	70	1.20	0.93-1.51	65	1.06	0.82-1.35	184	1.14	0.98-1.31
III	113	1.23	1.01-1.47	128	1.13	0.94-1.33	115	1.09	0.90-1.30	356	1.14	1.03-1.27
IV	52	1.39	1.04-1.83	58	1.24	0.94-1.61	54	1.38	1.03-1.80	164	1.33	1.13-1.54
Total	229	1.26	1.10-1.43	266	1.14	1.01-1.28	257	1.16	1.02-1.30	752	1.18	1.10-1.27

Pancreas

Males												
I	47	1.08	0.79-1.43	41	0.81	0.58-1.10	60	1.03	0.78-1.32	148	0.97	0.82-1.13
II	117	0.93	0.77-1.10	124	0.89	0.74-1.05	159	1.07	0.91-1.24	400	0.96	0.87-1.06
III	335	1.04	0.93-1.16	345	1.05	0.94-1.16	326	0.98	0.88-1.09	1006	1.02	0.96-1.09
IV	119	1.12	0.93-1.33	121	1.23	1.02-1.46	97	1.11	0.90-1.35	337	1.15	1.03-1.28
Total	618	1.03	0.95-1.12	631	1.02	0.94-1.10	642	1.02	0.95-1.10	1891	1.03	0.98-1.07
Females												
I	31	1.23	0.84-1.75	31	1.16	0.79-1.65	40	1.26	0.90-1.72	102	1.22	1.00-1.47
II	107	1.11	0.91-1.33	97	0.91	0.74-1.12	150	1.21	1.03-1.42	354	1.09	0.98-1.20
III	213	1.00	0.87-1.14	221	1.06	0.93-1.21	187	0.87	0.75-1.00	621	0.98	0.90-1.05
IV	105	1.21	0.99-1.45	92	1.07	0.86-1.31	76	0.94	0.74-1.17	273	1.07	0.95-1.21
Total	456	1.08	0.98-1.18	441	1.03	0.94-1.13	453	1.00	0.91-1.10	1350	1.04	0.98-1.09

Appendix Table B

Primary site Sex Social class	1971-75			1976-80			1981-85			1971-85		
	Obs.	SIR	95% CI	Obs.	SIR	95% CI	Obs.	SIR	95% CI	Obs.	SIR	95% CI

Nose, nasal sinuses

Males												
I	3	0.74	0.15-2.18	3	0.68	0.14-1.98	1	0.26	0.01-1.47	7	0.57	0.23-1.18
II	7	0.61	0.25-1.26	15	1.26	0.71-2.09	8	0.86	0.37-1.70	30	0.92	0.62-1.32
III	35	1.26	0.88-1.75	23	0.83	0.53-1.25	22	1.06	0.66-1.61	80	1.05	0.83-1.31
IV	8	0.92	0.40-1.82	15	1.88	1.05-3.11	9	1.69	0.77-3.21	32	1.46	1.00-2.06
Total	53	1.02	0.77-1.34	56	1.08	0.81-1.40	40	1.02	0.73-1.39	149	1.04	0.88-1.22
Females												
I	-	-	0.00-2.95	2	1.11	0.13-4.00	1	0.53	0.01-2.94	3	0.61	0.12-1.77
II	10	2.10	1.01-3.87	5	0.76	0.25-1.76	7	0.95	0.38-1.95	22	1.17	0.74-1.78
III	15	1.79	1.00-2.94	14	1.28	0.70-2.16	14	1.11	0.61-1.86	43	1.35	0.97-1.81
IV	5	1.56	0.51-3.65	8	2.10	0.91-4.14	3	0.63	0.13-1.85	16	1.36	0.78-2.21
Total	30	1.70	1.15-2.43	29	1.25	0.84-1.80	25	0.94	0.61-1.38	84	1.25	0.99-1.54

Larynx

Males												
I	25	0.75	0.49-1.11	20	0.66	0.40-1.02	20	0.62	0.38-0.95	65	0.68	0.52-0.86
II	83	0.87	0.69-1.07	60	0.72	0.55-0.93	70	0.85	0.66-1.07	213	0.82	0.71-0.93
III	296	1.24	1.10-1.38	228	1.17	1.02-1.33	209	1.14	0.99-1.30	733	1.19	1.10-1.27
IV	105	1.35	1.10-1.62	85	1.47	1.18-1.82	68	1.41	1.09-1.78	258	1.40	1.24-1.58
Total	509	1.14	1.04-1.24	393	1.07	0.97-1.18	367	1.06	0.95-1.17	1269	1.09	1.04-1.16
Females												
I	-	-	0.00-2.29	4	1.61	0.44-4.12	2	0.91	0.11-3.29	6	0.95	0.35-2.08
II	8	1.27	0.55-2.51	8	0.81	0.35-1.60	5	0.60	0.19-1.39	21	0.86	0.53-1.31
III	16	1.23	0.71-2.00	18	0.95	0.56-1.50	18	1.31	0.78-2.07	52	1.14	0.85-1.49
IV	10	1.88	0.90-3.46	6	0.77	0.28-1.68	9	1.82	0.83-3.45	25	1.39	0.90-2.05
Total	34	1.30	0.90-1.81	36	0.92	0.65-1.28	34	1.16	0.80-1.62	104	1.10	0.90-1.32

Lung, trachea

Males												
I	159	0.45	0.38-0.52	187	0.47	0.41-0.54	180	0.45	0.38-0.51	526	0.46	0.42-0.50
II	850	0.83	0.77-0.88	867	0.79	0.73-0.84	797	0.76	0.71-0.81	2514	0.79	0.76-0.82
III	3312	1.26	1.21-1.30	2985	1.15	1.11-1.19	2667	1.13	1.09-1.18	8964	1.18	1.16-1.21
IV	1365	1.55	1.47-1.63	1204	1.54	1.46-1.63	1040	1.64	1.54-1.74	3609	1.57	1.52-1.62
Total	5686	1.16	1.13-1.19	5243	1.08	1.05-1.11	4684	1.05	1.02-1.08	15613	1.10	1.08-1.12
Females												
I	30	0.92	0.62-1.32	51	1.21	0.90-1.59	42	0.81	0.59-1.10	123	0.97	0.81-1.15
II	138	1.11	0.93-1.30	184	1.11	0.95-1.27	206	1.04	0.90-1.18	528	1.08	0.99-1.17
III	231	0.85	0.74-0.96	305	0.95	0.85-1.06	302	0.89	0.79-0.99	838	0.90	0.84-0.96
IV	103	0.94	0.76-1.13	132	1.01	0.85-1.20	144	1.14	0.96-1.33	379	1.03	0.93-1.14
Total	502	0.93	0.85-1.01	672	1.02	0.94-1.10	694	0.97	0.90-1.04	1868	0.98	0.93-1.02

Primary site Sex Social class	1971-75			1976-80			1981-85			1971-85		
	Obs.	SIR	95% CI	Obs.	SIR	95% CI	Obs.	SIR	95% CI	Obs.	SIR	95% CI

Lung, adenocarcinoma

Males												
I	23	0.70	0.45-1.06	22	0.51	0.32-0.78	32	0.53	0.36-0.75	77	0.57	0.45-0.71
II	93	0.99	0.80-1.21	92	0.78	0.63-0.95	121	0.78	0.65-0.92	306	0.83	0.74-0.93
III	276	1.16	1.03-1.30	310	1.11	0.99-1.24	391	1.13	1.02-1.24	977	1.13	1.06-1.20
IV	85	1.09	0.87-1.34	111	1.33	1.10-1.59	131	1.42	1.19-1.68	327	1.29	1.15-1.43
Total	477	1.08	0.98-1.17	535	1.02	0.94-1.11	675	1.03	0.95-1.11	1687	1.04	0.99-1.09
Females												
I	7	0.90	0.36-1.85	19	1.48	0.89-2.31	20	1.08	0.66-1.66	46	1.17	0.86-1.56
II	36	1.20	0.84-1.66	56	1.12	0.85-1.46	78	1.10	0.87-1.37	170	1.13	0.96-1.30
III	61	1.01	0.77-1.30	88	0.95	0.76-1.17	105	0.87	0.71-1.04	254	0.93	0.82-1.04
IV	18	0.75	0.44-1.18	35	0.95	0.66-1.32	42	0.94	0.68-1.27	95	0.90	0.73-1.10
Total	122	1.00	0.83-1.18	198	1.03	0.89-1.18	245	0.96	0.84-1.09	565	0.99	0.91-1.08

Lung, small cell carcinoma

Males												
I	23	0.44	0.28-0.67	39	0.55	0.39-0.76	33	0.42	0.29-0.59	95	0.47	0.38-0.58
II	118	0.79	0.66-0.94	152	0.78	0.66-0.91	155	0.77	0.65-0.89	425	0.78	0.71-0.86
III	442	1.18	1.07-1.29	494	1.09	1.00-1.19	504	1.11	1.02-1.21	1440	1.12	1.07-1.18
IV	173	1.40	1.20-1.62	197	1.47	1.27-1.68	182	1.51	1.30-1.73	552	1.46	1.34-1.58
Total	756	1.08	1.00-1.16	882	1.04	0.97-1.11	874	1.02	0.96-1.09	2512	1.04	1.00-1.09
Females												
I	2	0.44	0.05-1.58	5	0.97	0.31-2.26	5	0.45	0.15-1.05	12	0.58	0.30-1.01
II	12	0.68	0.35-1.19	29	1.42	0.95-2.04	43	1.01	0.73-1.36	84	1.04	0.83-1.29
III	35	0.92	0.64-1.28	46	1.16	0.85-1.54	59	0.82	0.62-1.05	140	0.93	0.78-1.09
IV	20	1.28	0.78-1.98	15	0.91	0.51-1.51	32	1.20	0.82-1.70	67	1.14	0.89-1.45
Total	69	0.91	0.71-1.15	95	1.16	0.94-1.42	139	0.91	0.77-1.07	303	0.98	0.87-1.09

Lung, squamous cell carcinoma

Males												
I	39	0.33	0.24-0.46	57	0.43	0.33-0.56	64	0.42	0.32-0.54	160	0.40	0.34-0.46
II	262	0.77	0.68-0.86	302	0.81	0.72-0.91	283	0.71	0.63-0.80	847	0.76	0.71-0.81
III	1107	1.27	1.20-1.35	995	1.14	1.07-1.21	1027	1.15	1.08-1.22	3129	1.19	1.14-1.23
IV	438	1.50	1.37-1.65	391	1.48	1.34-1.63	408	1.69	1.53-1.85	1237	1.55	1.47-1.64
Total	1846	1.14	1.09-1.19	1745	1.06	1.01-1.11	1782	1.06	1.01-1.11	5373	1.09	1.06-1.11
Females												
I	9	1.60	0.73-3.04	5	0.67	0.22-1.56	9	0.82	0.37-1.55	23	0.95	0.60-1.43
II	27	1.25	0.82-1.82	29	0.98	0.66-1.41	50	1.16	0.86-1.53	106	1.12	0.92-1.35
III	26	0.56	0.37-0.82	52	0.90	0.67-1.18	60	0.79	0.60-1.02	138	0.77	0.64-0.90
IV	16	0.86	0.49-1.39	28	1.19	0.79-1.71	35	1.20	0.83-1.67	79	1.11	0.88-1.38
Total	78	0.84	0.67-1.05	114	0.96	0.80-1.15	154	0.97	0.82-1.13	346	0.94	0.84-1.04

Appendix Table B

Primary site Sex		1971-75			1976-80			1981-85			1971-85		
Social class	Obs.	SIR	95% CI	Obs.	SIR	95% CI	Obs.	SIR	95% CI	Obs.	SIR	95% CI

Mesothelioma

Males													
I	4	3.00	0.82-7.69	9	2.62	1.20-4.98	8	1.13	0.49-2.22	21	1.77	1.10-2.71
II	4	1.09	0.30-2.80	6	0.66	0.24-1.43	14	0.80	0.43-1.33	24	0.79	0.51-1.17
III	7	0.79	0.32-1.63	19	0.89	0.54-1.40	47	1.21	0.89-1.61	73	1.06	0.83-1.33
IV	2	0.74	0.09-2.66	6	0.98	0.36-2.14	4	0.41	0.11-1.04	12	0.64	0.33-1.12
Total	17	1.03	0.60-1.65	40	1.00	0.72-1.36	73	0.99	0.78-1.25	130	1.00	0.84-1.18
Females													
I	-	-	0.00-5.79	2	0.95	0.11-3.42	2	0.91	0.11-3.28	4	0.81	0.22-2.07
II	5	2.25	0.73-5.26	7	0.85	0.34-1.74	7	0.83	0.34-1.72	19	1.01	0.61-1.57
III	3	0.88	0.18-2.57	11	0.69	0.35-1.24	17	1.23	0.72-1.97	31	0.94	0.64-1.33
IV	3	2.80	0.58-8.18	5	0.77	0.25-1.81	3	0.61	0.13-1.77	11	0.88	0.44-1.58
Total	11	1.50	0.75-2.68	25	0.76	0.49-1.13	29	0.99	0.66-1.42	65	0.94	0.72-1.19

Breast

Males													
I	3	2.29	0.47-6.69	-	-	0.00-2.91	4	2.69	0.73-6.88	7	1.72	0.69-3.55
II	1	0.26	0.01-1.46	5	1.41	0.46-3.29	2	0.55	0.07-2.00	8	0.73	0.31-1.43
III	11	1.10	0.55-1.97	7	0.82	0.33-1.69	8	1.02	0.44-2.00	26	0.99	0.64-1.44
IV	2	0.59	0.07-2.11	3	1.15	0.24-3.37	1	0.53	0.01-2.95	6	0.76	0.28-1.65
Total	17	0.92	0.53-1.47	15	0.94	0.53-1.55	15	1.01	0.56-1.66	47	0.95	0.70-1.27
Females													
I	414	1.51	1.37-1.66	481	1.42	1.30-1.55	571	1.30	1.20-1.41	1466	1.39	1.32-1.47
II	1229	1.17	1.11-1.24	1459	1.14	1.08-1.20	1836	1.13	1.08-1.18	4524	1.14	1.11-1.18
III	1791	0.86	0.82-0.90	1953	0.87	0.84-0.91	2123	0.85	0.82-0.89	5867	0.86	0.84-0.88
IV	643	0.78	0.72-0.84	644	0.77	0.71-0.83	638	0.78	0.72-0.84	1925	0.78	0.74-0.81
Total	4077	0.96	0.93-0.99	4537	0.97	0.94-1.00	5168	0.96	0.94-0.99	13782	0.96	0.95-0.98

Cervix uteri

I	30	0.50	0.34-0.71	34	0.81	0.56-1.13	27	0.86	0.57-1.26	91	0.68	0.55-0.84
II	195	0.84	0.73-0.97	138	0.86	0.72-1.01	99	0.84	0.68-1.02	432	0.85	0.77-0.93
III	477	1.01	0.92-1.10	280	0.96	0.85-1.08	179	0.96	0.82-1.11	936	0.99	0.92-1.05
IV	235	1.25	1.09-1.41	128	1.14	0.95-1.34	95	1.48	1.20-1.81	458	1.26	1.14-1.37
Total	937	0.98	0.92-1.05	580	0.96	0.88-1.04	400	1.00	0.90-1.10	1917	0.98	0.94-1.02

Corpus uteri

I	99	1.31	1.07-1.60	91	0.96	0.77-1.18	109	1.14	0.94-1.37	299	1.13	1.00-1.26
II	329	1.12	1.00-1.24	395	1.07	0.97-1.18	401	1.11	1.01-1.23	1125	1.10	1.04-1.17
III	580	0.95	0.87-1.02	632	0.94	0.87-1.02	585	0.98	0.90-1.06	1797	0.96	0.91-1.00
IV	201	0.81	0.70-0.92	219	0.83	0.73-0.95	201	0.94	0.81-1.07	621	0.85	0.79-0.92
Total	1209	0.98	0.93-1.04	1337	0.96	0.91-1.01	1296	1.02	0.97-1.08	3842	0.99	0.96-1.02

Primary site Sex Social class	1971-75			1976-80			1981-85			1971-85		
	Obs.	SIR	95% CI	Obs.	SIR	95% CI	Obs.	SIR	95% CI	Obs.	SIR	95% CI
Ovary												
I	70	0.94	0.74-1.19	73	0.87	0.69-1.10	89	0.94	0.76-1.16	232	0.92	0.81-1.04
II	316	1.12	1.00-1.24	334	1.04	0.94-1.16	339	0.95	0.86-1.06	989	1.03	0.97-1.10
III	500	0.86	0.79-0.94	508	0.88	0.81-0.96	549	0.98	0.90-1.06	1557	0.91	0.86-0.95
IV	201	0.87	0.76-1.00	202	0.91	0.79-1.04	185	0.96	0.82-1.10	588	0.91	0.84-0.99
Total	1087	0.93	0.88-0.99	1117	0.93	0.88-0.99	1162	0.96	0.91-1.02	3366	0.94	0.91-0.97
Vulva												
I	6	1.46	0.54-3.18	4	0.71	0.19-1.82	7	1.12	0.45-2.31	17	1.06	0.62-1.70
II	29	1.91	1.28-2.74	28	1.30	0.86-1.88	28	1.17	0.77-1.69	85	1.40	1.12-1.73
III	33	1.00	0.69-1.41	44	1.11	0.80-1.49	43	1.09	0.79-1.47	120	1.07	0.89-1.27
IV	22	1.71	1.07-2.59	17	1.10	0.64-1.76	13	0.92	0.49-1.57	52	1.22	0.91-1.60
Total	90	1.38	1.11-1.70	93	1.13	0.91-1.38	91	1.09	0.87-1.33	274	1.18	1.05-1.33
Vagina												
I	1	0.33	0.01-1.84	2	0.67	0.08-2.41	-	-	0.00-1.48	3	0.35	0.07-1.03
II	8	0.69	0.30-1.36	6	0.50	0.18-1.10	8	0.85	0.37-1.67	22	0.67	0.42-1.01
III	19	0.75	0.45-1.16	16	0.70	0.40-1.13	13	0.91	0.48-1.55	48	0.76	0.56-1.01
IV	9	0.87	0.40-1.64	15	1.60	0.90-2.64	9	1.90	0.87-3.61	33	1.35	0.93-1.89
Total	37	0.73	0.52-1.01	39	0.83	0.59-1.13	30	0.97	0.65-1.38	106	0.82	0.67-0.99
Prostate												
I	89	1.32	1.06-1.63	102	1.20	0.98-1.44	125	1.21	1.01-1.43	316	1.24	1.10-1.38
II	220	1.10	0.96-1.25	253	1.02	0.90-1.15	287	1.03	0.92-1.16	760	1.05	0.97-1.12
III	523	0.97	0.89-1.06	582	0.98	0.90-1.06	616	0.99	0.92-1.07	1721	0.98	0.94-1.03
IV	160	0.84	0.72-0.98	178	0.95	0.81-1.09	135	0.78	0.66-0.92	473	0.86	0.78-0.94
Total	992	1.00	0.93-1.06	1115	1.00	0.94-1.06	1163	0.99	0.93-1.05	3270	1.00	0.96-1.03
Testis												
I	19	3.46	2.08-5.40	8	1.32	0.57-2.60	11	1.62	0.81-2.90	38	2.07	1.47-2.84
II	19	1.35	0.81-2.10	12	0.89	0.46-1.56	17	1.11	0.65-1.78	48	1.12	0.83-1.48
III	21	0.64	0.39-0.97	32	1.07	0.73-1.51	29	0.90	0.60-1.29	82	0.86	0.68-1.07
IV	4	0.43	0.12-1.10	7	0.99	0.40-2.04	5	0.73	0.24-1.71	16	0.69	0.39-1.12
Total	63	1.02	0.78-1.30	59	1.04	0.79-1.35	62	1.01	0.78-1.30	184	1.02	0.88-1.18
Penis												
I	3	1.09	0.22-3.19	4	1.25	0.34-3.21	2	0.58	0.07-2.08	9	0.96	0.44-1.82
II	6	0.77	0.28-1.68	9	1.11	0.51-2.11	10	1.18	0.57-2.18	25	1.03	0.67-1.52
III	25	1.30	0.84-1.92	18	0.96	0.57-1.51	17	0.92	0.53-1.47	60	1.06	0.81-1.36
IV	2	0.33	0.04-1.19	7	1.33	0.54-2.75	4	0.88	0.24-2.24	13	0.82	0.44-1.40
Total	36	1.00	0.70-1.39	38	1.07	0.76-1.48	33	0.94	0.65-1.32	107	1.01	0.83-1.21

Appendix Table B

Primary site Sex		1971-75			1976-80			1981-85			1971-85	
Social class	Obs.	SIR	95% CI	Obs.	SIR	95% CI	Obs.	SIR	95% CI	Obs.	SIR	95% CI

Kidney

Males												
I	58	1.37	1.04-1.78	73	1.42	1.11-1.78	69	1.03	0.80-1.31	200	1.25	1.08-1.42
II	149	1.24	1.05-1.44	145	1.04	0.88-1.22	180	1.08	0.93-1.24	474	1.11	1.01-1.21
III	272	0.90	0.80-1.01	329	1.02	0.91-1.13	374	1.01	0.91-1.11	975	0.98	0.92-1.04
IV	70	0.71	0.56-0.90	62	0.66	0.50-0.84	83	0.87	0.69-1.08	215	0.75	0.65-0.85
Total	549	0.98	0.90-1.06	609	1.00	0.92-1.08	706	1.01	0.94-1.09	1864	1.00	0.95-1.04
Females												
I	21	0.95	0.59-1.46	33	1.30	0.89-1.82	37	1.09	0.77-1.51	91	1.12	0.90-1.38
II	101	1.19	0.97-1.43	112	1.13	0.93-1.34	145	1.11	0.94-1.30	358	1.14	1.02-1.26
III	194	1.09	0.94-1.25	190	1.01	0.87-1.16	212	0.96	0.83-1.09	596	1.01	0.93-1.10
IV	63	0.88	0.67-1.12	68	0.90	0.70-1.14	93	1.13	0.92-1.39	224	0.98	0.85-1.11
Total	379	1.06	0.96-1.17	403	1.04	0.94-1.14	487	1.04	0.95-1.14	1269	1.05	0.99-1.10

Renal pelvis

Males												
I	3	1.01	0.21-2.94	2	0.77	0.09-2.79	3	0.91	0.19-2.66	8	0.90	0.39-1.78
II	10	1.18	0.57-2.17	3	0.42	0.09-1.23	5	0.61	0.20-1.43	18	0.76	0.45-1.20
III	25	1.18	0.76-1.74	25	1.52	0.98-2.24	20	1.11	0.68-1.72	70	1.26	0.98-1.59
IV	4	0.58	0.16-1.49	8	1.66	0.72-3.28	6	1.31	0.48-2.86	18	1.11	0.66-1.75
Total	42	1.06	0.76-1.43	38	1.23	0.87-1.68	34	1.00	0.69-1.40	114	1.09	0.90-1.30
Females												
I	2	2.15	0.26-7.76	3	2.44	0.50-7.12	6	4.88	1.79-10.63	11	3.24	1.62-5.80
II	6	1.62	0.59-3.53	4	0.83	0.23-2.14	6	1.23	0.45-2.67	16	1.20	0.68-1.94
III	10	1.20	0.58-2.21	8	0.82	0.35-1.62	5	0.61	0.20-1.41	23	0.87	0.55-1.31
IV	3	0.85	0.17-2.48	5	1.23	0.40-2.87	2	0.65	0.08-2.33	10	0.93	0.45-1.72
Total	21	1.27	0.79-1.95	20	1.01	0.62-1.56	19	1.09	0.65-1.70	60	1.12	0.85-1.44

Bladder, ureter, urethra

Males												
I	53	1.24	0.93-1.62	53	0.93	0.70-1.22	65	0.93	0.72-1.19	171	1.01	0.86-1.17
II	126	1.02	0.85-1.20	158	1.01	0.86-1.17	168	0.93	0.80-1.08	452	0.98	0.89-1.08
III	329	1.03	0.92-1.14	410	1.12	1.01-1.23	402	1.00	0.91-1.10	1141	1.05	0.99-1.11
IV	118	1.10	0.91-1.31	108	0.99	0.81-1.19	131	1.23	1.02-1.44	357	1.10	0.99-1.22
Total	626	1.05	0.97-1.14	729	1.06	0.98-1.14	766	1.01	0.94-1.08	2121	1.04	1.00-1.08
Females												
I	14	1.09	0.60-1.83	18	1.48	0.88-2.34	19	1.42	0.85-2.22	51	1.33	0.99-1.75
II	51	1.03	0.77-1.35	59	1.23	0.94-1.59	53	1.02	0.76-1.33	163	1.09	0.93-1.26
III	105	0.95	0.78-1.15	80	0.87	0.69-1.09	78	0.86	0.68-1.07	263	0.90	0.79-1.01
IV	27	0.60	0.39-0.87	38	1.02	0.72-1.40	22	0.64	0.40-0.97	87	0.74	0.60-0.92
Total	197	0.91	0.78-1.04	195	1.03	0.89-1.18	172	0.90	0.77-1.04	564	0.94	0.87-1.02

Primary site Sex Social class	1971-75			1976-80			1981-85			1971-85		
	Obs.	SIR	95% CI	Obs.	SIR	95% CI	Obs.	SIR	95% CI	Obs.	SIR	95% CI

Skin melanoma

Males												
I	38	1.65	1.17-2.26	51	1.54	1.15-2.03	75	1.44	1.14-1.81	164	1.52	1.29-1.76
II	73	1.16	0.91-1.46	110	1.32	1.08-1.58	123	0.99	0.82-1.17	306	1.13	1.01-1.26
III	138	0.90	0.75-1.05	158	0.83	0.70-0.96	266	0.98	0.86-1.10	562	0.91	0.84-0.99
IV	31	0.65	0.44-0.93	36	0.69	0.48-0.96	49	0.74	0.55-0.98	116	0.70	0.58-0.83
Total	280	0.98	0.86-1.09	355	0.99	0.89-1.09	513	1.00	0.91-1.08	1148	0.99	0.93-1.05
Females												
I	24	1.04	0.66-1.54	45	1.48	1.08-1.98	52	1.25	0.93-1.64	121	1.27	1.06-1.51
II	97	1.11	0.90-1.35	117	1.03	0.85-1.22	184	1.17	1.01-1.35	398	1.11	1.00-1.22
III	156	0.91	0.77-1.05	151	0.78	0.66-0.91	216	0.93	0.81-1.05	523	0.87	0.80-0.95
IV	64	0.96	0.74-1.22	73	1.03	0.81-1.30	55	0.73	0.55-0.95	192	0.90	0.78-1.03
Total	341	0.97	0.87-1.08	386	0.94	0.85-1.04	507	1.00	0.91-1.09	1234	0.97	0.92-1.03

Skin melanoma, head and neck

Males												
I	-	-	0.00-1.56	6	1.76	0.65-3.84	7	1.24	0.50-2.56	13	1.14	0.61-1.95
II	8	1.23	0.53-2.42	9	1.09	0.50-2.06	15	1.08	0.60-1.78	32	1.12	0.76-1.57
III	19	1.19	0.71-1.85	18	0.95	0.56-1.49	31	1.02	0.69-1.45	68	1.04	0.81-1.32
IV	6	1.20	0.44-2.61	7	1.38	0.55-2.84	4	0.52	0.14-1.34	17	0.96	0.56-1.54
Total	33	1.10	0.76-1.55	40	1.12	0.80-1.52	57	0.99	0.75-1.28	130	1.05	0.88-1.24
Females												
I	2	0.68	0.08-2.46	3	1.00	0.21-2.92	7	1.78	0.71-3.66	12	1.21	0.63-2.12
II	12	1.07	0.55-1.87	10	0.87	0.42-1.60	13	0.85	0.45-1.45	35	0.92	0.64-1.28
III	22	0.98	0.61-1.48	22	1.08	0.67-1.63	25	0.98	0.63-1.44	69	1.01	0.78-1.28
IV	14	1.59	0.87-2.67	6	0.77	0.28-1.68	15	1.59	0.89-2.63	35	1.35	0.94-1.87
Total	50	1.10	0.82-1.45	41	0.96	0.69-1.30	60	1.11	0.84-1.42	151	1.06	0.90-1.24

Skin melanoma, trunk

Males												
I	28	1.91	1.27-2.76	30	1.52	1.02-2.17	44	1.29	0.94-1.73	102	1.49	1.21-1.79
II	42	1.05	0.75-1.41	63	1.25	0.96-1.60	73	0.90	0.70-1.13	178	1.04	0.89-1.19
III	85	0.87	0.69-1.07	93	0.80	0.65-0.98	177	1.00	0.86-1.15	355	0.91	0.82-1.00
IV	20	0.66	0.41-1.02	19	0.59	0.36-0.93	37	0.87	0.61-1.20	76	0.73	0.57-0.91
Total	175	0.96	0.82-1.10	205	0.94	0.82-1.07	331	0.99	0.88-1.10	711	0.97	0.90-1.04
Females												
I	8	1.45	0.62-2.85	19	1.73	1.04-2.70	18	1.26	0.75-2.00	45	1.46	1.07-1.96
II	19	0.91	0.55-1.42	42	1.03	0.74-1.39	70	1.31	1.02-1.66	131	1.14	0.95-1.34
III	44	1.15	0.84-1.55	45	0.65	0.48-0.88	68	0.87	0.67-1.10	157	0.85	0.72-0.98
IV	15	1.03	0.58-1.71	25	1.01	0.65-1.49	9	0.36	0.16-0.68	49	0.76	0.56-1.01
Total	86	1.09	0.87-1.34	131	0.90	0.75-1.06	165	0.96	0.82-1.12	382	0.97	0.87-1.06

Appendix Table B

Primary site Sex Social class	1971-75			1976-80			1981-85			1971-85		
	Obs.	SIR	95% CI	Obs.	SIR	95% CI	Obs.	SIR	95% CI	Obs.	SIR	95% CI

Skin melanoma, limbs

Males												
I	7	1.48	0.60-3.05	15	1.73	0.97-2.85	20	1.99	1.22-3.08	42	1.79	1.29-2.42
II	18	1.42	0.84-2.24	32	1.48	1.01-2.09	33	1.36	0.93-1.91	83	1.42	1.13-1.76
III	29	0.94	0.63-1.35	40	0.81	0.58-1.10	42	0.79	0.57-1.07	111	0.83	0.69-1.00
IV	2	0.21	0.03-0.77	7	0.53	0.21-1.09	7	0.54	0.22-1.12	16	0.45	0.26-0.73
Total	56	0.97	0.73-1.26	94	1.01	0.82-1.24	102	1.02	0.83-1.23	252	1.00	0.88-1.13
Females												
I	13	0.94	0.50-1.61	23	1.49	0.94-2.23	23	1.06	0.67-1.59	59	1.16	0.88-1.49
II	62	1.18	0.91-1.52	62	1.07	0.82-1.38	94	1.14	0.92-1.40	218	1.13	0.99-1.29
III	85	0.81	0.65-1.00	80	0.81	0.65-1.01	115	0.96	0.79-1.14	280	0.87	0.77-0.97
IV	34	0.83	0.58-1.16	39	1.09	0.78-1.49	29	0.76	0.51-1.10	102	0.89	0.73-1.07
Total	194	0.92	0.79-1.05	204	0.98	0.85-1.12	261	1.00	0.88-1.12	659	0.97	0.90-1.04

Other skin (excluding melanoma and basa cell carcinoma)

Males												
I	20	1.05	0.64-1.62	19	0.94	0.56-1.46	28	1.27	0.84-1.84	67	1.09	0.85-1.39
II	50	0.92	0.68-1.21	45	0.82	0.60-1.09	59	1.06	0.80-1.36	154	0.93	0.79-1.08
III	144	1.03	0.87-1.21	141	1.09	0.92-1.27	121	0.98	0.81-1.16	406	1.03	0.94-1.14
IV	43	0.93	0.68-1.26	41	1.07	0.77-1.45	34	1.05	0.73-1.46	118	1.01	0.83-1.20
Total	257	0.99	0.87-1.12	246	1.01	0.89-1.14	242	1.03	0.91-1.17	745	1.01	0.94-1.09
Females												
I	10	0.97	0.47-1.79	15	1.31	0.73-2.16	21	1.46	0.90-2.23	46	1.27	0.93-1.70
II	38	0.98	0.69-1.35	43	0.96	0.70-1.29	51	0.92	0.69-1.21	132	0.95	0.80-1.12
III	97	1.14	0.92-1.39	92	1.08	0.87-1.33	99	1.06	0.86-1.29	288	1.09	0.97-1.22
IV	33	0.97	0.67-1.36	20	0.59	0.36-0.91	29	0.85	0.57-1.21	82	0.80	0.64-0.99
Total	178	1.06	0.91-1.22	170	0.97	0.83-1.12	200	1.01	0.88-1.16	548	1.01	0.93-1.10

Other skin, head and neck

Males												
I	14	1.31	0.72-2.20	8	0.70	0.30-1.39	12	0.93	0.48-1.63	34	0.97	0.68-1.36
II	24	0.78	0.50-1.17	28	0.90	0.60-1.30	37	1.12	0.79-1.54	89	0.94	0.75-1.15
III	78	0.98	0.78-1.23	85	1.15	0.92-1.42	70	0.95	0.74-1.20	233	1.03	0.90-1.16
IV	27	1.01	0.67-1.48	23	1.04	0.66-1.56	24	1.22	0.78-1.81	74	1.08	0.85-1.36
Total	143	0.97	0.82-1.14	144	1.04	0.88-1.22	143	1.02	0.86-1.20	430	1.01	0.92-1.11
Females												
I	5	0.87	0.28-2.02	11	1.52	0.76-2.71	10	1.21	0.58-2.23	26	1.22	0.80-1.79
II	26	1.20	0.78-1.75	31	1.09	0.74-1.54	23	0.72	0.45-1.07	80	0.97	0.77-1.21
III	59	1.19	0.91-1.54	56	1.02	0.77-1.32	61	1.07	0.82-1.37	176	1.09	0.93-1.26
IV	17	0.85	0.50-1.36	11	0.49	0.25-0.88	21	0.96	0.59-1.47	49	0.76	0.56-1.01
Total	107	1.10	0.91-1.32	109	0.96	0.79-1.15	115	0.96	0.80-1.15	331	1.01	0.90-1.12

Primary site Sex Social class	1971-75			1976-80			1981-85			1971-85		
	Obs.	SIR	95% CI	Obs.	SIR	95% CI	Obs.	SIR	95% CI	Obs.	SIR	95% CI

Other skin, trunk

Males												
I	2	0.86	0.10-3.10	5	1.67	0.54-3.91	5	1.45	0.47-3.38	12	1.37	0.71-2.39
II	11	1.67	0.84-2.99	10	1.27	0.61-2.33	8	0.95	0.41-1.88	29	1.27	0.85-1.82
III	15	0.92	0.51-1.51	13	0.71	0.38-1.21	22	1.19	0.74-1.80	50	0.94	0.70-1.24
IV	5	0.96	0.31-2.23	6	1.13	0.42-2.47	2	0.43	0.05-1.56	13	0.86	0.46-1.47
Total	33	1.08	0.74-1.52	34	0.98	0.68-1.37	37	1.06	0.74-1.46	104	1.04	0.85-1.25
Females												
I	2	1.07	0.13-3.86	1	0.72	0.02-4.03	5	2.39	0.78-5.58	8	1.50	0.65-2.95
II	3	0.42	0.09-1.23	5	0.94	0.31-2.20	9	1.10	0.50-2.08	17	0.82	0.48-1.32
III	16	1.20	0.69-1.95	11	1.16	0.58-2.08	10	0.77	0.37-1.41	37	1.03	0.73-1.42
IV	2	0.39	0.05-1.41	2	0.55	0.07-2.00	3	0.65	0.13-1.90	7	0.52	0.21-1.08
Total	23	0.84	0.53-1.26	19	0.96	0.58-1.50	27	0.96	0.64-1.40	69	0.92	0.71-1.16

Other skin, limbs

Males												
I	2	0.42	0.05-1.51	5	1.05	0.34-2.45	7	1.57	0.63-3.24	14	1.00	0.55-1.68
II	11	0.81	0.40-1.45	6	0.47	0.17-1.03	9	0.82	0.38-1.56	26	0.70	0.46-1.02
III	43	1.24	0.90-1.67	37	1.25	0.88-1.73	24	0.99	0.64-1.48	104	1.18	0.96-1.41
IV	7	0.61	0.25-1.26	7	0.82	0.33-1.70	6	0.98	0.36-2.13	20	0.77	0.47-1.18
Total	63	0.98	0.75-1.25	55	0.99	0.75-1.29	46	1.01	0.74-1.34	164	0.99	0.84-1.15
Females												
I	3	1.36	0.28-3.98	3	1.14	0.24-3.34	5	1.43	0.46-3.33	11	1.32	0.66-2.36
II	6	0.72	0.27-1.57	5	0.50	0.16-1.16	15	1.16	0.65-1.91	26	0.83	0.54-1.22
III	19	0.98	0.59-1.53	23	1.24	0.79-1.86	20	1.02	0.62-1.57	62	1.08	0.83-1.38
IV	12	1.53	0.79-2.68	6	0.83	0.30-1.80	5	0.78	0.25-1.81	23	1.07	0.68-1.60
Total	40	1.06	0.76-1.44	37	0.96	0.68-1.33	45	1.06	0.77-1.41	122	1.03	0.85-1.22

Eye

Males												
I	3	0.83	0.17-2.43	12	1.84	0.95-3.22	7	1.21	0.49-2.50	22	1.38	0.87-2.10
II	12	1.20	0.62-2.09	14	0.85	0.47-1.43	14	0.95	0.52-1.59	40	0.97	0.69-1.32
III	27	1.08	0.71-1.56	32	0.85	0.58-1.20	33	1.02	0.70-1.43	92	0.97	0.78-1.18
IV	9	1.12	0.51-2.13	14	1.35	0.74-2.27	4	0.48	0.13-1.22	27	1.01	0.67-1.47
Total	51	1.09	0.81-1.43	72	1.01	0.79-1.28	58	0.95	0.72-1.22	181	1.01	0.87-1.16
Females												
I	4	1.22	0.33-3.12	5	1.06	0.34-2.47	3	0.89	0.18-2.60	12	1.05	0.54-1.84
II	16	1.26	0.72-2.04	16	0.89	0.51-1.44	11	0.86	0.43-1.53	43	0.98	0.71-1.33
III	25	0.91	0.59-1.35	32	0.98	0.67-1.39	20	0.95	0.58-1.46	77	0.95	0.75-1.19
IV	12	1.08	0.56-1.88	16	1.28	0.73-2.08	11	1.46	0.73-2.60	39	1.25	0.89-1.71
Total	57	1.04	0.79-1.35	69	1.02	0.79-1.29	45	1.00	0.73-1.34	171	1.02	0.87-1.18

Appendix Table B

Primary site Sex Social class	1971-75			1976-80			1981-85			1971-85		
	Obs.	SIR	95% CI	Obs.	SIR	95% CI	Obs.	SIR	95% CI	Obs.	SIR	95% CI

Brain, nervous system

Males												
I	33	1.03	0.71-1.45	52	1.10	0.82-1.45	65	1.14	0.88-1.45	150	1.10	0.93-1.28
II	108	1.22	1.00-1.47	131	1.09	0.91-1.28	144	1.05	0.88-1.23	383	1.11	1.00-1.22
III	209	0.96	0.83-1.09	287	1.03	0.92-1.16	295	0.98	0.87-1.10	791	0.99	0.93-1.06
IV	62	0.91	0.70-1.17	55	0.72	0.54-0.93	63	0.86	0.66-1.10	180	0.83	0.71-0.95
Total	412	1.01	0.92-1.11	525	1.00	0.92-1.09	567	1.00	0.92-1.08	1504	1.00	0.95-1.06
Females												
I	46	1.39	1.02-1.85	51	1.12	0.83-1.47	63	1.08	0.83-1.38	160	1.17	0.99-1.36
II	134	1.05	0.88-1.24	205	1.20	1.04-1.37	236	1.08	0.94-1.22	575	1.11	1.02-1.20
III	249	0.97	0.86-1.10	297	1.00	0.89-1.12	351	1.05	0.94-1.16	897	1.01	0.95-1.08
IV	90	0.88	0.71-1.09	116	1.06	0.87-1.26	105	0.94	0.77-1.13	311	0.96	0.86-1.07
Total	519	1.00	0.92-1.09	669	1.07	0.99-1.16	755	1.04	0.97-1.12	1943	1.04	1.00-1.09

Nervous system, glioma

Males												
I	16	1.01	0.58-1.65	22	0.93	0.59-1.41	31	1.15	0.78-1.63	69	1.04	0.81-1.32
II	49	1.14	0.85-1.51	66	1.10	0.85-1.39	69	1.07	0.84-1.36	184	1.10	0.95-1.26
III	97	0.93	0.75-1.13	144	1.04	0.88-1.22	134	0.96	0.80-1.13	375	0.98	0.88-1.08
IV	25	0.78	0.51-1.15	27	0.71	0.47-1.03	29	0.87	0.58-1.25	81	0.78	0.62-0.97
Total	187	0.96	0.83-1.10	259	0.99	0.88-1.12	263	0.99	0.88-1.12	709	0.98	0.91-1.06
Females												
I	15	1.26	0.70-2.07	23	1.55	0.98-2.33	17	0.99	0.58-1.58	55	1.25	0.94-1.63
II	42	0.92	0.66-1.24	71	1.29	1.01-1.62	71	1.09	0.85-1.37	184	1.11	0.95-1.27
III	80	0.89	0.71-1.11	88	0.95	0.76-1.17	100	0.99	0.81-1.20	268	0.95	0.84-1.06
IV	27	0.77	0.50-1.11	32	0.96	0.66-1.35	40	1.17	0.84-1.60	99	0.96	0.78-1.17
Total	164	0.90	0.77-1.04	214	1.09	0.95-1.24	228	1.05	0.92-1.19	606	1.02	0.94-1.10

Nervous system, meningeoma

Males												
I	6	1.00	0.37-2.18	15	1.39	0.78-2.29	11	0.86	0.43-1.53	32	1.08	0.74-1.53
II	19	1.15	0.69-1.79	29	1.05	0.70-1.51	36	1.15	0.81-1.59	84	1.11	0.89-1.38
III	40	0.97	0.69-1.31	72	1.13	0.88-1.42	69	1.00	0.78-1.27	181	1.04	0.89-1.20
IV	11	0.84	0.42-1.50	10	0.57	0.27-1.05	16	0.93	0.53-1.50	37	0.77	0.54-1.06
Total	76	0.98	0.78-1.23	126	1.05	0.88-1.24	132	1.01	0.85-1.19	334	1.02	0.91-1.13
Females												
I	21	1.46	0.90-2.23	21	1.05	0.65-1.61	30	1.17	0.79-1.67	72	1.20	0.94-1.51
II	56	1.02	0.77-1.32	94	1.25	1.01-1.53	98	1.02	0.83-1.25	248	1.10	0.97-1.24
III	110	0.99	0.82-1.19	125	0.95	0.79-1.12	164	1.11	0.95-1.29	399	1.02	0.92-1.13
IV	35	0.80	0.56-1.11	53	1.07	0.80-1.40	37	0.75	0.53-1.04	125	0.88	0.73-1.04
Total	222	0.99	0.87-1.13	293	1.06	0.94-1.18	329	1.03	0.93-1.15	844	1.03	0.96-1.10

Primary site Sex Social class	1971-75			1976-80			1981-85			1971-85		
	Obs.	SIR	95% CI	Obs.	SIR	95% CI	Obs.	SIR	95% CI	Obs.	SIR	95% CI

Thyroid

Males												
I	8	0.99	0.43-1.95	9	1.04	0.48-1.97	11	1.03	0.51-1.84	28	1.02	0.68-1.48
II	26	1.17	0.77-1.72	24	1.08	0.69-1.60	34	1.31	0.91-1.83	84	1.19	0.95-1.48
III	55	1.01	0.76-1.31	56	1.09	0.82-1.42	54	0.95	0.71-1.24	165	1.01	0.87-1.18
IV	10	0.59	0.28-1.08	8	0.56	0.24-1.10	7	0.50	0.20-1.03	25	0.55	0.36-0.82
Total	99	0.97	0.79-1.19	97	1.00	0.81-1.22	106	0.99	0.81-1.18	302	0.99	0.88-1.10
Females												
I	13	0.71	0.38-1.22	36	1.38	0.96-1.90	46	1.30	0.95-1.73	95	1.19	0.96-1.45
II	68	0.98	0.76-1.24	113	1.14	0.94-1.36	134	1.01	0.85-1.19	315	1.05	0.93-1.17
III	133	0.98	0.82-1.16	164	0.95	0.81-1.10	200	1.06	0.92-1.21	497	1.00	0.91-1.09
IV	52	0.99	0.74-1.29	63	0.98	0.75-1.25	59	1.02	0.77-1.31	174	0.99	0.85-1.15
Total	266	0.97	0.85-1.08	376	1.04	0.94-1.15	439	1.06	0.96-1.16	1081	1.03	0.97-1.09

Thyroid, follicular

Males												
I	5	2.05	0.67-4.79	2	1.14	0.14-4.13	2	0.96	0.12-3.48	9	1.44	0.66-2.73
II	7	1.03	0.42-2.13	6	1.23	0.45-2.67	8	1.66	0.72-3.27	21	1.27	0.79-1.95
III	14	0.83	0.45-1.39	13	1.14	0.60-1.94	10	0.94	0.45-1.73	37	0.95	0.67-1.31
IV	4	0.75	0.20-1.92	2	0.58	0.07-2.10	1	0.39	0.01-2.19	7	0.62	0.25-1.27
Total	30	0.96	0.65-1.37	23	1.07	0.68-1.60	21	1.05	0.65-1.60	74	1.01	0.80-1.27
Females												
I	4	0.72	0.19-1.83	4	0.73	0.20-1.87	5	0.90	0.29-2.09	13	0.78	0.42-1.33
II	25	1.17	0.76-1.73	21	1.01	0.62-1.54	20	0.96	0.59-1.48	66	1.05	0.81-1.33
III	47	1.16	0.85-1.54	37	1.00	0.71-1.38	42	1.32	0.95-1.78	126	1.15	0.96-1.36
IV	24	1.52	0.97-2.26	14	1.00	0.55-1.69	13	1.24	0.66-2.11	51	1.27	0.94-1.67
Total	100	1.20	0.98-1.45	76	0.99	0.78-1.23	80	1.16	0.92-1.45	256	1.12	0.98-1.26

Thyroid, papillary

Males												
I	1	0.31	0.01-1.72	5	1.20	0.39-2.80	7	1.09	0.44-2.25	13	0.94	0.50-1.61
II	12	1.36	0.70-2.37	13	1.26	0.67-2.16	18	1.16	0.69-1.83	43	1.24	0.90-1.67
III	22	1.03	0.65-1.57	24	1.02	0.65-1.52	33	0.98	0.67-1.37	79	1.01	0.80-1.25
IV	2	0.31	0.04-1.12	3	0.48	0.10-1.40	4	0.49	0.13-1.25	9	0.43	0.20-0.82
Total	37	0.93	0.65-1.28	45	1.02	0.74-1.36	62	0.97	0.74-1.24	144	0.97	0.82-1.14
Females												
I	8	0.93	0.40-1.83	29	1.68	1.12-2.41	38	1.44	1.02-1.97	75	1.43	1.13-1.80
II	30	0.93	0.62-1.32	75	1.15	0.91-1.45	101	1.03	0.84-1.24	206	1.05	0.91-1.20
III	49	0.78	0.58-1.04	97	0.87	0.71-1.06	139	1.04	0.87-1.21	285	0.92	0.82-1.04
IV	21	0.87	0.54-1.33	35	0.85	0.59-1.19	32	0.83	0.56-1.16	88	0.85	0.68-1.04
Total	108	0.85	0.69-1.01	236	1.01	0.88-1.14	310	1.04	0.93-1.16	654	0.99	0.92-1.07

Primary site Sex Social class	1971-75			1976-80			1981-85			1971-85		
	Obs.	SIR	95% CI	Obs.	SIR	95% CI	Obs.	SIR	95% CI	Obs.	SIR	95% CI

Other endocrine glands

Males

I	3	1.38	0.28-4.02	-	-	0.00-1.03	2	0.51	0.06-1.85	5	0.52	0.17-1.21
II	2	0.33	0.04-1.19	8	0.83	0.36-1.64	9	0.91	0.42-1.73	19	0.74	0.45-1.16
III	21	1.41	0.88-2.16	22	0.98	0.61-1.48	27	1.23	0.81-1.79	70	1.18	0.92-1.49
IV	2	0.43	0.05-1.55	9	1.37	0.62-2.59	6	1.05	0.39-2.28	17	1.00	0.58-1.60
Total	28	1.01	0.67-1.46	39	0.92	0.65-1.26	44	1.06	0.77-1.42	111	1.00	0.82-1.19

Females

I	2	1.68	0.20-6.06	1	0.52	0.01-2.90	-	-	0.00-1.71	3	0.57	0.12-1.66
II	2	0.44	0.05-1.58	7	0.98	0.39-2.01	12	1.45	0.75-2.54	21	1.05	0.65-1.60
III	10	1.09	0.52-2.00	11	0.88	0.44-1.57	16	1.15	0.66-1.87	37	1.04	0.73-1.43
IV	4	1.09	0.30-2.79	6	1.29	0.47-2.81	4	0.79	0.21-2.02	14	1.04	0.57-1.75
Total	18	0.97	0.57-1.53	25	0.95	0.62-1.40	32	1.09	0.74-1.54	75	1.01	0.79-1.27

Bone

Males

I	7	1.60	0.64-3.29	5	1.20	0.39-2.80	7	1.37	0.55-2.82	19	1.39	0.84-2.17
II	12	1.01	0.52-1.76	12	1.10	0.57-1.93	10	0.81	0.39-1.49	34	0.97	0.67-1.35
III	29	1.00	0.67-1.44	26	1.04	0.68-1.53	30	1.13	0.76-1.62	85	1.06	0.85-1.31
IV	9	1.02	0.47-1.94	6	0.86	0.31-1.87	3	0.47	0.10-1.38	18	0.81	0.48-1.28
Total	57	1.06	0.80-1.37	49	1.04	0.77-1.38	50	0.99	0.74-1.31	156	1.03	0.88-1.20

Females

I	1	0.47	0.01-2.61	2	1.06	0.13-3.83	3	1.34	0.28-3.92	6	0.96	0.35-2.09
II	9	1.08	0.49-2.05	10	1.40	0.67-2.58	15	1.73	0.97-2.85	34	1.41	0.98-1.97
III	17	1.09	0.64-1.75	13	1.00	0.53-1.71	12	0.88	0.45-1.53	42	0.99	0.72-1.34
IV	7	1.15	0.46-2.36	3	0.60	0.12-1.76	3	0.63	0.13-1.84	13	0.82	0.44-1.40
Total	34	1.06	0.73-1.48	28	1.04	0.69-1.50	33	1.12	0.77-1.58	95	1.07	0.87-1.31

Soft tissue

Males

I	12	1.38	0.71-2.40	6	0.67	0.24-1.45	9	0.90	0.41-1.70	27	0.97	0.64-1.41
II	19	0.78	0.47-1.22	21	0.94	0.58-1.43	27	1.09	0.72-1.59	67	0.94	0.73-1.19
III	52	0.86	0.65-1.13	57	1.11	0.84-1.44	55	1.02	0.77-1.32	164	0.99	0.84-1.15
IV	25	1.31	0.85-1.94	10	0.72	0.35-1.33	15	1.11	0.62-1.83	50	1.08	0.80-1.42
Total	108	0.96	0.79-1.15	94	0.97	0.79-1.19	106	1.03	0.85-1.24	308	0.99	0.88-1.10

Females

I	10	1.57	0.75-2.89	8	1.06	0.46-2.09	11	1.21	0.60-2.16	29	1.26	0.84-1.81
II	28	1.14	0.76-1.64	34	1.20	0.83-1.68	25	0.71	0.46-1.05	87	0.99	0.79-1.22
III	49	0.95	0.70-1.26	56	1.15	0.87-1.50	52	0.93	0.70-1.22	157	1.01	0.86-1.17
IV	21	1.00	0.62-1.54	9	0.50	0.23-0.96	18	0.92	0.55-1.46	48	0.82	0.61-1.09
Total	108	1.04	0.86-1.25	107	1.05	0.86-1.25	106	0.89	0.73-1.06	321	0.99	0.88-1.10

Primary site Sex Social class	1971-75			1976-80			1981-85			1971-85		
	Obs.	SIR	95% CI	Obs.	SIR	95% CI	Obs.	SIR	95% CI	Obs.	SIR	95% CI

Unspecified

Males												
I	13	0.54	0.29-0.92	14	0.68	0.37-1.15	19	0.94	0.56-1.46	46	0.71	0.52-0.95
II	67	0.96	0.75-1.22	52	0.92	0.68-1.20	48	0.92	0.68-1.22	167	0.94	0.80-1.08
III	191	1.08	0.93-1.24	143	1.07	0.90-1.26	127	1.09	0.91-1.29	461	1.08	0.98-1.18
IV	92	1.56	1.26-1.92	51	1.28	0.95-1.68	40	1.30	0.93-1.77	183	1.41	1.22-1.63
Total	363	1.10	0.99-1.22	260	1.04	0.92-1.17	234	1.07	0.93-1.21	857	1.07	1.00-1.15
Females												
I	15	0.75	0.42-1.24	14	0.79	0.43-1.33	17	0.97	0.56-1.55	46	0.83	0.61-1.11
II	76	1.00	0.79-1.25	79	1.15	0.91-1.43	61	0.90	0.69-1.15	216	1.01	0.88-1.15
III	162	0.95	0.81-1.10	124	0.94	0.78-1.11	137	1.19	1.00-1.40	423	1.01	0.92-1.11
IV	78	1.12	0.88-1.40	60	1.12	0.86-1.44	43	1.01	0.73-1.36	181	1.09	0.94-1.26
Total	331	0.98	0.88-1.09	277	1.02	0.90-1.14	258	1.06	0.94-1.20	866	1.02	0.95-1.08

Non-Hodgkin's lymphoma

Males												
I	36	1.30	0.91-1.80	40	1.07	0.76-1.46	47	0.97	0.71-1.28	123	1.08	0.90-1.28
II	83	1.06	0.85-1.32	109	1.10	0.90-1.31	123	1.02	0.85-1.21	315	1.06	0.94-1.18
III	212	1.09	0.95-1.24	232	1.00	0.88-1.14	260	0.98	0.86-1.10	704	1.02	0.94-1.09
IV	48	0.77	0.57-1.02	63	0.95	0.73-1.21	75	1.12	0.88-1.40	186	0.95	0.82-1.09
Total	379	1.04	0.94-1.15	444	1.02	0.93-1.12	505	1.01	0.92-1.10	1328	1.02	0.97-1.08
Females												
I	24	1.64	1.05-2.44	20	0.84	0.51-1.30	30	0.92	0.62-1.32	74	1.04	0.82-1.31
II	65	1.14	0.88-1.46	91	0.99	0.80-1.21	131	1.05	0.88-1.24	287	1.05	0.93-1.18
III	126	1.06	0.88-1.25	175	1.01	0.87-1.17	215	1.05	0.91-1.19	516	1.04	0.95-1.13
IV	46	0.95	0.70-1.27	62	0.90	0.69-1.16	64	0.87	0.67-1.11	172	0.90	0.77-1.04
Total	261	1.09	0.96-1.23	348	0.97	0.87-1.08	440	1.01	0.92-1.11	1049	1.02	0.96-1.08

Non-Hodgkin's lymphoma, nodal

Males												
I	30	1.48	1.00-2.11	30	1.10	0.74-1.56	29	0.90	0.60-1.29	89	1.11	0.89-1.37
II	59	1.02	0.78-1.32	82	1.12	0.89-1.39	76	0.95	0.75-1.19	217	1.03	0.90-1.17
III	154	1.07	0.90-1.24	163	0.96	0.82-1.11	178	1.01	0.87-1.17	495	1.01	0.92-1.10
IV	42	0.90	0.65-1.22	46	0.93	0.68-1.24	52	1.17	0.88-1.54	140	1.00	0.84-1.17
Total	285	1.06	0.94-1.19	321	1.00	0.90-1.12	335	1.01	0.90-1.12	941	1.02	0.96-1.09
Females												
I	17	1.76	1.02-2.81	15	0.92	0.52-1.52	19	0.84	0.50-1.31	51	1.05	0.78-1.38
II	49	1.30	0.96-1.72	68	1.08	0.84-1.36	98	1.13	0.92-1.38	215	1.15	1.00-1.31
III	95	1.24	1.00-1.51	123	1.04	0.86-1.23	153	1.09	0.92-1.27	371	1.10	0.99-1.22
IV	26	0.84	0.55-1.22	41	0.87	0.62-1.18	42	0.84	0.61-1.14	109	0.85	0.70-1.02
Total	187	1.21	1.04-1.38	247	1.01	0.88-1.14	312	1.04	0.93-1.16	746	1.06	0.99-1.14

Appendix Table B

Primary site Sex	1971-75			1976-80			1981-85			1971-85		
Social class	Obs.	SIR	95% CI	Obs.	SIR	95% CI	Obs.	SIR	95% CI	Obs.	SIR	95% CI

Non-Hodgkin's lymphoma, extranodal

Males												
I	6	0.81	0.30-1.75	10	1.00	0.48-1.84	18	1.11	0.66-1.75	34	1.01	0.70-1.41
II	24	1.17	0.75-1.74	27	1.03	0.68-1.49	47	1.16	0.85-1.54	98	1.12	0.91-1.37
III	58	1.14	0.87-1.48	69	1.14	0.88-1.44	82	0.92	0.73-1.14	209	1.04	0.90-1.19
IV	6	0.38	0.14-0.82	17	0.99	0.57-1.58	23	1.01	0.64-1.51	46	0.82	0.60-1.10
Total	94	0.99	0.80-1.22	123	1.08	0.89-1.27	170	1.00	0.86-1.16	387	1.02	0.92-1.13
Females												
I	7	1.41	0.57-2.91	5	0.67	0.22-1.57	11	1.12	0.56-2.01	23	1.04	0.66-1.55
II	16	0.83	0.48-1.36	23	0.80	0.50-1.19	33	0.88	0.60-1.23	72	0.84	0.66-1.06
III	31	0.74	0.50-1.04	52	0.96	0.72-1.26	62	0.96	0.74-1.24	145	0.90	0.76-1.06
IV	20	1.16	0.71-1.79	21	0.98	0.60-1.49	22	0.92	0.58-1.40	63	1.01	0.77-1.29
Total	74	0.89	0.70-1.11	101	0.90	0.73-1.09	128	0.94	0.79-1.11	303	0.92	0.81-1.02

Hodgkin's disease

Males												
I	14	1.12	0.61-1.88	11	0.83	0.41-1.49	18	1.27	0.75-2.00	43	1.08	0.78-1.45
II	23	0.67	0.43-1.01	30	0.91	0.61-1.30	43	1.30	0.94-1.75	96	0.96	0.78-1.17
III	96	1.14	0.93-1.40	79	1.04	0.83-1.30	56	0.79	0.60-1.02	231	1.00	0.88-1.13
IV	19	0.73	0.44-1.14	27	1.32	0.87-1.92	12	0.74	0.38-1.29	58	0.92	0.70-1.19
Total	152	0.97	0.82-1.13	147	1.03	0.87-1.21	129	0.96	0.80-1.13	428	0.99	0.90-1.08
Females												
I	6	0.93	0.34-2.02	9	1.32	0.60-2.50	7	1.20	0.48-2.47	22	1.15	0.72-1.74
II	22	0.90	0.56-1.36	30	1.17	0.79-1.66	25	1.12	0.72-1.65	77	1.06	0.84-1.33
III	49	1.01	0.75-1.33	37	0.82	0.58-1.13	31	0.94	0.64-1.33	117	0.92	0.76-1.10
IV	18	0.95	0.56-1.50	12	0.71	0.37-1.25	15	1.40	0.78-2.31	45	0.97	0.71-1.29
Total	95	0.96	0.78-1.18	88	0.93	0.75-1.15	78	1.08	0.86-1.35	261	0.99	0.87-1.11

Multiple myeloma

Males												
I	14	1.03	0.57-1.74	9	0.56	0.26-1.06	14	0.81	0.44-1.35	37	0.79	0.56-1.09
II	39	1.02	0.72-1.39	51	1.15	0.86-1.52	56	1.26	0.95-1.64	146	1.15	0.97-1.34
III	100	1.04	0.84-1.25	100	0.96	0.78-1.16	88	0.89	0.71-1.09	288	0.96	0.85-1.08
IV	32	1.02	0.70-1.44	33	1.07	0.74-1.50	27	1.03	0.68-1.50	92	1.04	0.84-1.28
Total	185	1.03	0.89-1.18	193	0.99	0.86-1.13	185	0.99	0.85-1.14	563	1.00	0.92-1.09
Females												
I	9	0.88	0.40-1.68	9	0.73	0.33-1.38	7	0.62	0.25-1.28	25	0.74	0.48-1.09
II	38	0.98	0.69-1.34	43	0.88	0.64-1.18	46	1.06	0.78-1.42	127	0.97	0.81-1.14
III	94	1.11	0.90-1.36	91	0.96	0.78-1.18	83	1.13	0.90-1.40	268	1.06	0.94-1.19
IV	27	0.79	0.52-1.15	50	1.30	0.96-1.71	35	1.28	0.89-1.78	112	1.12	0.92-1.34
Total	168	1.00	0.85-1.16	193	0.99	0.86-1.14	171	1.10	0.94-1.27	532	1.03	0.94-1.12

Primary site	1971-75			1976-80			1981-85			1971-85		
Sex												
Social class	Obs.	SIR	95% CI	Obs.	SIR	95% CI	Obs.	SIR	95% CI	Obs.	SIR	95% CI

Leukaemia

Males												
I	31	0.97	0.66-1.38	47	1.40	1.03-1.87	33	0.99	0.68-1.40	111	1.13	0.93-1.35
II	106	1.18	0.96-1.41	70	0.79	0.61-0.99	88	1.07	0.85-1.31	264	1.01	0.89-1.13
III	231	1.02	0.89-1.15	218	1.05	0.92-1.20	186	1.02	0.88-1.17	635	1.03	0.95-1.11
IV	55	0.75	0.56-0.97	54	0.91	0.68-1.18	44	0.94	0.68-1.26	153	0.85	0.72-0.99
Total	423	1.00	0.91-1.10	389	1.00	0.90-1.10	351	1.02	0.91-1.12	1163	1.01	0.95-1.06
Females												
I	25	1.18	0.76-1.74	12	0.51	0.26-0.89	18	0.93	0.55-1.47	55	0.86	0.65-1.12
II	86	1.06	0.85-1.31	93	1.02	0.82-1.25	76	1.04	0.82-1.31	255	1.04	0.92-1.17
III	169	1.00	0.85-1.15	177	1.06	0.91-1.23	127	1.08	0.90-1.27	473	1.04	0.95-1.14
IV	83	1.23	0.98-1.52	60	0.93	0.71-1.19	41	0.99	0.71-1.34	184	1.06	0.91-1.22
Total	363	1.07	0.96-1.18	342	0.99	0.89-1.10	262	1.04	0.92-1.17	967	1.03	0.97-1.10

Chronic lymphocytic leukaemia

Males												
I	13	1.17	0.62-1.99	15	1.34	0.75-2.22	13	1.20	0.64-2.04	41	1.24	0.89-1.68
II	41	1.27	0.91-1.72	25	0.80	0.52-1.18	29	1.03	0.69-1.48	95	1.04	0.84-1.27
III	79	0.96	0.76-1.20	78	1.06	0.84-1.33	65	1.03	0.80-1.32	222	1.02	0.89-1.15
IV	21	0.77	0.47-1.17	17	0.77	0.45-1.24	17	1.01	0.59-1.62	55	0.83	0.63-1.08
Total	154	1.01	0.85-1.17	135	0.98	0.82-1.15	124	1.05	0.87-1.24	413	1.01	0.91-1.11
Females												
I	5	0.85	0.28-1.98	4	0.69	0.19-1.77	6	1.61	0.59-3.50	15	0.97	0.54-1.60
II	24	1.07	0.68-1.59	29	1.28	0.85-1.83	19	1.32	0.79-2.06	72	1.21	0.94-1.52
III	39	0.74	0.53-1.02	49	1.12	0.83-1.48	32	1.32	0.90-1.86	120	1.00	0.83-1.18
IV	25	1.16	0.75-1.72	13	0.73	0.39-1.25	8	0.90	0.39-1.77	46	0.96	0.70-1.28
Total	93	0.91	0.73-1.11	95	1.06	0.85-1.29	65	1.27	0.98-1.62	253	1.04	0.91-1.17

Acute myelocytic leukaemia

Males												
I	10	0.99	0.48-1.83	21	1.92	1.19-2.94	11	0.98	0.49-1.75	42	1.30	0.94-1.76
II	37	1.30	0.92-1.80	19	0.68	0.41-1.07	23	0.84	0.53-1.25	79	0.94	0.75-1.18
III	59	0.83	0.63-1.06	67	1.04	0.81-1.33	65	1.07	0.83-1.37	191	0.97	0.84-1.12
IV	18	0.78	0.46-1.23	18	1.01	0.60-1.60	16	1.05	0.60-1.71	52	0.93	0.69-1.21
Total	124	0.93	0.77-1.10	125	1.04	0.86-1.22	115	1.00	0.83-1.19	364	0.99	0.89-1.09
Females												
I	9	1.17	0.53-2.21	3	0.35	0.07-1.03	10	1.17	0.56-2.16	22	0.89	0.56-1.35
II	32	1.10	0.75-1.55	32	0.97	0.66-1.37	33	1.04	0.71-1.46	97	1.03	0.84-1.26
III	72	1.23	0.96-1.55	57	0.92	0.70-1.20	48	0.94	0.69-1.25	177	1.03	0.89-1.19
IV	25	1.09	0.71-1.61	21	0.86	0.53-1.31	18	1.02	0.60-1.61	64	0.98	0.76-1.26
Total	138	1.17	0.98-1.37	113	0.89	0.73-1.06	109	1.00	0.82-1.20	360	1.01	0.91-1.12

Appendix Table B

Primary site	1971-75			1976-80			1981-85			1971-85		
Sex												
Social class	Obs.	SIR	95% CI	Obs.	SIR	95% CI	Obs.	SIR	95% CI	Obs.	SIR	95% CI

Other leukaemia

Males												
I	8	0.75	0.32-1.48	11	0.96	0.48-1.72	9	0.81	0.37-1.54	28	0.85	0.56-1.22
II	28	0.95	0.63-1.38	26	0.87	0.57-1.27	36	1.33	0.93-1.85	90	1.04	0.84-1.28
III	93	1.28	1.03-1.56	73	1.05	0.82-1.32	56	0.94	0.71-1.22	222	1.10	0.96-1.25
IV	16	0.70	0.40-1.13	19	0.96	0.58-1.51	11	0.74	0.37-1.33	46	0.80	0.59-1.07
Total	145	1.07	0.90-1.25	129	0.99	0.83-1.17	112	1.00	0.82-1.19	386	1.02	0.92-1.12
Females												
I	11	1.44	0.72-2.58	5	0.54	0.17-1.25	2	0.28	0.03-1.03	18	0.75	0.44-1.19
II	30	1.02	0.69-1.46	32	0.91	0.62-1.28	24	0.90	0.58-1.34	86	0.94	0.75-1.16
III	58	0.99	0.76-1.29	71	1.17	0.91-1.47	47	1.11	0.81-1.47	176	1.09	0.93-1.26
IV	33	1.43	0.98-2.00	26	1.15	0.75-1.69	15	1.01	0.57-1.67	74	1.22	0.96-1.54
Total	132	1.11	0.93-1.31	134	1.05	0.88-1.23	88	0.97	0.78-1.19	354	1.05	0.94-1.16

Not included above:

Cervix uteri, carcinoma in situ

I	34	0.63	0.44-0.88	20	0.67	0.41-1.03	21	0.69	0.42-1.05	75	0.65	0.51-0.82
II	177	0.89	0.76-1.02	84	0.78	0.63-0.97	110	0.96	0.79-1.15	371	0.88	0.80-0.97
III	345	1.02	0.91-1.13	173	1.04	0.89-1.20	148	0.99	0.84-1.16	666	1.02	0.94-1.09
IV	141	1.16	0.97-1.36	66	1.21	0.94-1.54	55	1.35	1.01-1.75	262	1.21	1.06-1.36
Total	697	0.97	0.90-1.05	343	0.96	0.86-1.06	334	1.00	0.89-1.11	1374	0.98	0.93-1.03

Skin, basal cell carcinoma

Males												
I	188	1.43	1.23-1.64	272	1.62	1.43-1.82	371	1.54	1.38-1.70	831	1.54	1.43-1.64
II	418	1.12	1.01-1.23	494	1.09	1.00-1.19	678	1.12	1.03-1.20	1590	1.11	1.05-1.16
III	871	0.92	0.86-0.98	995	0.94	0.88-1.00	1233	0.92	0.86-0.97	3099	0.92	0.89-0.96
IV	244	0.79	0.69-0.89	239	0.77	0.68-0.87	260	0.75	0.66-0.84	743	0.77	0.71-0.82
Total	1721	0.98	0.93-1.02	2000	1.01	0.96-1.05	2542	1.00	0.96-1.04	6263	0.99	0.97-1.02
Females												
I	164	1.41	1.21-1.64	209	1.41	1.22-1.60	296	1.37	1.22-1.53	669	1.39	1.29-1.50
II	506	1.14	1.04-1.24	653	1.13	1.05-1.22	894	1.08	1.01-1.15	2053	1.11	1.06-1.16
III	972	1.01	0.95-1.08	1061	0.98	0.92-1.04	1262	0.93	0.88-0.98	3295	0.97	0.94-1.00
IV	362	0.93	0.84-1.03	381	0.88	0.80-0.98	458	0.94	0.85-1.03	1201	0.92	0.87-0.97
Total	2004	1.05	1.01-1.10	2304	1.03	0.99-1.07	2910	1.01	0.97-1.04	7218	1.03	1.00-1.05

Appendix tables C1-C42

Numbers of cancer cases (Obs.) and crude and social class adjusted standardised incidence ratios (SIR) with 95% confidence intervals (95% CI) for all occupational branches and specific occupational categories with at least 5 expected cases or with a SIR significantly different from 1.0 in 1971-85, by primary site and sex. Ages 35-64 years. Reference: Economically active population.

Stars (*) at the end of lines indicate that either crude or social class adjusted SIR or both are statistically significant (p<0.05). If observed number of cases is zero, the expected number (Exp) is given in SIR column (-/Exp).

C1.	Lip cancer, ♂	C22.	Prostate cancer
C2.	Lip cancer, ♀	C23.	Kidney cancer, ♂
C3.	Oesophageal cancer, ♂	C24.	Kidney cancer, ♀
C4.	Oesophageal cancer, ♀	C25.	Cancer of the bladder, ureter and urethra, ♂
C5.	Stomach cancer, ♂	C26.	Cancer of the bladder, ureter and urethra, ♀
C6.	Stomach cancer, ♀	C27.	Skin melanoma, ♂
C7.	Colon cancer, ♂	C28.	Skin melanoma, ♀
C8.	Colon cancer, ♀	C29.	Non-melanoma skin cancer, ♂
C9.	Rectal cancer, ♂	C30.	Non-melanoma skin cancer, ♀
C10.	Rectal cancer, ♀	C31.	Basal cell carcinoma of the skin, ♂
C11.	Cancer of the pancreas, ♂	C32.	Basal cell carcinoma of the skin, ♀
C12.	Cancer of the pancreas, ♀	C33.	Cancer of the brain and nervous system, ♂
C13.	Laryngeal cancer, ♂	C34.	Cancer of the brain and nervous system, ♀
C14.	Laryngeal cancer, ♀	C35.	Non-Hodgkin lymphoma, ♂
C15.	Lung cancer, ♂	C36.	Non-Hodgkin lymphoma, ♀
C16.	Lung cancer, ♀	C37.	Multiple myeloma, ♂
C17.	Breast cancer, ♂	C38.	Multiple myeloma, ♀
C18.	Breast cancer, ♀	C39.	Leukaemia, ♂
C19.	Cervical cancer	C40.	Leukaemia, ♀
C20.	Cancer of the corpus uteri	C41.	Cancer of all sites, ♂
C21.	Ovarian cancer	C42.	Cancer of all sites, ♀

C1. Lip cancer, males

Occupation	Obs.	Crude SIR	95% CI	Adjusted SIR	95% CI	
WHOLE POPULATION	1046	1.05	0.98-1.11	1.03	0.97-1.10	
ECONOMICALLY ACTIVE PERSONS	874	1.00	0.93-1.07	1.00	0.93-1.07	
0 Technical, humanistic, etc. work	29	0.36	0.24-0.51	0.69	0.46-0.98	*
00 Technical professions	4	0.44	0.12-1.12	1.43	0.39-3.67	
01 Technical work	12	0.40	0.21-0.71	0.56	0.29-0.99	*
010 Civil engineering technicians	10	0.91	0.44-1.67	1.28	0.61-2.35	
013 Mechanical technicians	1	0:13	0.00-0.72	0.18	0.00-1.00	*
02 Chemical/physical/biological work	-	-/5.2	0.00-0.71	-/2.6	0.00-1.40	*
05 Teaching	6	0.35	0.13-0.76	0.98	0.36-2.13	*
052 Primary school teachers	2	0.30	0.04-1.07	1.09	0.13-3.95	
08 Artistic and literary professions	3	0.56	0.11-1.63	1.30	0.27-3.79	
09 Humanistic and social work etc.	2	0.39	0.05-1.41	0.80	0.10-2.87	
1 Administrative and clerical work	17	0.32	0.19-0.51	0.66	0.38-1.06	*
10 Public administration	3	0.59	0.12-1.73	1.77	0.36-5.16	
11 Corporate administration	3	0.12	0.02-0.35	0.36	0.07-1.05	*
110 Corporate managers	2	0.17	0.02-0.62	0.50	0.06-1.82	*
112 Commercial managers	1	0.16	0.00-0.91	0.55	0.01-3.04	*
14/15 Clerical work NOS	10	0.50	0.24-0.91	0.71	0.34-1.31	*
150 Property managers, warehousemen	4	0.40	0.11-1.01	0.56	0.15-1.42	
2 Sales professions	17	0.41	0.24-0.65	0.50	0.29-0.79	*
20 Wholesale and retail dealers	5	0.41	0.13-0.97	0.59	0.19-1.38	*
201 Retailers	5	0.43	0.14-1.01	0.61	0.20-1.43	
22 Sales representatives	1	0.12	0.00-0.64	0.16	0.00-0.90	*
220 Commercial travellers, etc.	1	0.13	0.00-0.70	0.18	0.00-0.98	*
23 Sales work	11	0.61	0.31-1.10	0.62	0.31-1.12	
231 Shop personnel	7	0.63	0.25-1.29	0.55	0.22-1.14	
3 Farming, forestry and fishing	402	1.60	1.45-1.76	1.45	1.31-1.59	*
30 Agricultural/forestry management	323	1.55	1.39-1.73	1.48	1.32-1.64	*
300 Farmers, silviculturists	306	1.56	1.39-1.73	1.46	1.30-1.63	*
302 Forestry managers	11	1.50	0.75-2.68	2.11	1.05-3.77	*
31 Farming, animal husbandry	31	2.42	1.64-3.43	1.88	1.28-2.67	*
310 Agricultural workers	27	2.80	1.84-4.07	2.22	1.47-3.23	*
33 Fishing	8	3.56	1.54-7.01	3.13	1.35-6.17	*
330 Fishermen	8	3.69	1.59-7.27	3.24	1.40-6.39	*
34 Forestry work	40	1.40	1.00-1.91	0.99	0.71-1.35	*
4 Mining and quarrying	7	1.43	0.57-2.94	1.29	0.52-2.66	
5 Transport and communications	77	0.93	0.74-1.17	0.98	0.77-1.23	
54 Road transport	53	1.05	0.79-1.37	1.09	0.81-1.42	
540 Motor-vehicle and tram drivers	53	1.05	0.79-1.38	1.09	0.82-1.43	
55 Transport services	8	0.99	0.43-1.95	0.98	0.42-1.92	
550 Railway staff	8	1.01	0.43-1.98	0.99	0.43-1.95	
58 Postal services/couriers	1	0.19	0.00-1.05	0.17	0.00-0.94	*
6/7 Industrial and construction work	297	0.93	0.83-1.04	0.80	0.71-0.90	*
63 Smelting, metal and foundry work	9	1.02	0.47-1.94	0.94	0.43-1.78	
65 Machine shop/steelworkers	37	0.59	0.42-0.81	0.53	0.38-0.74	*
650 Turners, machinists	4	0.29	0.08-0.74	0.26	0.07-0.67	*
651 Fitter-assemblers etc.	5	0.82	0.27-1.92	0.73	0.24-1.70	
652 Machine and motor repairers	11	0.76	0.38-1.35	0.70	0.35-1.25	
653 Sheetmetalworkers	4	0.70	0.19-1.79	0.64	0.17-1.64	
654 Plumbers	3	0.37	0.08-1.07	0.33	0.07-0.97	*
655 Welders and flame cutters	3	0.48	0.10-1.40	0.42	0.09-1.22	
659 Machine shop/steelworkers NOS	3	0.52	0.11-1.52	0.47	0.10-1.38	
66 Electrical work	9	0.48	0.22-0.90	0.42	0.19-0.80	*
660 Electricians (indoors)	6	0.58	0.21-1.27	0.52	0.19-1.13	
67 Woodwork	73	1.13	0.89-1.42	1.03	0.81-1.30	
670 Round-timber workers	5	3.42	1.11-7.97	3.06	0.99-7.13	*
671 Timber workers	19	2.36	1.42-3.68	2.15	1.29-3.35	*
673 Construction carpenters	43	1.06	0.77-1.43	0.96	0.69-1.29	

Occupation	Obs.	Crude SIR	95% CI	Adjusted SIR	95% CI	
675 Bench carpenters	-	-/3.7	0.00-0.99	-/3.7	0.00-1.00	*
68 Painting and lacquering	6	0.50	0.18-1.08	0.46	0.17-1.01	
680 Painters	6	0.54	0.20-1.17	0.50	0.18-1.09	
69 Construction work NOS	68	1.32	1.02-1.67	0.99	0.77-1.25	*
690 Bricklayers and tile setters	5	0.76	0.25-1.77	0.68	0.22-1.60	
697 Building hands	24	1.15	0.73-1.71	0.80	0.51-1.18	
698 Roadbuilding hands	25	1.80	1.17-2.66	1.24	0.80-1.83	*
70 Printing	-	-/4.2	0.00-0.87	-/4.8	0.00-0.77	*
72 Food industry	8	1.17	0.51-2.31	1.08	0.46-2.12	
73 Chemical process/paper making	11	1.03	0.52-1.85	0.91	0.45-1.62	
75 Industrial work NOS	8	1.15	0.49-2.26	1.06	0.46-2.10	
77 Machinists	22	0.92	0.57-1.39	0.82	0.52-1.25	
772 Construction machinery operator	11	1.40	0.70-2.50	1.32	0.66-2.37	
773 Operators of stationary engine	3	0.50	0.10-1.45	0.44	0.09-1.28	
78 Dock and warehouse work	21	1.11	0.69-1.70	0.84	0.52-1.28	
780 Dockers	5	1.09	0.35-2.55	0.94	0.30-2.19	
782 Warehousemen	12	1.04	0.54-1.82	0.76	0.39-1.33	
79 Labourers not classified elsewhere	18	1.64	0.97-2.59	1.14	0.68-1.81	
8 Services	24	0.68	0.44-1.02	0.68	0.43-1.01	
80 Watchmen, security guards	10	0.66	0.31-1.21	0.71	0.34-1.30	
801 Policemen	2	0.33	0.04-1.19	0.45	0.05-1.61	
804 Civilian guards	4	0.86	0.23-2.19	0.70	0.19-1.79	
83 Caretakers and cleaners	13	0.87	0.46-1.49	0.78	0.41-1.33	
830 Caretakers	10	0.75	0.36-1.38	0.67	0.32-1.23	
9 Work not classified elsewhere	4	0.71	0.19-1.82	0.93	0.25-2.38	
ECONOMICALLY INACTIVE PERSONS	172	1.36	1.17-1.57	1.24	1.06-1.43	*

C2. Lip cancer, females

Occupation	Obs.	Crude SIR	95% CI	Adjusted SIR	95% CI	
WHOLE POPULATION	86	1.17	0.93-1.44	1.22	0.98-1.51	
ECONOMICALLY ACTIVE PERSONS	43	1.00	0.72-1.35	1.00	0.72-1.35	
0 Technical, humanistic, etc. work	2	0.40	0.05-1.44	0.74	0.09-2.66	
1 Administrative and clerical work	2	0.40	0.05-1.44	1.04	0.13-3.77	
2 Sales professions	2	0.48	0.06-1.75	0.56	0.07-2.03	
3 Farming, forestry and fishing	18	1.73	1.02-2.73	1.54	0.91-2.43	*
30 Agricultural/forestry management	7	2.53	1.02-5.20	2.09	0.84-4.30	*
300 Farmers, silviculturists	7	2.59	1.04-5.34	2.13	0.86-4.39	*
31 Farming, animal husbandry	11	1.44	0.72-2.58	1.32	0.66-2.36	
312 Livestock workers	7	1.07	0.43-2.20	1.00	0.40-2.06	
4 Mining and quarrying	-	-/0.0	0.00-287	-/0.0	0.00-297	
5 Transport and communications	-	-/1.5	0.00-2.46	-/1.1	0.00-3.30	
6/7 Industrial and construction work	7	0.91	0.36-1.87	0.85	0.34-1.75	
676 Cabinetmakers etc.	1	54.5	1.38-303	55.0	1.39-306	*
734 Pulp mill workers	1	43.9	1.11-245	44.4	1.12-247	*
781 Freight handlers	1	62.0	1.57-346	38.9	0.98-216	*
8 Services	12	1.32	0.68-2.31	0.88	0.46-1.54	
811 Chefs, cooks etc.	4	5.06	1.38-12.9	5.19	1.42-13.3	*
83 Caretakers and cleaners	4	0.95	0.26-2.44	0.53	0.14-1.35	
831 Cleaners	4	1.07	0.29-2.73	0.56	0.15-1.43	
9 Work not classified elsewhere	-	-/0.1	0.00-39.0	-/0.1	0.00-40.4	
ECONOMICALLY INACTIVE PERSONS	43	1.41	1.02-1.89	1.56	1.13-2.10	*

C3. Oesophageal cancer, males

Occupation	Obs.	Crude SIR	95% CI	Adjusted SIR	95% CI	
WHOLE POPULATION	599	1.17	1.08-1.27	1.16	1.07-1.26	*
ECONOMICALLY ACTIVE PERSONS	444	1.00	0.91-1.10	1.00	0.91-1.10	
0 Technical, humanistic, etc. work	23	0.57	0.36-0.85	0.72	0.45-1.08	*
01 Technical work	8	0.54	0.23-1.06	0.64	0.28-1.26	
010 Civil engineering technicians	3	0.54	0.11-1.58	0.65	0.13-1.90	
05 Teaching	2	0.24	0.03-0.87	0.32	0.04-1.17	*
1 Administrative and clerical work	29	1.07	0.71-1.53	1.38	0.92-1.98	
11 Corporate administration	10	0.78	0.37-1.43	1.05	0.51-1.94	
110 Corporate managers	6	1.00	0.37-2.17	1.36	0.50-2.96	
14/15 Clerical work NOS	13	1.26	0.67-2.15	1.51	0.81-2.59	
150 Property managers, warehousemen	5	0.96	0.31-2.24	1.16	0.38-2.71	
2 Sales professions	17	0.82	0.48-1.31	0.92	0.53-1.47	
20 Wholesale and retail dealers	5	0.80	0.26-1.88	0.98	0.32-2.30	
201 Retailers	4	0.67	0.18-1.72	0.82	0.22-2.10	
23 Sales work	8	0.90	0.39-1.78	0.94	0.41-1.85	
231 Shop personnel	5	0.91	0.30-2.13	0.89	0.29-2.08	
3 Farming, forestry and fishing	120	0.92	0.76-1.09	0.87	0.72-1.03	
30 Agricultural/forestry management	97	0.89	0.72-1.09	0.87	0.71-1.06	
300 Farmers, silviculturists	91	0.88	0.71-1.08	0.86	0.69-1.05	
31 Farming, animal husbandry	4	0.63	0.17-1.61	0.52	0.14-1.34	
310 Agricultural workers	4	0.84	0.23-2.15	0.71	0.19-1.81	
34 Forestry work	19	1.34	0.81-2.09	1.04	0.63-1.62	
4 Mining and quarrying	8	3.25	1.40-6.40	3.13	1.35-6.17	*
41 Deep drilling	2	8.92	1.08-32.2	8.84	1.07-31.9	*
5 Transport and communications	38	0.93	0.66-1.27	0.98	0.70-1.35	
54 Road transport	22	0.89	0.56-1.35	0.94	0.59-1.43	
540 Motor-vehicle and tram drivers	22	0.89	0.56-1.35	0.95	0.59-1.43	
6/7 Industrial and construction work	189	1.18	1.02-1.35	1.10	0.95-1.26	*
65 Machine shop/steelworkers	26	0.83	0.55-1.22	0.82	0.53-1.20	
650 Turners, machinists	6	0.86	0.31-1.86	0.83	0.30-1.80	
652 Machine and motor repairers	2	0.28	0.03-1.00	0.28	0.03-0.99	*
66 Electrical work	13	1.39	0.74-2.38	1.35	0.72-2.31	
660 Electricians (indoors)	12	2.38	1.23-4.16	2.31	1.20-4.04	*
67 Woodwork	37	1.11	0.78-1.53	1.08	0.76-1.48	
673 Construction carpenters	21	1.00	0.62-1.53	0.96	0.60-1.47	
676 Cabinetmakers etc.	5	4.11	1.34-9.60	4.11	1.33-9.59	*
68 Painting and lacquering	11	1.82	0.91-3.25	1.81	0.90-3.23	
680 Painters	11	1.96	0.98-3.50	1.95	0.97-3.48	
69 Construction work NOS	40	1.53	1.09-2.08	1.26	0.90-1.72	*
697 Building hands	21	1.99	1.23-3.04	1.54	0.95-2.35	*
698 Roadbuilding hands	7	0.97	0.39-2.00	0.75	0.30-1.55	
73 Chemical process/paper making	3	0.56	0.12-1.65	0.54	0.11-1.58	
77 Machinists	17	1.44	0.84-2.30	1.40	0.82-2.24	
774 Greasers	4	4.37	1.19-11.2	4.27	1.16-10.9	*
78 Dock and warehouse work	10	1.04	0.50-1.91	0.86	0.41-1.57	
782 Warehousemen	6	1.02	0.37-2.22	0.81	0.30-1.77	
79 Labourers not classified elsewhere	11	1.95	0.97-3.49	1.51	0.75-2.70	
8 Services	15	0.83	0.46-1.36	0.83	0.47-1.38	
80 Watchmen, security guards	4	0.50	0.14-1.29	0.53	0.15-1.37	
83 Caretakers and cleaners	6	0.78	0.29-1.71	0.75	0.27-1.63	
830 Caretakers	6	0.87	0.32-1.90	0.84	0.31-1.82	
9 Work not classified elsewhere	5	1.82	0.59-4.24	1.97	0.64-4.60	
91 Occupation not specified	5	4.45	1.44-10.4	4.34	1.41-10.1	*
ECONOMICALLY INACTIVE PERSONS	155	2.29	1.94-2.66	2.17	1.85-2.53	*

Occupation	Obs.	Crude SIR	95% CI	Adjusted SIR	95% CI

C4. Oesophageal cancer, females

Occupation	Obs.	Crude SIR	95% CI	Adjusted SIR	95% CI
WHOLE POPULATION	462	1.05	0.96-1.15	1.07	0.97-1.17
ECONOMICALLY ACTIVE PERSONS	243	1.00	0.88-1.13	1.00	0.88-1.13
0 Technical, humanistic, etc. work	17	0.64	0.37-1.03	0.96	0.56-1.53
03 Medical work and nursing	9	0.81	0.37-1.53	0.93	0.43-1.77
036 Auxiliary nurses	4	0.81	0.22-2.07	0.79	0.21-2.01
05 Teaching	4	0.50	0.13-1.27	1.05	0.29-2.69
1 Administrative and clerical work	21	0.79	0.49-1.20	1.03	0.64-1.58
12 Clerical work	6	0.93	0.34-2.02	1.20	0.44-2.60
14/15 Clerical work NOS	10	0.60	0.29-1.11	0.77	0.37-1.41
144 Office clerks	8	0.71	0.31-1.40	0.90	0.39-1.78
2 Sales professions	20	0.91	0.56-1.40	0.97	0.59-1.49
23 Sales work	18	1.02	0.60-1.61	1.04	0.62-1.64
231 Shop personnel	17	1.02	0.60-1.64	1.03	0.60-1.65
3 Farming, forestry and fishing	63	1.01	0.78-1.29	0.95	0.73-1.21
30 Agricultural/forestry management	14	0.75	0.41-1.26	0.69	0.37-1.15
300 Farmers, silviculturists	14	0.77	0.42-1.29	0.70	0.38-1.18
31 Farming, animal husbandry	48	1.10	0.81-1.46	1.04	0.77-1.39
312 Livestock workers	39	1.05	0.75-1.43	1.00	0.71-1.37
4 Mining and quarrying	-	-/0.1	0.00-44.8	-/0.1	0.00-43.9
5 Transport and communications	6	0.74	0.27-1.61	0.80	0.29-1.73
6/7 Industrial and construction work	57	1.33	1.01-1.72	1.28	0.97-1.66 *
60 Textiles	10	1.88	0.90-3.46	1.89	0.91-3.47
61 Cutting/sewing etc.	15	1.71	0.96-2.82	1.77	0.99-2.92
612 Furriers	2	11.5	1.39-41.6	12.2	1.48-44.2 *
69 Construction work NOS	6	3.27	1.20-7.11	2.40	0.88-5.22 *
697 Building hands	6	3.93	1.44-8.56	2.85	1.05-6.21 *
72 Food industry	5	0.98	0.32-2.28	0.96	0.31-2.25
8 Services	59	1.10	0.83-1.41	0.91	0.69-1.17
81 Housekeeping, domestic work, etc.	17	0.90	0.53-1.44	0.78	0.46-1.25
812 Kitchen assistants	6	1.24	0.45-2.69	0.91	0.33-1.97
813 Domestic servants	4	0.73	0.20-1.88	0.58	0.16-1.49
83 Caretakers and cleaners	33	1.31	0.90-1.84	0.99	0.68-1.39
831 Cleaners	30	1.33	0.89-1.89	0.97	0.66-1.39
9 Work not classified elsewhere	-	-/0.6	0.00-6.62	-/0.6	0.00-6.54
ECONOMICALLY INACTIVE PERSONS	219	1.11	0.97-1.27	1.15	1.00-1.31 *

C5. Stomach cancer, males

Occupation	Obs.	Crude SIR	95% CI	Adjusted SIR	95% CI
WHOLE POPULATION	4364	1.03	1.00-1.06	1.02	0.99-1.05
ECONOMICALLY ACTIVE PERSONS	3669	1.00	0.97-1.03	1.00	0.97-1.03
0 Technical, humanistic, etc. work	244	0.72	0.63-0.81	0.95	0.84-1.07 *
00 Technical professions	23	0.61	0.38-0.91	0.98	0.62-1.47 *
001 Civil engineers	4	0.49	0.13-1.26	0.79	0.22-2.03
002 Electrical engineers	4	0.79	0.21-2.02	1.26	0.34-3.22
004 Mechanical engineers	10	0.89	0.43-1.63	1.43	0.68-2.63
01 Technical work	101	0.82	0.67-0.99	0.94	0.76-1.13 *
010 Civil engineering technicians	39	0.85	0.61-1.17	0.97	0.69-1.33
011 Power technicians	7	0.70	0.28-1.45	0.81	0.33-1.67
012 Teletechnicians	3	0.54	0.11-1.59	0.63	0.13-1.83
013 Mechanical technicians	23	0.72	0.45-1.08	0.82	0.52-1.23

Occupation	Obs.	Crude		Adjusted	
		SIR	95% CI	SIR	95% CI
016 Technicians NOS	14	1.11	0.61-1.87	1.27	0.70-2.13
018 Draughtsmen, survey assistants	5	0.75	0.24-1.76	0.87	0.28-2.02
02 Chemical/physical/biological work	15	0.70	0.39-1.15	0.94	0.53-1.55
021 Physicists	2	5.88	0.71-21.3	9.55	1.16-34.5 *
027 Consultancy, agriculture	6	0.98	0.36-2.14	1.20	0.44-2.61
028 Consultancy, forestry	6	0.59	0.21-1.27	0.79	0.29-1.71
03 Medical work and nursing	10	0.59	0.28-1.08	0.79	0.38-1.46
030 Medical doctors	3	0.32	0.07-0.93	0.51	0.10-1.49 *
04 Health-care related work	5	0.90	0.29-2.11	1.14	0.37-2.67
05 Teaching	47	0.66	0.49-0.88	0.99	0.73-1.32 *
050 University teachers	5	0.78	0.25-1.82	1.25	0.41-2.92
051 Subject teachers	11	0.80	0.40-1.43	1.26	0.63-2.26
052 Primary school teachers	16	0.58	0.33-0.95	0.93	0.53-1.51 *
054 Vocational teachers	11	0.67	0.33-1.20	0.87	0.44-1.56
06 Religious professions	8	0.90	0.39-1.78	1.27	0.55-2.51
060 Clergy and lay preachers	8	0.99	0.43-1.96	1.42	0.61-2.80
07 Legal professions	5	0.48	0.16-1.12	0.71	0.23-1.66
08 Artistic and literary professions	18	0.80	0.47-1.26	1.13	0.67-1.79
084 Journalists	3	0.40	0.08-1.18	0.60	0.12-1.77
087 Musicians	4	0.71	0.19-1.82	0.97	0.27-2.49
088 Film and radio producers	3	3.61	0.74-10.6	5.91	1.22-17.3 *
09 Humanistic and social work etc.	12	0.55	0.29-0.97	0.75	0.39-1.31 *
091 Social workers	5	0.97	0.32-2.27	1.22	0.40-2.84
096 PR officers	5	0.63	0.20-1.47	0.80	0.26-1.88
1 Administrative and clerical work	173	0.77	0.66-0.89	1.05	0.90-1.22 *
10 Public administration	8	0.37	0.16-0.73	0.59	0.25-1.15 *
11 Corporate administration	72	0.68	0.53-0.86	1.08	0.84-1.36 *
110 Corporate managers	40	0.82	0.59-1.12	1.29	0.92-1.75
111 Technical managers	4	0.43	0.12-1.11	0.69	0.19-1.76
112 Commercial managers	13	0.52	0.28-0.89	0.82	0.44-1.41 *
113 Administrative managers	5	0.92	0.30-2.15	1.47	0.48-3.42
119 Private sector managers NOS	9	0.73	0.33-1.39	1.16	0.53-2.21
12 Clerical work	13	1.39	0.74-2.37	1.69	0.90-2.89
120 Book-keepers, accountants	13	1.64	0.87-2.80	2.02	1.08-3.46 *
14/15 Clerical work NOS	79	0.93	0.73-1.16	1.06	0.84-1.32
144 Office clerks	10	0.72	0.34-1.32	0.81	0.39-1.49
145 Bank clerks	3	0.59	0.12-1.72	0.78	0.16-2.27
150 Property managers, warehousemen	47	1.10	0.81-1.46	1.24	0.91-1.64
159 Clerical workers NOS	9	0.89	0.41-1.68	1.00	0.46-1.90
2 Sales professions	128	0.74	0.61-0.87	0.79	0.66-0.94 *
20 Wholesale and retail dealers	42	0.83	0.60-1.12	0.93	0.67-1.26
201 Retailers	40	0.82	0.59-1.12	0.92	0.66-1.26
21 Real estate, services, securities	12	0.93	0.48-1.63	1.10	0.57-1.93
210 Insurance salesmen	6	0.80	0.29-1.74	0.91	0.34-1.99
22 Sales representatives	25	0.70	0.45-1.03	0.81	0.52-1.19
220 Commercial travellers, etc.	21	0.64	0.40-0.98	0.74	0.46-1.14 *
23 Sales work	49	0.66	0.49-0.87	0.66	0.49-0.87 *
230 Buyers, office sales staff	11	0.79	0.39-1.41	0.93	0.47-1.67
231 Shop personnel	27	0.58	0.39-0.85	0.54	0.36-0.79 *
232 Door-to-door salesmen	8	1.60	0.69-3.15	1.76	0.76-3.47
233 Service station attendants	2	0.36	0.04-1.31	0.42	0.05-1.51
3 Farming, forestry and fishing	1158	1.08	1.02-1.14	1.03	0.97-1.09 *
30 Agricultural/forestry management	924	1.04	0.97-1.11	1.01	0.94-1.07
300 Farmers, silviculturists	881	1.04	0.98-1.11	1.01	0.94-1.08
302 Forestry managers	24	0.78	0.50-1.16	0.88	0.57-1.31
305 Fur-bearing animal breeders	6	1.26	0.46-2.75	1.19	0.44-2.60
31 Farming, animal husbandry	54	0.99	0.75-1.30	0.89	0.67-1.17
310 Agricultural workers	37	0.90	0.64-1.25	0.82	0.58-1.13
311 Gardeners	4	0.61	0.16-1.55	0.52	0.14-1.33
312 Livestock workers	10	1.96	0.94-3.61	1.78	0.85-3.27
33 Fishing	11	1.13	0.57-2.03	1.07	0.54-1.92
330 Fishermen	11	1.18	0.59-2.10	1.11	0.55-1.98
34 Forestry work	169	1.43	1.22-1.66	1.22	1.04-1.41 *
4 Mining and quarrying	30	1.47	0.99-2.10	1.39	0.94-1.98
40 Mining and quarrying	24	1.90	1.22-2.83	1.80	1.15-2.68 *

Appendix Table C

Occupation	Obs.	Crude SIR	95% CI	Adjusted SIR	95% CI
5 Transport and communications	326	0.96	0.86-1.07	0.97	0.87-1.08
50 Ship's officers	12	0.81	0.42-1.42	0.99	0.51-1.74
500 Ship's masters and mates	3	0.45	0.09-1.33	0.61	0.13-1.80
502 Chief engineers in ships	7	1.32	0.53-2.72	1.49	0.60-3.07
51 Deck and engine-room crew	10	1.10	0.53-2.02	1.02	0.49-1.88
510 Deck crew	7	1.13	0.45-2.32	1.05	0.42-2.16
53 Engine drivers	8	0.54	0.23-1.07	0.50	0.22-0.98 *
54 Road transport	206	0.99	0.86-1.13	0.99	0.86-1.13
540 Motor-vehicle and tram drivers	206	1.00	0.86-1.14	1.00	0.87-1.14
55 Transport services	30	0.91	0.61-1.30	0.89	0.60-1.26
550 Railway staff	30	0.93	0.62-1.32	0.90	0.61-1.28
56 Traffic supervisors	11	0.57	0.28-1.02	0.70	0.35-1.26
562 Railway traffic supervisors	4	0.42	0.11-1.07	0.50	0.14-1.29
563 Road transport supervisors	5	0.74	0.24-1.73	0.95	0.31-2.22
57 Post and telecommunications	8	0.81	0.35-1.60	0.92	0.40-1.81
570 Post/telecommunications officials	7	0.91	0.36-1.87	1.02	0.41-2.11
58 Postal services/couriers	30	1.34	0.91-1.92	1.26	0.85-1.80
580 Postmen	19	1.40	0.85-2.19	1.30	0.78-2.03
581 Caretakers/messengers	11	1.25	0.62-2.23	1.20	0.60-2.14
59 Communication work NOS	10	1.17	0.56-2.16	1.10	0.53-2.03
599 Communication workers NOS	7	1.08	0.43-2.22	1.01	0.41-2.08
6/7 Industrial and construction work	1435	1.08	1.02-1.14	1.00	0.95-1.05 *
60 Textiles	9	0.73	0.33-1.38	0.69	0.31-1.31
61 Cutting/sewing etc.	9	0.72	0.33-1.37	0.72	0.33-1.36
62 Shoes and leather	8	0.75	0.33-1.48	0.75	0.32-1.48
63 Smelting, metal and foundry work	44	1.19	0.86-1.59	1.13	0.82-1.51
630 Smelter furnacemen	5	0.80	0.26-1.86	0.74	0.24-1.74
634 Blacksmiths	13	1.31	0.70-2.24	1.30	0.69-2.23
635 Founders	12	1.13	0.59-1.98	1.06	0.55-1.84
639 Metalworkers NOS	8	1.28	0.55-2.52	1.20	0.52-2.36
64 Precision mechanical work	10	0.70	0.33-1.28	0.70	0.33-1.28
65 Machine shop/steelworkers	280	1.08	0.95-1.21	1.02	0.90-1.14
650 Turners, machinists	50	0.87	0.64-1.15	0.82	0.61-1.08
651 Fitter-assemblers etc.	20	0.80	0.49-1.23	0.75	0.46-1.15
652 Machine and motor repairers	69	1.14	0.89-1.45	1.09	0.85-1.38
653 Sheetmetalworkers	29	1.21	0.81-1.73	1.14	0.77-1.64
654 Plumbers	39	1.16	0.82-1.58	1.10	0.78-1.50
655 Welders and flame cutters	38	1.47	1.04-2.02	1.37	0.97-1.88 *
656 Plate/constructional steel work	5	0.65	0.21-1.53	0.61	0.20-1.42
659 Machine shop/steelworkers NOS	27	1.12	0.74-1.62	1.06	0.70-1.54
66 Electrical work	83	1.06	0.85-1.32	1.00	0.79-1.23
660 Electricians (indoors)	50	1.18	0.88-1.56	1.11	0.82-1.46
661 Electric machine operators	4	0.67	0.18-1.71	0.62	0.17-1.60
664 Telephone installers and repair	8	0.68	0.29-1.34	0.63	0.27-1.24
665 Linemen	9	1.15	0.52-2.17	1.07	0.49-2.02
67 Woodwork	303	1.12	1.00-1.25	1.06	0.94-1.18
670 Round-timber workers	10	1.63	0.78-3.00	1.54	0.74-2.82
671 Timber workers	36	1.06	0.74-1.47	1.01	0.70-1.39
672 Plywood makers	15	1.63	0.91-2.69	1.52	0.85-2.51
673 Construction carpenters	199	1.17	1.02-1.34	1.11	0.96-1.26 *
674 Boatbuilders etc.	5	0.78	0.25-1.82	0.76	0.25-1.78
675 Bench carpenters	17	1.08	0.63-1.73	1.07	0.62-1.71
676 Cabinetmakers etc.	7	0.70	0.28-1.45	0.68	0.27-1.39
677 Woodworking machine operators e	13	0.86	0.46-1.47	0.82	0.43-1.39
68 Painting and lacquering	53	1.04	0.78-1.37	1.00	0.75-1.31
680 Painters	50	1.06	0.79-1.40	1.02	0.76-1.35
69 Construction work NOS	246	1.14	1.00-1.29	1.01	0.89-1.14 *
690 Bricklayers and tile setters	29	1.06	0.71-1.52	1.00	0.67-1.44
692 Reinforcing iron workers	3	0.46	0.09-1.34	0.43	0.09-1.25
693 Concrete/cement shutterers	21	1.18	0.73-1.81	1.11	0.69-1.70
695 Insulators	9	1.71	0.78-3.25	1.62	0.74-3.07
697 Building hands	102	1.17	0.96-1.41	1.00	0.82-1.20
698 Roadbuilding hands	61	1.03	0.79-1.33	0.89	0.68-1.14
699 Construction workers NOS	15	1.68	0.94-2.77	1.63	0.91-2.69
70 Printing	15	0.84	0.47-1.38	0.78	0.44-1.29
700 Typographers etc.	10	1.42	0.68-2.62	1.32	0.64-2.44
701 Printers	1	0.19	0.00-1.04	0.17	0.00-0.97 *
71 Glass and ceramic work	14	1.60	0.88-2.69	1.51	0.82-2.53
72 Food industry	33	1.15	0.79-1.62	1.10	0.76-1.54
721 Bakers and pastry chiefs	2	0.30	0.04-1.08	0.29	0.04-1.05

Occupation	Obs.	Crude SIR	95% CI	Adjusted SIR	95% CI
725 Butchers and sausage makers	12	1.61	0.83-2.81	1.50	0.78-2.63
73 Chemical process/paper making	41	0.92	0.66-1.25	0.86	0.62-1.17
734 Pulp mill workers	11	0.90	0.45-1.61	0.84	0.42-1.50
735 Paper and board mill workers	15	0.90	0.50-1.48	0.84	0.47-1.38
739 Chemical process workers NOS	7	0.87	0.35-1.80	0.81	0.33-1.68
75 Industrial work NOS	29	0.99	0.67-1.43	0.95	0.64-1.37
752 Plastics	9	1.68	0.77-3.19	1.58	0.72-3.00
76 Packing and labelling	14	1.19	0.65-2.00	1.11	0.61-1.87
77 Machinists	107	1.08	0.88-1.29	1.02	0.83-1.22
770 Crane and hoist operators	9	1.29	0.59-2.45	1.19	0.54-2.26
771 Forklift operators	15	1.07	0.60-1.77	0.99	0.55-1.63
772 Construction machinery operator	37	1.15	0.81-1.59	1.12	0.79-1.54
773 Operators of stationary engine	20	0.79	0.48-1.21	0.74	0.45-1.14
774 Greasers	10	1.29	0.62-2.37	1.22	0.58-2.24
775 Industrial personnel, riggers	16	1.23	0.70-2.00	1.15	0.66-1.86
78 Dock and warehouse work	75	0.94	0.74-1.18	0.82	0.65-1.03
780 Dockers	19	0.99	0.60-1.55	0.92	0.56-1.44
781 Freight handlers	14	1.19	0.65-2.00	1.02	0.55-1.70
782 Warehousemen	42	0.86	0.62-1.17	0.74	0.54-1.01
79 Labourers not classified elsewhere	62	1.33	1.02-1.70	1.13	0.87-1.45 *
8 Services	151	1.02	0.86-1.19	1.01	0.85-1.17
80 Watchmen, security guards	68	1.05	0.82-1.34	1.09	0.85-1.38
800 Firemen	5	0.80	0.26-1.87	0.83	0.27-1.94
801 Policemen	24	0.94	0.60-1.40	1.07	0.69-1.60
802 Customs/border control	6	0.91	0.33-1.98	1.07	0.39-2.32
803 Prison guards	7	1.33	0.53-2.73	1.27	0.51-2.61
804 Civilian guards	26	1.25	0.81-1.83	1.14	0.74-1.67
83 Caretakers and cleaners	71	1.13	0.88-1.43	1.06	0.83-1.34
830 Caretakers	62	1.10	0.85-1.42	1.04	0.80-1.33
89 Services NOS	7	1.01	0.41-2.08	0.94	0.38-1.94
890 Hotel porters	6	1.04	0.38-2.27	0.98	0.36-2.12
9 Work not classified elsewhere	24	1.03	0.66-1.54	1.19	0.76-1.77
90 Military occupations	11	0.79	0.40-1.42	1.08	0.54-1.93
900 Officers etc.	4	0.65	0.18-1.65	1.09	0.30-2.79
901 Non-commissioned officers	7	0.96	0.39-1.98	1.14	0.46-2.34
91 Occupation not specified	13	1.38	0.74-2.36	1.31	0.70-2.24
ECONOMICALLY INACTIVE PERSONS	695	1.20	1.11-1.29	1.15	1.07-1.24 *

C6. Stomach cancer, females

	Obs.	Crude SIR	95% CI	Adjusted SIR	95% CI
WHOLE POPULATION	2698	1.06	1.02-1.10	1.06	1.02-1.11 *
ECONOMICALLY ACTIVE PERSONS	1461	1.00	0.95-1.05	1.00	0.95-1.05
0 Technical, humanistic, etc. work	157	0.87	0.74-1.01	0.99	0.84-1.15
01 Technical work	9	1.04	0.48-1.98	1.11	0.51-2.10
019 Laboratory assistants	7	1.26	0.51-2.59	1.34	0.54-2.75
03 Medical work and nursing	86	1.10	0.88-1.36	1.11	0.89-1.37
032 Nurses	25	1.12	0.72-1.65	1.21	0.78-1.79
035 Psychiatric nurses	9	1.66	0.76-3.16	1.75	0.80-3.32
036 Auxiliary nurses	34	1.00	0.69-1.39	0.92	0.64-1.29
04 Health-care related work	8	0.75	0.32-1.48	0.94	0.40-1.84
040 Pharmacists	6	0.93	0.34-2.01	1.30	0.48-2.82
05 Teaching	34	0.63	0.43-0.88	0.84	0.58-1.17 *
051 Subject teachers	5	0.38	0.12-0.89	0.57	0.18-1.32 *
052 Primary school teachers	19	0.74	0.45-1.16	1.03	0.62-1.62
053 Teachers of practical subjects	4	0.58	0.16-1.48	0.68	0.18-1.73
08 Artistic and literary professions	2	0.31	0.04-1.14	0.40	0.05-1.43
09 Humanistic and social work etc.	7	0.51	0.20-1.04	0.60	0.24-1.24
091 Social workers	5	0.78	0.25-1.83	0.89	0.29-2.08
092 Librarians, museum officials	-	-/4.2	0.00-0.87	-/3.5	0.00-1.04 *
1 Administrative and clerical work	166	0.93	0.80-1.08	1.00	0.85-1.15
11 Corporate administration	10	2.10	1.01-3.86	2.76	1.32-5.07 *

Appendix Table C

Occupation	Obs.	Crude SIR	95% CI	Adjusted SIR	95% CI
110 Corporate managers	7	3.59	1.44-7.40	4.46	1.79-9.18 *
12 Clerical work	34	0.83	0.57-1.16	0.87	0.60-1.22
120 Book-keepers, accountants	7	0.36	0.15-0.74	0.38	0.15-0.78 *
121 Office cashiers	7	0.86	0.34-1.76	0.90	0.36-1.85
123 Shop and restaurant cashiers	16	1.53	0.87-2.48	1.61	0.92-2.62
13 Stenographers and typists	13	0.81	0.43-1.39	0.87	0.46-1.48
130 Private secretaries	6	0.68	0.25-1.49	0.73	0.27-1.59
131 Typists	7	0.97	0.39-2.00	1.03	0.41-2.12
14/15 Clerical work NOS	109	0.97	0.79-1.16	1.02	0.84-1.23
144 Office clerks	74	0.98	0.77-1.23	1.04	0.81-1.30
145 Bank clerks	7	0.54	0.22-1.11	0.58	0.23-1.20
159 Clerical workers NOS	14	1.37	0.75-2.31	1.44	0.79-2.42
2 Sales professions	139	0.98	0.83-1.15	0.95	0.80-1.11
20 Wholesale and retail dealers	21	0.97	0.60-1.48	1.00	0.62-1.54
201 Retailers	20	0.92	0.56-1.43	0.96	0.59-1.49
23 Sales work	113	0.97	0.80-1.16	0.92	0.76-1.10
231 Shop personnel	107	0.97	0.80-1.17	0.92	0.76-1.10
3 Farming, forestry and fishing	343	1.00	0.90-1.11	0.98	0.88-1.09
30 Agricultural/forestry management	104	1.13	0.92-1.35	1.10	0.90-1.33
300 Farmers, silviculturists	101	1.12	0.92-1.35	1.10	0.90-1.33
31 Farming, animal husbandry	238	0.96	0.84-1.08	0.94	0.82-1.06
310 Agricultural workers	26	1.03	0.68-1.52	1.02	0.67-1.50
311 Gardeners	6	0.65	0.24-1.42	0.62	0.23-1.35
312 Livestock workers	203	0.95	0.82-1.09	0.93	0.81-1.07
4 Mining and quarrying	-	-/0.5	0.00-8.12	-/0.5	0.00-8.01
5 Transport and communications	41	0.83	0.59-1.12	0.84	0.60-1.13
57 Post and telecommunications	21	0.81	0.50-1.24	0.85	0.53-1.30
570 Post/telecommunications officials	7	0.63	0.26-1.31	0.66	0.27-1.37
571 Telephone operators	8	0.86	0.37-1.69	0.89	0.39-1.76
58 Postal services/couriers	10	0.67	0.32-1.24	0.65	0.31-1.19
580 Postmen	10	0.78	0.37-1.43	0.75	0.36-1.37
6/7 Industrial and construction work	281	1.08	0.96-1.21	1.04	0.92-1.16
60 Textiles	27	0.88	0.58-1.29	0.86	0.56-1.25
601 Spinners etc.	8	1.18	0.51-2.33	1.14	0.49-2.25
602 Weavers	7	0.67	0.27-1.38	0.66	0.26-1.35
61 Cutting/sewing etc.	63	1.19	0.91-1.52	1.14	0.88-1.46
611 Dressmakers	13	1.15	0.61-1.97	1.17	0.62-1.99
616 Garment workers	34	1.15	0.80-1.60	1.09	0.75-1.52
62 Shoes and leather	11	1.14	0.57-2.03	1.09	0.54-1.95
65 Machine shop/steelworkers	6	0.61	0.22-1.32	0.58	0.21-1.26
659 Machine shop/steelworkers NOS	5	0.83	0.27-1.94	0.79	0.26-1.84
66 Electrical work	5	1.03	0.34-2.41	0.96	0.31-2.24
67 Woodwork	20	0.91	0.56-1.41	0.87	0.53-1.35
672 Plywood makers	14	1.38	0.75-2.31	1.31	0.72-2.20
69 Construction work NOS	19	1.80	1.09-2.82	1.75	1.05-2.73 *
697 Building hands	13	1.49	0.79-2.54	1.44	0.77-2.47
70 Printing	10	1.03	0.49-1.89	0.99	0.47-1.81
703 Bookbinders	7	1.47	0.59-3.03	1.41	0.57-2.91
72 Food industry	30	0.97	0.65-1.38	0.93	0.63-1.33
721 Bakers and pastry chiefs	11	0.77	0.38-1.37	0.74	0.37-1.33
726 Dairy workers	6	0.97	0.36-2.12	0.91	0.33-1.98
73 Chemical process/paper making	9	1.05	0.48-2.00	1.01	0.46-1.92
75 Industrial work NOS	18	1.17	0.69-1.84	1.11	0.66-1.76
76 Packing and labelling	30	1.26	0.85-1.79	1.19	0.80-1.70
77 Machinists	7	1.34	0.54-2.75	1.28	0.52-2.64
78 Dock and warehouse work	11	0.95	0.48-1.70	0.92	0.46-1.65
782 Warehousemen	10	1.03	0.49-1.90	1.00	0.48-1.83
8 Services	333	1.09	0.97-1.21	1.05	0.94-1.17
81 Housekeeping, domestic work, etc.	116	1.10	0.91-1.31	1.07	0.89-1.28
810 Housekeepers	6	0.59	0.22-1.28	0.61	0.23-1.34
811 Chefs, cooks etc.	33	1.24	0.86-1.75	1.21	0.83-1.69
812 Kitchen assistants	30	1.05	0.71-1.50	1.02	0.69-1.45
813 Domestic servants	29	1.04	0.70-1.50	0.99	0.66-1.42
814 Communal home-help services	7	1.07	0.43-2.20	1.09	0.44-2.24
82 Waiters	33	1.09	0.75-1.52	1.05	0.72-1.47

Occupation	Obs.	Crude		Adjusted	
		SIR	95% CI	SIR	95% CI
820 Waiters in restaurants	18	1.28	0.76-2.03	1.22	0.72-1.93
821 Waiters in cafés etc.	15	0.92	0.51-1.51	0.89	0.50-1.47
83 Caretakers and cleaners	151	1.08	0.91-1.25	1.03	0.87-1.20
830 Caretakers	13	0.86	0.46-1.47	0.81	0.43-1.39
831 Cleaners	138	1.11	0.93-1.30	1.06	0.89-1.24
84 Hygiene and beauty services	11	0.78	0.39-1.39	0.79	0.39-1.41
840 Hairdressers and barbers	10	0.90	0.43-1.66	0.92	0.44-1.69
85 Laundry and pressing	14	1.13	0.62-1.90	1.11	0.61-1.86
850 Launderers	10	0.97	0.46-1.78	0.95	0.45-1.74
9 Work not classified elsewhere	1	0.32	0.01-1.76	0.31	0.01-1.70
ECONOMICALLY INACTIVE PERSONS	1237	1.13	1.07-1.19	1.15	1.09-1.22 *

C7. Colon cancer, males

Occupation	Obs.	Crude		Adjusted	
		SIR	95% CI	SIR	95% CI
WHOLE POPULATION	1744	1.02	0.97-1.07	1.02	0.98-1.07
ECONOMICALLY ACTIVE PERSONS	1517	1.00	0.95-1.05	1.00	0.95-1.05
0 Technical, humanistic, etc. work	185	1.27	1.09-1.46	1.05	0.90-1.20 *
00 Technical professions	26	1.54	1.01-2.26	1.16	0.76-1.70 *
004 Mechanical engineers	5	1.00	0.32-2.33	0.75	0.24-1.74
007 Engineers NOS	4	4.00	1.09-10.2	2.93	0.80-7.50 *
01 Technical work	76	1.44	1.13-1.80	1.32	1.04-1.65 *
010 Civil engineering technicians	29	1.50	1.01-2.16	1.37	0.92-1.97 *
013 Mechanical technicians	18	1.30	0.77-2.05	1.20	0.71-1.90
016 Technicians NOS	6	1.12	0.41-2.43	1.02	0.38-2.22
02 Chemical/physical/biological work	8	0.87	0.38-1.72	0.68	0.30-1.35
028 Consultancy, forestry	3	0.69	0.14-2.03	0.53	0.11-1.55
03 Medical work and nursing	7	0.96	0.39-1.97	0.78	0.31-1.60
030 Medical doctors	7	1.75	0.70-3.60	1.29	0.52-2.65
05 Teaching	31	1.01	0.69-1.43	0.79	0.54-1.12
051 Subject teachers	8	1.36	0.59-2.68	1.06	0.46-2.08
052 Primary school teachers	10	0.83	0.40-1.53	0.64	0.31-1.18
054 Vocational teachers	9	1.26	0.58-2.39	1.04	0.47-1.97
07 Legal professions	5	1.19	0.39-2.77	0.85	0.28-1.98
08 Artistic and literary professions	16	1.68	0.96-2.73	1.30	0.74-2.11
09 Humanistic and social work etc.	10	1.08	0.52-1.99	0.87	0.42-1.61
1 Administrative and clerical work	128	1.38	1.15-1.63	1.07	0.89-1.26 *
10 Public administration	10	1.14	0.55-2.09	0.80	0.38-1.46
11 Corporate administration	71	1.60	1.25-2.02	1.14	0.89-1.43 *
110 Corporate managers	33	1.64	1.13-2.30	1.14	0.78-1.60 *
111 Technical managers	6	1.51	0.55-3.29	1.08	0.40-2.36
112 Commercial managers	18	1.67	0.99-2.64	1.24	0.73-1.95
119 Private sector managers NOS	6	1.16	0.43-2.52	0.82	0.30-1.78
14/15 Clerical work NOS	41	1.16	0.84-1.58	1.04	0.75-1.41
144 Office clerks	7	1.22	0.49-2.52	1.10	0.44-2.27
150 Property managers, warehousemen	20	1.15	0.70-1.78	1.03	0.63-1.59
2 Sales professions	93	1.26	1.01-1.54	1.18	0.96-1.45 *
20 Wholesale and retail dealers	28	1.36	0.90-1.96	1.21	0.80-1.74
201 Retailers	27	1.37	0.90-1.99	1.22	0.80-1.78
21 Real estate, services, securities	4	0.73	0.20-1.87	0.65	0.18-1.67
22 Sales representatives	16	1.03	0.59-1.67	0.96	0.55-1.56
220 Commercial travellers, etc.	15	1.05	0.59-1.72	0.98	0.55-1.62
23 Sales work	45	1.40	1.02-1.87	1.38	1.01-1.85 *
230 Buyers, office sales staff	7	1.17	0.47-2.42	1.05	0.42-2.16
231 Shop personnel	28	1.38	0.92-2.00	1.43	0.95-2.07
239 Sales staff NOS	5	3.16	1.03-7.38	3.24	1.05-7.56 *
3 Farming, forestry and fishing	298	0.70	0.62-0.78	0.74	0.66-0.83 *
30 Agricultural/forestry management	249	0.71	0.63-0.80	0.74	0.65-0.84 *
300 Farmers, silviculturists	228	0.69	0.60-0.78	0.72	0.63-0.82 *
302 Forestry managers	10	0.78	0.38-1.44	0.71	0.34-1.30
31 Farming, animal husbandry	19	0.84	0.50-1.31	0.97	0.58-1.52

Occupation	Obs.	Crude SIR	95% CI	Adjusted SIR	95% CI
310 Agricultural workers	16	0.93	0.53-1.51	1.06	0.61-1.73
34 Forestry work	28	0.56	0.37-0.82	0.68	0.45-0.98 *
4 Mining and quarrying	9	1.05	0.48-2.00	1.11	0.51-2.10
40 Mining and quarrying	5	0.96	0.31-2.23	1.00	0.33-2.34
5 Transport and communications	153	1.06	0.89-1.23	1.03	0.87-1.20
50 Ship's officers	4	0.66	0.18-1.68	0.56	0.15-1.42
53 Engine drivers	8	1.21	0.52-2.39	1.29	0.56-2.54
54 Road transport	95	1.07	0.86-1.30	1.05	0.85-1.28
540 Motor-vehicle and tram drivers	95	1.07	0.87-1.31	1.05	0.85-1.29
55 Transport services	19	1.34	0.81-2.10	1.36	0.82-2.12
550 Railway staff	19	1.37	0.82-2.14	1.38	0.83-2.16
56 Traffic supervisors	8	1.00	0.43-1.98	0.83	0.36-1.64
58 Postal services/couriers	10	1.08	0.52-1.98	1.13	0.54-2.09
580 Postmen	3	0.52	0.11-1.51	0.55	0.11-1.60
6/7 Industrial and construction work	575	1.04	0.96-1.13	1.12	1.03-1.21 *
60 Textiles	6	1.18	0.43-2.57	1.23	0.45-2.69
61 Cutting/sewing etc.	8	1.61	0.69-3.17	1.59	0.68-3.12
63 Smelting, metal and foundry work	18	1.18	0.70-1.86	1.22	0.72-1.93
64 Precision mechanical work	10	1.64	0.79-3.01	1.61	0.77-2.97
644 Goldsmiths, silversmiths etc.	5	3.52	1.14-8.21	3.48	1.13-8.11 *
65 Machine shop/steelworkers	116	1.05	0.86-1.24	1.09	0.90-1.29
650 Turners, machinists	23	0.95	0.60-1.43	1.00	0.64-1.50
651 Fitter-assemblers etc.	6	0.56	0.20-1.22	0.58	0.21-1.27
652 Machine and motor repairers	35	1.35	0.94-1.88	1.39	0.97-1.93
653 Sheetmetalworkers	12	1.17	0.61-2.05	1.21	0.62-2.11
654 Plumbers	15	1.04	0.58-1.72	1.08	0.60-1.78
655 Welders and flame cutters	9	0.78	0.36-1.48	0.81	0.37-1.54
659 Machine shop/steelworkers NOS	12	1.19	0.62-2.09	1.25	0.65-2.18
66 Electrical work	45	1.34	0.97-1.79	1.39	1.02-1.87 *
660 Electricians (indoors)	32	1.76	1.20-2.48	1.83	1.25-2.58 *
664 Telephone installers and repair	7	1.36	0.55-2.81	1.43	0.57-2.94
67 Woodwork	106	0.96	0.78-1.15	1.01	0.82-1.21
671 Timber workers	13	0.93	0.50-1.60	0.98	0.52-1.67
673 Construction carpenters	59	0.86	0.65-1.10	0.91	0.69-1.17
675 Bench carpenters	7	1.10	0.44-2.26	1.10	0.44-2.26
677 Woodworking machine operators e	7	1.12	0.45-2.31	1.17	0.47-2.42
68 Painting and lacquering	22	1.05	0.66-1.60	1.08	0.68-1.64
680 Painters	21	1.09	0.68-1.67	1.12	0.69-1.71
69 Construction work NOS	76	0.86	0.68-1.08	1.02	0.80-1.28
690 Bricklayers and tile setters	9	0.80	0.37-1.53	0.85	0.39-1.61
693 Concrete/cement shutterers	3	0.40	0.08-1.17	0.42	0.09-1.23
697 Building hands	36	1.01	0.70-1.39	1.25	0.87-1.72
698 Roadbuilding hands	14	0.60	0.33-1.00	0.78	0.43-1.31
70 Printing	16	2.09	1.19-3.39	2.17	1.24-3.53 *
72 Food industry	13	1.09	0.58-1.86	1.12	0.60-1.91
73 Chemical process/paper making	17	0.91	0.53-1.45	0.96	0.56-1.53
734 Pulp mill workers	8	1.57	0.68-3.09	1.66	0.72-3.27
735 Paper and board mill workers	2	0.28	0.03-1.02	0.30	0.04-1.07
75 Industrial work NOS	14	1.14	0.62-1.92	1.17	0.64-1.97
76 Packing and labelling	5	1.01	0.33-2.35	1.06	0.35-2.48
77 Machinists	41	0.96	0.69-1.30	1.00	0.72-1.36
771 Forklift operators	4	0.65	0.18-1.66	0.68	0.18-1.73
772 Construction machinery operator	11	0.78	0.39-1.39	0.79	0.40-1.42
773 Operators of stationary engine	15	1.44	0.80-2.37	1.52	0.85-2.52
775 Industrial personnel, riggers	7	1.28	0.51-2.64	1.35	0.54-2.79
78 Dock and warehouse work	38	1.16	0.82-1.60	1.38	0.97-1.89
780 Dockers	11	1.42	0.71-2.53	1.53	0.77-2.74
782 Warehousemen	21	1.05	0.65-1.61	1.28	0.79-1.96
79 Labourers not classified elsewhere	13	0.71	0.38-1.21	0.92	0.49-1.57
8 Services	65	1.06	0.82-1.36	1.09	0.84-1.39
80 Watchmen, security guards	25	0.93	0.60-1.37	0.92	0.60-1.36
801 Policemen	15	1.34	0.75-2.22	1.24	0.69-2.04
804 Civilian guards	4	0.52	0.14-1.33	0.62	0.17-1.58
83 Caretakers and cleaners	28	1.10	0.73-1.59	1.18	0.78-1.70
830 Caretakers	24	1.06	0.68-1.57	1.12	0.72-1.67
9 Work not classified elsewhere	11	1.07	0.53-1.91	0.99	0.49-1.76

Occupation	Obs.	Crude SIR	95% CI	Adjusted SIR	95% CI
90 Military occupations	8	1.23	0.53-2.43	1.06	0.46-2.10
ECONOMICALLY INACTIVE PERSONS	227	1.15	1.00-1.30	1.23	1.08-1.40 *

C8. Colon cancer, females

Occupation	Obs.	Crude SIR	95% CI	Adjusted SIR	95% CI
WHOLE POPULATION	2031	0.97	0.93-1.01	0.97	0.93-1.01
ECONOMICALLY ACTIVE PERSONS	1217	1.00	0.94-1.06	1.00	0.94-1.06
0 Technical, humanistic, etc. work	174	1.14	0.98-1.31	1.03	0.88-1.19
001 Civil engineers	2	31.7	3.84-114	21.1	2.55-76.1 *
01 Technical work	11	1.49	0.75-2.67	1.26	0.63-2.26
019 Laboratory assistants	6	1.27	0.46-2.76	1.07	0.39-2.32
03 Medical work and nursing	69	1.04	0.81-1.31	1.01	0.78-1.27
032 Nurses	24	1.26	0.81-1.87	1.08	0.69-1.61
035 Psychiatric nurses	7	1.52	0.61-3.13	1.26	0.51-2.60
036 Auxiliary nurses	29	1.00	0.67-1.44	1.14	0.76-1.63
04 Health-care related work	7	0.78	0.31-1.60	0.67	0.27-1.37
040 Pharmacists	5	0.91	0.29-2.12	0.78	0.25-1.83
05 Teaching	58	1.27	0.97-1.64	1.11	0.84-1.43
050 University teachers	4	5.56	1.52-14.2	4.57	1.24-11.7 *
051 Subject teachers	10	0.89	0.43-1.64	0.76	0.36-1.39
052 Primary school teachers	27	1.26	0.83-1.83	1.14	0.75-1.66
053 Teachers of practical subjects	11	1.89	0.94-3.39	1.60	0.80-2.87
08 Artistic and literary professions	4	0.74	0.20-1.90	0.63	0.17-1.61
09 Humanistic and social work etc.	15	1.29	0.72-2.12	1.10	0.62-1.82
091 Social workers	7	1.30	0.52-2.68	1.14	0.46-2.34
1 Administrative and clerical work	174	1.16	0.99-1.34	0.97	0.84-1.13
12 Clerical work	33	0.96	0.66-1.34	0.79	0.55-1.11
120 Book-keepers, accountants	12	0.74	0.38-1.29	0.61	0.32-1.07
121 Office cashiers	5	0.73	0.24-1.71	0.60	0.20-1.40
123 Shop and restaurant cashiers	12	1.36	0.70-2.37	1.14	0.59-1.98
13 Stenographers and typists	17	1.25	0.73-2.00	1.06	0.62-1.70
130 Private secretaries	10	1.33	0.64-2.45	1.14	0.55-2.10
131 Typists	7	1.14	0.46-2.35	0.97	0.39-1.99
14/15 Clerical work NOS	115	1.21	1.00-1.44	1.01	0.84-1.21
144 Office clerks	79	1.24	0.98-1.55	1.04	0.82-1.30
145 Bank clerks	16	1.43	0.82-2.32	1.24	0.71-2.01
159 Clerical workers NOS	10	1.18	0.56-2.16	0.97	0.46-1.78
2 Sales professions	130	1.09	0.91-1.29	1.11	0.93-1.31
20 Wholesale and retail dealers	19	1.07	0.64-1.66	0.86	0.52-1.34
201 Retailers	19	1.07	0.65-1.67	0.86	0.52-1.34
23 Sales work	110	1.12	0.92-1.34	1.19	0.98-1.43
231 Shop personnel	102	1.10	0.90-1.32	1.19	0.97-1.43
3 Farming, forestry and fishing	224	0.80	0.70-0.90	0.83	0.73-0.95 *
30 Agricultural/forestry management	48	0.65	0.48-0.86	0.69	0.51-0.91 *
300 Farmers, silviculturists	48	0.67	0.49-0.88	0.71	0.52-0.94 *
31 Farming, animal husbandry	176	0.85	0.73-0.98	0.89	0.76-1.02 *
310 Agricultural workers	20	0.97	0.59-1.49	0.99	0.60-1.52
311 Gardeners	3	0.40	0.08-1.16	0.45	0.09-1.31
312 Livestock workers	151	0.85	0.72-0.99	0.88	0.75-1.03 *
4 Mining and quarrying	-	-/0.4	0.00-9.84	-/0.3	0.00-10.6
5 Transport and communications	60	1.45	1.10-1.86	1.33	1.01-1.71 *
54 Road transport	5	3.24	1.05-7.56	2.84	0.92-6.63 *
540 Motor-vehicle and tram drivers	5	3.40	1.10-7.93	2.95	0.96-6.87 *
57 Post and telecommunications	34	1.56	1.08-2.18	1.29	0.89-1.80 *
570 Post/telecommunications officials	16	1.71	0.98-2.78	1.42	0.81-2.30
571 Telephone operators	9	1.15	0.53-2.18	0.94	0.43-1.78
572 Switchboard operators	8	2.36	1.02-4.66	1.96	0.84-3.85 *
58 Postal services/couriers	13	1.06	0.56-1.81	1.17	0.62-2.00
580 Postmen	11	1.03	0.51-1.84	1.14	0.57-2.04

Appendix Table C

Occupation	Obs.	Crude SIR	95% CI	Adjusted SIR	95% CI
6/7 Industrial and construction work	211	0.98	0.85-1.11	1.06	0.92-1.21
60 Textiles	18	0.71	0.42-1.13	0.77	0.46-1.22
601 Spinners etc.	3	0.54	0.11-1.57	0.59	0.12-1.73
602 Weavers	7	0.82	0.33-1.68	0.85	0.34-1.76
61 Cutting/sewing etc.	47	1.06	0.78-1.41	1.11	0.81-1.47
611 Dressmakers	4	0.43	0.12-1.11	0.38	0.10-0.97 *
616 Garment workers	31	1.25	0.85-1.78	1.39	0.94-1.97
62 Shoes and leather	7	0.86	0.35-1.78	0.94	0.38-1.94
65 Machine shop/steelworkers	10	1.21	0.58-2.22	1.33	0.64-2.45
659 Machine shop/steelworkers NOS	7	1.39	0.56-2.86	1.54	0.62-3.18
67 Woodwork	14	0.76	0.42-1.28	0.85	0.46-1.42
672 Plywood makers	4	0.47	0.13-1.20	0.52	0.14-1.34
69 Construction work NOS	6	0.69	0.25-1.49	0.76	0.28-1.66
697 Building hands	5	0.69	0.22-1.61	0.77	0.25-1.79
70 Printing	10	1.23	0.59-2.26	1.37	0.66-2.52
72 Food industry	23	0.89	0.56-1.34	0.98	0.62-1.47
721 Bakers and pastry chiefs	12	1.01	0.52-1.77	1.09	0.56-1.90
726 Dairy workers	3	0.58	0.12-1.68	0.65	0.13-1.89
73 Chemical process/paper making	10	1.40	0.67-2.58	1.55	0.74-2.86
75 Industrial work NOS	14	1.08	0.59-1.82	1.20	0.65-2.01
76 Packing and labelling	21	1.05	0.65-1.60	1.18	0.73-1.80
78 Dock and warehouse work	11	1.15	0.57-2.05	1.26	0.63-2.25
782 Warehousemen	8	0.99	0.43-1.96	1.10	0.47-2.16
8 Services	243	0.96	0.84-1.08	1.02	0.90-1.16
81 Housekeeping, domestic work, etc.	74	0.85	0.67-1.07	0.89	0.70-1.12
810 Housekeepers	10	1.19	0.57-2.18	0.97	0.47-1.79
811 Chefs, cooks etc.	15	0.69	0.38-1.13	0.75	0.42-1.24
812 Kitchen assistants	26	1.10	0.72-1.61	1.20	0.78-1.76
813 Domestic servants	14	0.62	0.34-1.04	0.70	0.38-1.17
814 Communal home-help services	6	1.08	0.40-2.35	1.04	0.38-2.26
82 Waiters	35	1.36	0.95-1.90	1.39	0.97-1.93
820 Waiters in restaurants	14	1.18	0.65-1.98	1.27	0.69-2.12
821 Waiters in cafés etc.	21	1.52	0.94-2.32	1.49	0.92-2.28
83 Caretakers and cleaners	109	0.94	0.77-1.13	1.06	0.87-1.27
830 Caretakers	13	1.02	0.55-1.75	1.14	0.61-1.96
831 Cleaners	95	0.93	0.75-1.13	1.04	0.85-1.28
84 Hygiene and beauty services	12	1.02	0.53-1.78	0.91	0.47-1.59
840 Hairdressers and barbers	11	1.18	0.59-2.12	1.03	0.51-1.84
85 Laundry and pressing	8	0.78	0.34-1.54	0.82	0.36-1.62
850 Launderers	6	0.70	0.26-1.53	0.73	0.27-1.60
9 Work not classified elsewhere	1	0.38	0.01-2.13	0.42	0.01-2.32
ECONOMICALLY INACTIVE PERSONS	814	0.92	0.86-0.99	0.93	0.87-1.00 *

C9. Rectal cancer, males

Occupation	Obs.	Crude SIR	95% CI	Adjusted SIR	95% CI
WHOLE POPULATION	1678	1.00	0.95-1.05	1.00	0.96-1.05
ECONOMICALLY ACTIVE PERSONS	1461	1.00	0.95-1.05	1.00	0.95-1.05
0 Technical, humanistic, etc. work	167	1.23	1.05-1.42	1.12	0.95-1.29 *
00 Technical professions	15	0.99	0.56-1.64	0.90	0.50-1.49
01 Technical work	67	1.36	1.05-1.72	1.19	0.92-1.52 *
010 Civil engineering technicians	23	1.26	0.80-1.89	1.10	0.70-1.65
013 Mechanical technicians	23	1.79	1.14-2.69	1.58	1.00-2.37 *
016 Technicians NOS	3	0.59	0.12-1.73	0.52	0.11-1.51
02 Chemical/physical/biological work	8	0.92	0.40-1.82	0.87	0.37-1.71
028 Consultancy, forestry	-	-/4.2	0.00-0.89	-/4.4	0.00-0.85 *
03 Medical work and nursing	4	0.59	0.16-1.51	0.55	0.15-1.42
05 Teaching	24	0.85	0.54-1.26	0.77	0.49-1.14
051 Subject teachers	7	1.28	0.52-2.64	1.14	0.46-2.35
052 Primary school teachers	6	0.55	0.20-1.19	0.49	0.18-1.07
054 Vocational teachers	5	0.75	0.24-1.75	0.69	0.22-1.62
08 Artistic and literary professions	22	2.46	1.54-3.72	2.33	1.46-3.52 *
080 Sculptors, painters, etc.	6	5.47	2.01-11.9	5.45	2.00-11.9 *

Occupation	Obs.	Crude		Adjusted	
		SIR	95% CI	SIR	95% CI
09 Humanistic and social work etc.	17	1.97	1.15-3.16	1.79	1.04-2.86 *
1 Administrative and clerical work	92	1.03	0.83-1.26	0.97	0.78-1.18
10 Public administration	12	1.40	0.72-2.45	1.42	0.74-2.49
11 Corporate administration	36	0.85	0.60-1.18	0.84	0.59-1.17
110 Corporate managers	16	0.82	0.47-1.33	0.84	0.48-1.36
112 Commercial managers	12	1.19	0.62-2.09	1.13	0.58-1.98
119 Private sector managers NOS	4	0.81	0.22-2.07	0.80	0.22-2.04
14/15 Clerical work NOS	40	1.18	0.84-1.60	1.02	0.73-1.39
144 Office clerks	3	0.54	0.11-1.58	0.47	0.10-1.37
150 Property managers, warehousemen	21	1.23	0.76-1.88	1.05	0.65-1.61
2 Sales professions	81	1.17	0.93-1.45	1.08	0.85-1.34
20 Wholesale and retail dealers	25	1.23	0.80-1.82	1.06	0.69-1.57
201 Retailers	25	1.29	0.83-1.90	1.11	0.72-1.63
21 Real estate, services, securities	8	1.55	0.67-3.06	1.36	0.59-2.67
22 Sales representatives	14	0.99	0.54-1.66	0.89	0.49-1.49
220 Commercial travellers, etc.	14	1.08	0.59-1.81	0.97	0.53-1.64
23 Sales work	34	1.15	0.79-1.60	1.13	0.78-1.58
230 Buyers, office sales staff	9	1.62	0.74-3.07	1.43	0.65-2.71
231 Shop personnel	20	1.08	0.66-1.67	1.14	0.69-1.76
3 Farming, forestry and fishing	371	0.87	0.79-0.96	0.89	0.80-0.98 *
30 Agricultural/forestry management	319	0.90	0.81-1.01	0.90	0.81-1.01
300 Farmers, silviculturists	301	0.90	0.80-1.00	0.91	0.81-1.01
302 Forestry managers	12	0.97	0.50-1.69	0.83	0.43-1.45
31 Farming, animal husbandry	13	0.61	0.32-1.04	0.66	0.35-1.14
310 Agricultural workers	11	0.69	0.34-1.23	0.75	0.37-1.33
34 Forestry work	38	0.81	0.57-1.11	0.91	0.65-1.25
4 Mining and quarrying	7	0.86	0.35-1.77	0.89	0.36-1.83
40 Mining and quarrying	5	0.99	0.32-2.31	1.03	0.33-2.40
5 Transport and communications	158	1.16	0.99-1.35	1.13	0.96-1.31
50 Ship's officers	7	1.18	0.48-2.44	1.06	0.43-2.18
53 Engine drivers	4	0.67	0.18-1.72	0.69	0.19-1.77
54 Road transport	107	1.29	1.06-1.55	1.25	1.03-1.50 *
540 Motor-vehicle and tram drivers	107	1.30	1.06-1.55	1.26	1.03-1.51 *
55 Transport services	10	0.74	0.36-1.37	0.72	0.35-1.33
550 Railway staff	10	0.76	0.36-1.39	0.74	0.35-1.35
56 Traffic supervisors	10	1.29	0.62-2.37	1.17	0.56-2.15
58 Postal services/couriers	9	1.01	0.46-1.92	1.05	0.48-1.99
580 Postmen	6	1.12	0.41-2.43	1.17	0.43-2.56
6/7 Industrial and construction work	511	0.97	0.88-1.05	1.01	0.93-1.10
61 Cutting/sewing etc.	5	1.02	0.33-2.38	0.99	0.32-2.31
63 Smelting, metal and foundry work	21	1.42	0.88-2.17	1.46	0.90-2.22
64 Precision mechanical work	9	1.57	0.72-2.98	1.52	0.69-2.88
65 Machine shop/steelworkers	98	0.95	0.77-1.15	0.98	0.80-1.19
650 Turners, machinists	30	1.31	0.88-1.86	1.35	0.91-1.93
651 Fitter-assemblers etc.	10	1.00	0.48-1.84	1.05	0.50-1.93
652 Machine and motor repairers	20	0.83	0.51-1.29	0.85	0.52-1.32
653 Sheetmetalworkers	6	0.63	0.23-1.36	0.65	0.24-1.41
654 Plumbers	15	1.12	0.63-1.85	1.15	0.65-1.90
655 Welders and flame cutters	7	0.68	0.27-1.40	0.72	0.29-1.48
659 Machine shop/steelworkers NOS	9	0.94	0.43-1.78	0.96	0.44-1.83
66 Electrical work	30	0.96	0.65-1.37	1.00	0.68-1.43
660 Electricians (indoors)	16	0.95	0.54-1.54	0.99	0.56-1.60
67 Woodwork	107	0.99	0.81-1.19	1.02	0.83-1.22
671 Timber workers	15	1.11	0.62-1.83	1.14	0.64-1.88
673 Construction carpenters	63	0.93	0.71-1.19	0.96	0.74-1.23
675 Bench carpenters	7	1.12	0.45-2.31	1.09	0.44-2.26
677 Woodworking machine operators e	8	1.33	0.58-2.63	1.37	0.59-2.71
68 Painting and lacquering	13	0.65	0.34-1.11	0.66	0.35-1.12
680 Painters	13	0.70	0.37-1.19	0.71	0.38-1.21
69 Construction work NOS	80	0.93	0.74-1.16	1.02	0.81-1.27
690 Bricklayers and tile setters	10	0.92	0.44-1.69	0.94	0.45-1.73
693 Concrete/cement shutterers	6	0.84	0.31-1.83	0.87	0.32-1.89
697 Building hands	32	0.92	0.63-1.31	1.04	0.71-1.47
698 Roadbuilding hands	25	1.06	0.69-1.57	1.20	0.78-1.77
70 Printing	8	1.13	0.49-2.22	1.19	0.51-2.35

Occupation	Obs.	Crude		Adjusted	
		SIR	95% CI	SIR	95% CI
72 Food industry	8	0.70	0.30-1.39	0.72	0.31-1.42
73 Chemical process/paper making	19	1.07	0.65-1.67	1.13	0.68-1.76
735 Paper and board mill workers	3	0.45	0.09-1.32	0.48	0.10-1.39
75 Industrial work NOS	10	0.86	0.41-1.59	0.88	0.42-1.61
77 Machinists	35	0.88	0.62-1.23	0.92	0.64-1.28
771 Forklift operators	3	0.54	0.11-1.57	0.57	0.12-1.66
772 Construction machinery operator	7	0.55	0.22-1.13	0.56	0.22-1.15
773 Operators of stationary engine	10	0.99	0.47-1.81	1.03	0.49-1.90
775 Industrial personnel, riggers	10	1.93	0.93-3.56	2.02	0.97-3.72
78 Dock and warehouse work	35	1.11	0.77-1.54	1.21	0.84-1.68
780 Dockers	7	0.93	0.37-1.91	0.97	0.39-2.00
782 Warehousemen	24	1.24	0.79-1.84	1.37	0.88-2.04
79 Labourers not classified elsewhere	18	0.98	0.58-1.55	1.11	0.66-1.75
8 Services	62	1.04	0.80-1.34	1.03	0.79-1.32
80 Watchmen, security guards	31	1.19	0.81-1.69	1.13	0.77-1.60
801 Policemen	18	1.70	1.01-2.69	1.44	0.85-2.28 *
804 Civilian guards	7	0.86	0.35-1.78	0.93	0.37-1.91
83 Caretakers and cleaners	22	0.88	0.55-1.33	0.92	0.57-1.39
830 Caretakers	21	0.94	0.58-1.43	0.98	0.60-1.49
9 Work not classified elsewhere	12	1.30	0.67-2.27	1.25	0.64-2.18
90 Military occupations	7	1.26	0.51-2.60	1.16	0.47-2.39
ECONOMICALLY INACTIVE PERSONS	217	1.01	0.88-1.15	1.03	0.90-1.18

C10. Rectal cancer, females

Occupation	Obs.	Crude		Adjusted	
		SIR	95% CI	SIR	95% CI
WHOLE POPULATION	1588	1.02	0.97-1.07	1.02	0.97-1.07
ECONOMICALLY ACTIVE PERSONS	893	1.00	0.94-1.07	1.00	0.94-1.07
0 Technical, humanistic, etc. work	127	1.17	0.98-1.39	1.12	0.94-1.33
01 Technical work	7	1.36	0.55-2.81	1.33	0.54-2.75
03 Medical work and nursing	59	1.26	0.96-1.62	1.25	0.95-1.61
032 Nurses	22	1.67	1.05-2.53	1.60	1.01-2.43 *
036 Auxiliary nurses	21	1.02	0.63-1.56	1.06	0.65-1.62
04 Health-care related work	7	1.08	0.44-2.23	1.05	0.42-2.16
05 Teaching	33	1.02	0.70-1.43	0.93	0.64-1.31
051 Subject teachers	4	0.52	0.14-1.34	0.50	0.14-1.27
052 Primary school teachers	17	1.09	0.63-1.74	0.96	0.56-1.54
09 Humanistic and social work etc.	7	0.84	0.34-1.73	0.79	0.32-1.62
1 Administrative and clerical work	103	0.96	0.78-1.16	0.93	0.76-1.12
12 Clerical work	26	1.04	0.68-1.52	1.01	0.66-1.48
120 Book-keepers, accountants	15	1.27	0.71-2.09	1.23	0.69-2.02
121 Office cashiers	6	1.20	0.44-2.62	1.17	0.43-2.54
123 Shop and restaurant cashiers	3	0.48	0.10-1.39	0.46	0.10-1.36
13 Stenographers and typists	9	0.95	0.43-1.80	0.92	0.42-1.76
130 Private secretaries	6	1.16	0.43-2.52	1.13	0.41-2.46
14/15 Clerical work NOS	64	0.95	0.73-1.21	0.92	0.71-1.18
144 Office clerks	43	0.95	0.69-1.28	0.92	0.67-1.24
145 Bank clerks	7	0.92	0.37-1.90	0.89	0.36-1.84
159 Clerical workers NOS	6	0.96	0.35-2.10	0.94	0.34-2.04
2 Sales professions	87	1.01	0.81-1.25	1.03	0.83-1.27
20 Wholesale and retail dealers	10	0.74	0.36-1.37	0.73	0.35-1.34
201 Retailers	9	0.67	0.31-1.28	0.66	0.30-1.25
23 Sales work	73	1.03	0.81-1.30	1.06	0.83-1.33
231 Shop personnel	69	1.03	0.80-1.31	1.06	0.83-1.35
3 Farming, forestry and fishing	167	0.79	0.67-0.91	0.80	0.69-0.93 *
30 Agricultural/forestry management	49	0.86	0.64-1.13	0.88	0.65-1.16
300 Farmers, silviculturists	48	0.86	0.64-1.15	0.88	0.65-1.17
31 Farming, animal husbandry	118	0.77	0.63-0.91	0.78	0.65-0.93 *
310 Agricultural workers	16	1.03	0.59-1.68	1.05	0.60-1.70
311 Gardeners	10	1.75	0.84-3.23	1.73	0.83-3.18

Occupation	Obs.	Crude		Adjusted	
		SIR	95% CI	SIR	95% CI
312 Livestock workers	92	0.70	0.56-0.85	0.71	0.57-0.87 *
4 Mining and quarrying	-	-/0.3	0.00-13.0	-/0.3	0.00-13.8
5 Transport and communications	29	0.95	0.64-1.37	0.94	0.63-1.36
57 Post and telecommunications	16	1.01	0.57-1.63	0.98	0.56-1.59
570 Post/telecommunications officials	6	0.88	0.32-1.92	0.86	0.31-1.87
571 Telephone operators	6	1.04	0.38-2.27	1.01	0.37-2.20
58 Postal services/couriers	7	0.76	0.31-1.57	0.78	0.31-1.60
580 Postmen	6	0.75	0.28-1.64	0.77	0.28-1.67
6/7 Industrial and construction work	159	1.00	0.85-1.16	1.03	0.88-1.20
60 Textiles	18	0.96	0.57-1.51	0.99	0.59-1.57
602 Weavers	8	1.24	0.54-2.45	1.28	0.55-2.53
61 Cutting/sewing etc.	29	0.89	0.60-1.28	0.92	0.62-1.32
611 Dressmakers	9	1.29	0.59-2.46	1.28	0.59-2.44
616 Garment workers	14	0.78	0.43-1.30	0.81	0.44-1.36
62 Shoes and leather	4	0.67	0.18-1.73	0.70	0.19-1.79
65 Machine shop/steelworkers	12	1.98	1.02-3.45	2.06	1.06-3.60 *
67 Woodwork	13	0.96	0.51-1.65	1.00	0.54-1.72
672 Plywood makers	8	1.28	0.55-2.52	1.33	0.58-2.63
69 Construction work NOS	6	0.92	0.34-1.99	0.90	0.33-1.96
697 Building hands	4	0.74	0.20-1.88	0.72	0.20-1.85
70 Printing	7	1.18	0.47-2.43	1.22	0.49-2.52
72 Food industry	11	0.58	0.29-1.04	0.61	0.30-1.08
721 Bakers and pastry chiefs	5	0.57	0.19-1.33	0.59	0.19-1.39
73 Chemical process/paper making	6	1.14	0.42-2.48	1.20	0.44-2.60
75 Industrial work NOS	14	1.48	0.81-2.49	1.54	0.84-2.59
76 Packing and labelling	16	1.10	0.63-1.78	1.14	0.65-1.85
78 Dock and warehouse work	8	1.12	0.49-2.21	1.11	0.48-2.18
782 Warehousemen	7	1.17	0.47-2.42	1.15	0.46-2.36
8 Services	217	1.15	1.00-1.31	1.14	0.99-1.30 *
81 Housekeeping, domestic work, etc.	75	1.16	0.91-1.45	1.15	0.90-1.44
810 Housekeepers	9	1.44	0.66-2.73	1.39	0.64-2.64
811 Chefs, cooks etc.	15	0.92	0.51-1.52	0.97	0.54-1.60
812 Kitchen assistants	16	0.91	0.52-1.48	0.88	0.50-1.43
813 Domestic servants	21	1.23	0.76-1.88	1.20	0.74-1.84
82 Waiters	26	1.41	0.92-2.06	1.43	0.93-2.09
820 Waiters in restaurants	8	0.94	0.41-1.85	0.97	0.42-1.91
821 Waiters in cafés etc.	18	1.81	1.07-2.85	1.80	1.07-2.85 *
83 Caretakers and cleaners	98	1.13	0.92-1.38	1.11	0.90-1.35
830 Caretakers	5	0.55	0.18-1.28	0.57	0.19-1.34
831 Cleaners	91	1.18	0.95-1.45	1.15	0.93-1.41
84 Hygiene and beauty services	10	1.17	0.56-2.15	1.15	0.55-2.11
840 Hairdressers and barbers	7	1.04	0.42-2.14	1.02	0.41-2.10
85 Laundry and pressing	5	0.65	0.21-1.52	0.65	0.21-1.52
850 Launderers	4	0.63	0.17-1.60	0.62	0.17-1.58
9 Work not classified elsewhere	4	2.07	0.56-5.29	2.18	0.59-5.59
ECONOMICALLY INACTIVE PERSONS	695	1.05	0.97-1.13	1.06	0.98-1.14

C11. Cancer of the pancreas, males

WHOLE POPULATION	1891	1.03	0.98-1.07	1.02	0.98-1.07
ECONOMICALLY ACTIVE PERSONS	1606	1.00	0.95-1.05	1.00	0.95-1.05
0 Technical, humanistic, etc. work	134	0.90	0.76-1.06	0.96	0.80-1.13
00 Technical professions	14	0.84	0.46-1.42	0.89	0.49-1.49
01 Technical work	62	1.15	0.88-1.47	1.23	0.94-1.57
010 Civil engineering technicians	26	1.29	0.84-1.89	1.38	0.90-2.02
013 Mechanical technicians	14	0.99	0.54-1.67	1.07	0.58-1.79
016 Technicians NOS	6	1.09	0.40-2.36	1.16	0.42-2.52
02 Chemical/physical/biological work	8	0.84	0.36-1.65	0.88	0.38-1.73
03 Medical work and nursing	6	0.81	0.30-1.77	0.84	0.31-1.83

Occupation	Obs.	Crude		Adjusted	
		SIR	95% CI	SIR	95% CI
05 Teaching	23	0.75	0.47-1.12	0.79	0.50-1.19
051 Subject teachers	7	1.19	0.48-2.45	1.27	0.51-2.62
052 Primary school teachers	4	0.33	0.09-0.86	0.36	0.10-0.92 *
054 Vocational teachers	6	0.82	0.30-1.79	0.87	0.32-1.90
06 Religious professions	-	-/3.8	0.00-0.96	-/3.6	0.00-1.02 *
08 Artistic and literary professions	7	0.71	0.29-1.47	0.75	0.30-1.55
09 Humanistic and social work etc.	9	0.95	0.44-1.81	1.01	0.46-1.92
1 Administrative and clerical work	104	1.06	0.87-1.27	1.12	0.91-1.34
10 Public administration	7	0.74	0.30-1.53	0.77	0.31-1.59
11 Corporate administration	51	1.09	0.81-1.44	1.14	0.85-1.50
110 Corporate managers	26	1.20	0.79-1.76	1.25	0.81-1.83
112 Commercial managers	14	1.27	0.70-2.14	1.35	0.74-2.27
119 Private sector managers NOS	5	0.92	0.30-2.15	0.95	0.31-2.22
14/15 Clerical work NOS	39	1.05	0.74-1.43	1.12	0.79-1.53
144 Office clerks	7	1.15	0.46-2.37	1.24	0.50-2.55
150 Property managers, warehousemen	20	1.07	0.65-1.65	1.14	0.69-1.75
2 Sales professions	77	1.01	0.80-1.27	1.06	0.84-1.32
20 Wholesale and retail dealers	27	1.21	0.80-1.76	1.28	0.85-1.87
201 Retailers	27	1.26	0.83-1.84	1.34	0.88-1.95
21 Real estate, services, securities	5	0.88	0.29-2.06	0.94	0.31-2.20
22 Sales representatives	11	0.71	0.35-1.27	0.76	0.38-1.37
220 Commercial travellers, etc.	11	0.78	0.39-1.39	0.84	0.42-1.50
23 Sales work	34	1.05	0.72-1.46	1.06	0.74-1.48
230 Buyers, office sales staff	6	0.98	0.36-2.14	1.05	0.39-2.29
231 Shop personnel	22	1.09	0.68-1.65	1.08	0.68-1.63
3 Farming, forestry and fishing	397	0.85	0.77-0.93	0.84	0.76-0.92 *
30 Agricultural/forestry management	319	0.82	0.73-0.91	0.82	0.73-0.91 *
300 Farmers, silviculturists	294	0.80	0.71-0.89	0.80	0.71-0.89 *
302 Forestry managers	16	1.17	0.67-1.90	1.24	0.71-2.02
303 Horticultural managers	5	3.14	1.02-7.34	3.37	1.09-7.87 *
31 Farming, animal husbandry	20	0.86	0.52-1.32	0.81	0.49-1.25
310 Agricultural workers	15	0.86	0.48-1.41	0.81	0.46-1.34
34 Forestry work	55	1.07	0.80-1.39	0.96	0.73-1.26
4 Mining and quarrying	14	1.56	0.86-2.62	1.56	0.85-2.61
40 Mining and quarrying	9	1.63	0.74-3.09	1.63	0.74-3.09
5 Transport and communications	172	1.15	0.98-1.33	1.17	1.00-1.35 *
50 Ship's officers	5	0.77	0.25-1.81	0.82	0.27-1.92
53 Engine drivers	7	1.04	0.42-2.14	1.03	0.41-2.12
54 Road transport	105	1.15	0.94-1.39	1.18	0.96-1.41
540 Motor-vehicle and tram drivers	104	1.15	0.94-1.38	1.17	0.95-1.40
55 Transport services	24	1.61	1.03-2.39	1.62	1.04-2.41 *
550 Railway staff	24	1.63	1.05-2.43	1.65	1.05-2.45 *
56 Traffic supervisors	9	1.05	0.48-2.00	1.11	0.51-2.12
58 Postal services/couriers	10	1.02	0.49-1.88	1.01	0.49-1.87
580 Postmen	4	0.68	0.18-1.73	0.67	0.18-1.71
6/7 Industrial and construction work	614	1.06	0.97-1.14	1.03	0.95-1.12
60 Textiles	6	1.12	0.41-2.44	1.11	0.41-2.42
61 Cutting/sewing etc.	7	1.30	0.52-2.67	1.32	0.53-2.73
619 Cutting/sewing workers NOS	2	8.99	1.09-32.5	9.04	1.09-32.7 *
63 Smelting, metal and foundry work	13	0.80	0.43-1.37	0.80	0.43-1.37
64 Precision mechanical work	4	0.63	0.17-1.62	0.64	0.18-1.65
65 Machine shop/steelworkers	134	1.18	0.99-1.39	1.17	0.98-1.38
650 Turners, machinists	14	0.55	0.30-0.93	0.55	0.30-0.92 *
651 Fitter-assemblers etc.	15	1.37	0.77-2.26	1.36	0.76-2.24
652 Machine and motor repairers	27	1.02	0.67-1.49	1.02	0.67-1.48
653 Sheetmetalworkers	12	1.15	0.59-2.01	1.14	0.59-2.00
654 Plumbers	32	2.17	1.49-3.07	2.16	1.48-3.05 *
655 Welders and flame cutters	17	1.51	0.88-2.42	1.49	0.87-2.39
656 Plate/constructional steel work	12	3.57	1.85-6.24	3.54	1.83-6.19 *
659 Machine shop/steelworkers NOS	5	0.47	0.15-1.10	0.47	0.15-1.10
66 Electrical work	33	0.96	0.66-1.35	0.96	0.66-1.34
660 Electricians (indoors)	18	0.97	0.58-1.54	0.96	0.57-1.52
664 Telephone installers and repair	5	0.97	0.31-2.26	0.96	0.31-2.23
67 Woodwork	110	0.92	0.76-1.10	0.92	0.76-1.10
671 Timber workers	15	1.01	0.56-1.66	1.01	0.56-1.66

Occupation	Obs.	Crude		Adjusted	
		SIR	95% CI	SIR	95% CI
673 Construction carpenters	68	0.91	0.70-1.15	0.90	0.70-1.15
675 Bench carpenters	5	0.72	0.24-1.69	0.74	0.24-1.72
677 Woodworking machine operators e	8	1.21	0.52-2.39	1.21	0.52-2.38
68 Painting and lacquering	32	1.45	0.99-2.05	1.46	1.00-2.06
680 Painters	29	1.42	0.95-2.04	1.43	0.95-2.05
69 Construction work NOS	99	1.05	0.85-1.27	0.98	0.79-1.19
690 Bricklayers and tile setters	9	0.75	0.34-1.42	0.74	0.34-1.41
693 Concrete/cement shutterers	3	0.38	0.08-1.11	0.38	0.08-1.11
697 Building hands	51	1.34	0.99-1.76	1.21	0.90-1.59
698 Roadbuilding hands	27	1.05	0.69-1.52	0.95	0.62-1.38
70 Printing	7	0.91	0.37-1.88	0.90	0.36-1.85
72 Food industry	18	1.45	0.86-2.29	1.45	0.86-2.29
73 Chemical process/paper making	16	0.82	0.47-1.34	0.82	0.47-1.32
734 Pulp mill workers	4	0.75	0.20-1.91	0.74	0.20-1.90
735 Paper and board mill workers	10	1.38	0.66-2.54	1.36	0.65-2.51
75 Industrial work NOS	12	0.94	0.49-1.65	0.94	0.49-1.64
76 Packing and labelling	7	1.36	0.55-2.81	1.35	0.54-2.78
77 Machinists	40	0.92	0.66-1.26	0.92	0.66-1.25
771 Forklift operators	7	1.15	0.46-2.36	1.13	0.45-2.33
772 Construction machinery operator	13	0.93	0.49-1.58	0.93	0.50-1.59
773 Operators of stationary engine	8	0.72	0.31-1.41	0.71	0.31-1.41
775 Industrial personnel, riggers	1	0.18	0.00-0.98	0.17	0.00-0.97 *
78 Dock and warehouse work	46	1.32	0.97-1.76	1.23	0.90-1.64
780 Dockers	6	0.72	0.26-1.56	0.71	0.26-1.54
781 Freight handlers	8	1.56	0.67-3.07	1.41	0.61-2.79
782 Warehousemen	32	1.51	1.03-2.13	1.38	0.95-1.95 *
79 Labourers not classified elsewhere	17	0.84	0.49-1.34	0.76	0.44-1.22
8 Services	83	1.27	1.01-1.58	1.29	1.02-1.59 *
80 Watchmen, security guards	37	1.30	0.91-1.79	1.33	0.93-1.83
801 Policemen	14	1.21	0.66-2.03	1.28	0.70-2.15
804 Civilian guards	11	1.24	0.62-2.22	1.20	0.60-2.15
83 Caretakers and cleaners	30	1.09	0.74-1.56	1.08	0.73-1.55
830 Caretakers	28	1.14	0.75-1.64	1.13	0.75-1.63
84 Hygiene and beauty services	5	8.86	2.88-20.7	9.45	3.07-22.1 *
840 Hairdressers and barbers	3	7.80	1.61-22.8	8.31	1.71-24.3 *
843 Sauna attendants etc.	2	11.2	1.36-40.6	12.1	1.46-43.6 *
9 Work not classified elsewhere	11	1.09	0.54-1.94	1.13	0.56-2.02
90 Military occupations	6	0.99	0.36-2.15	1.06	0.39-2.31
ECONOMICALLY INACTIVE PERSONS	285	1.20	1.06-1.34	1.18	1.05-1.32 *

C12. Cancer of the pancreas, females

Occupation	Obs.	Crude		Adjusted	
		SIR	95% CI	SIR	95% CI
WHOLE POPULATION	1350	1.04	0.98-1.09	1.05	0.99-1.10
ECONOMICALLY ACTIVE PERSONS	731	1.00	0.93-1.07	1.00	0.93-1.07
0 Technical, humanistic, etc. work	83	0.98	0.78-1.22	0.92	0.73-1.14
03 Medical work and nursing	28	0.78	0.52-1.12	0.77	0.51-1.11
032 Nurses	8	0.80	0.35-1.57	0.74	0.32-1.45
036 Auxiliary nurses	12	0.75	0.39-1.31	0.82	0.42-1.44
04 Health-care related work	6	1.17	0.43-2.56	1.03	0.38-2.24
05 Teaching	32	1.26	0.86-1.78	1.14	0.78-1.61
050 University teachers	3	7.92	1.63-23.2	6.92	1.43-20.2 *
051 Subject teachers	5	0.88	0.29-2.06	0.80	0.26-1.86
052 Primary school teachers	16	1.28	0.73-2.09	1.17	0.67-1.90
09 Humanistic and social work etc.	6	0.90	0.33-1.97	0.82	0.30-1.77
1 Administrative and clerical work	103	1.22	0.99-1.47	1.10	0.90-1.32
12 Clerical work	19	0.95	0.57-1.48	0.85	0.51-1.32
120 Book-keepers, accountants	7	0.73	0.29-1.50	0.65	0.26-1.34
123 Shop and restaurant cashiers	10	2.01	0.96-3.70	1.80	0.86-3.32
13 Stenographers and typists	10	1.36	0.65-2.51	1.24	0.59-2.28
14/15 Clerical work NOS	70	1.32	1.03-1.67	1.19	0.93-1.50 *
144 Office clerks	46	1.29	0.94-1.71	1.15	0.85-1.54

Occupation	Obs.	Crude		Adjusted	
		SIR	95% CI	SIR	95% CI
145 Bank clerks	7	1.25	0.50-2.58	1.16	0.47-2.39
159 Clerical workers NOS	10	1.97	0.95-3.62	1.75	0.84-3.23
2 Sales professions	60	0.87	0.67-1.12	0.89	0.68-1.15
20 Wholesale and retail dealers	11	0.96	0.48-1.72	0.85	0.42-1.52
201 Retailers	10	0.88	0.42-1.62	0.78	0.37-1.43
23 Sales work	48	0.86	0.63-1.14	0.91	0.67-1.21
231 Shop personnel	43	0.82	0.59-1.10	0.87	0.63-1.17
3 Farming, forestry and fishing	158	0.88	0.75-1.02	0.91	0.77-1.06
30 Agricultural/forestry management	40	0.79	0.57-1.08	0.82	0.58-1.11
300 Farmers, silviculturists	39	0.79	0.56-1.08	0.82	0.58-1.12
31 Farming, animal husbandry	118	0.92	0.76-1.09	0.95	0.78-1.13
310 Agricultural workers	17	1.30	0.76-2.08	1.33	0.78-2.13
312 Livestock workers	96	0.87	0.70-1.06	0.90	0.73-1.10
4 Mining and quarrying	-	-/0.2	0.00-15.5	-/0.2	0.00-16.9
5 Transport and communications	32	1.28	0.88-1.81	1.23	0.84-1.73
57 Post and telecommunications	23	1.80	1.14-2.70	1.60	1.01-2.40 *
570 Post/telecommunications officials	12	2.21	1.14-3.86	1.96	1.01-3.42 *
571 Telephone operators	5	1.07	0.35-2.49	0.95	0.31-2.21
58 Postal services/couriers	4	0.52	0.14-1.34	0.55	0.15-1.42
580 Postmen	2	0.30	0.04-1.09	0.32	0.04-1.15
6/7 Industrial and construction work	117	0.90	0.75-1.07	0.97	0.80-1.15
60 Textiles	10	0.64	0.31-1.18	0.70	0.33-1.28
602 Weavers	2	0.37	0.04-1.34	0.40	0.05-1.43
61 Cutting/sewing etc.	19	0.72	0.43-1.12	0.76	0.46-1.18
611 Dressmakers	4	0.68	0.18-1.73	0.64	0.17-1.64
616 Garment workers	14	0.97	0.53-1.62	1.06	0.58-1.79
655 Welders and flame cutters	2	9.41	1.14-34.0	10.4	1.26-37.7 *
67 Woodwork	11	1.00	0.50-1.78	1.10	0.55-1.97
672 Plywood makers	6	1.18	0.43-2.58	1.31	0.48-2.85
681 Lacquerers	3	7.32	1.51-21.4	7.93	1.64-23.2 *
69 Construction work NOS	4	0.73	0.20-1.88	0.72	0.20-1.85
72 Food industry	18	1.17	0.69-1.84	1.28	0.76-2.02
721 Bakers and pastry chiefs	5	0.69	0.23-1.62	0.75	0.24-1.76
73 Chemical process/paper making	9	2.07	0.95-3.94	2.30	1.05-4.37 *
75 Industrial work NOS	6	0.79	0.29-1.72	0.86	0.32-1.87
76 Packing and labelling	8	0.68	0.30-1.35	0.76	0.33-1.49
78 Dock and warehouse work	3	0.51	0.11-1.49	0.52	0.11-1.51
8 Services	178	1.13	0.97-1.31	1.13	0.97-1.30
81 Housekeeping, domestic work, etc.	53	0.98	0.73-1.28	0.98	0.74-1.29
810 Housekeepers	3	0.57	0.12-1.68	0.51	0.11-1.49
811 Chefs, cooks etc.	18	1.32	0.78-2.08	1.46	0.87-2.31
812 Kitchen assistants	11	0.76	0.38-1.36	0.75	0.38-1.35
813 Domestic servants	17	1.15	0.67-1.84	1.14	0.66-1.83
82 Waiters	20	1.35	0.83-2.09	1.39	0.85-2.14
820 Waiters in restaurants	9	1.32	0.60-2.50	1.42	0.65-2.69
821 Waiters in cafés etc.	11	1.38	0.69-2.47	1.37	0.68-2.44
83 Caretakers and cleaners	81	1.11	0.88-1.38	1.10	0.88-1.37
830 Caretakers	3	0.41	0.08-1.20	0.45	0.09-1.32
831 Cleaners	77	1.18	0.93-1.48	1.16	0.91-1.45
84 Hygiene and beauty services	15	2.14	1.20-3.52	1.99	1.11-3.28 *
840 Hairdressers and barbers	11	2.00	1.00-3.58	1.84	0.92-3.29
843 Sauna attendants etc.	4	3.68	1.00-9.42	3.65	1.00-9.35 *
85 Laundry and pressing	7	1.09	0.44-2.25	1.10	0.44-2.27
850 Launderers	6	1.12	0.41-2.44	1.11	0.41-2.42
9 Work not classified elsewhere	-	-/1.6	0.00-2.28	-/1.5	0.00-2.53
ECONOMICALLY INACTIVE PERSONS	619	1.09	1.00-1.18	1.11	1.03-1.20 *

Occupation	Obs.	Crude		Adjusted		
		SIR	95% CI	SIR	95% CI	

C13. Laryngeal cancer, males

Occupation	Obs.	SIR	95% CI	SIR	95% CI	
WHOLE POPULATION	1269	1.09	1.04-1.16	1.09	1.03-1.15	*
ECONOMICALLY ACTIVE PERSONS	1015	1.00	0.94-1.06	1.00	0.94-1.06	
0 Technical, humanistic, etc. work	53	0.56	0.42-0.74	0.80	0.60-1.04	*
00 Technical professions	6	0.57	0.21-1.25	0.99	0.36-2.15	
01 Technical work	16	0.47	0.27-0.76	0.59	0.34-0.96	*
010 Civil engineering technicians	6	0.47	0.17-1.02	0.59	0.22-1.29	
013 Mechanical technicians	4	0.45	0.12-1.15	0.57	0.15-1.45	
02 Chemical/physical/biological work	3	0.50	0.10-1.45	0.71	0.15-2.09	
05 Teaching	9	0.46	0.21-0.88	0.72	0.33-1.36	*
052 Primary school teachers	2	0.26	0.03-0.95	0.43	0.05-1.55	*
08 Artistic and literary professions	9	1.45	0.66-2.75	2.14	0.98-4.06	
09 Humanistic and social work etc.	4	0.67	0.18-1.72	0.97	0.26-2.49	
1 Administrative and clerical work	48	0.77	0.57-1.03	1.10	0.81-1.46	
10 Public administration	3	0.51	0.10-1.48	0.78	0.16-2.27	
11 Corporate administration	26	0.88	0.58-1.29	1.39	0.91-2.04	
110 Corporate managers	13	0.95	0.51-1.63	1.47	0.78-2.52	
112 Commercial managers	6	0.86	0.31-1.86	1.39	0.51-3.02	
14/15 Clerical work NOS	18	0.77	0.45-1.21	0.97	0.57-1.53	
148 Travel agents	2	39.0	4.72-141	48.3	5.84-174	*
150 Property managers, warehousemen	7	0.59	0.24-1.22	0.74	0.30-1.52	
2 Sales professions	59	1.23	0.93-1.58	1.41	1.07-1.82	*
20 Wholesale and retail dealers	15	1.06	0.59-1.75	1.33	0.74-2.19	
201 Retailers	15	1.11	0.62-1.83	1.38	0.77-2.28	
22 Sales representatives	12	1.22	0.63-2.13	1.57	0.81-2.73	
220 Commercial travellers, etc.	9	1.00	0.46-1.90	1.29	0.59-2.44	
23 Sales work	29	1.41	0.94-2.02	1.44	0.96-2.07	
231 Shop personnel	21	1.64	1.02-2.51	1.52	0.94-2.32	*
3 Farming, forestry and fishing	234	0.80	0.70-0.90	0.75	0.66-0.85	*
30 Agricultural/forestry management	178	0.73	0.63-0.84	0.71	0.61-0.82	*
300 Farmers, silviculturists	172	0.75	0.64-0.86	0.72	0.62-0.83	*
302 Forestry managers	4	0.46	0.13-1.18	0.58	0.16-1.48	
31 Farming, animal husbandry	13	0.89	0.47-1.52	0.75	0.40-1.28	
310 Agricultural workers	11	1.00	0.50-1.79	0.86	0.43-1.53	
34 Forestry work	43	1.31	0.95-1.76	1.00	0.73-1.35	
4 Mining and quarrying	7	1.23	0.49-2.53	1.16	0.47-2.38	
5 Transport and communications	117	1.23	1.01-1.46	1.27	1.05-1.51	*
50 Ship's officers	8	1.97	0.85-3.88	2.57	1.11-5.05	*
501 Ship pilots	4	5.04	1.37-12.9	6.31	1.72-16.2	*
54 Road transport	76	1.31	1.03-1.64	1.35	1.07-1.69	*
540 Motor-vehicle and tram drivers	76	1.32	1.04-1.65	1.36	1.07-1.70	*
55 Transport services	10	1.04	0.50-1.91	1.03	0.49-1.90	
550 Railway staff	9	0.95	0.43-1.80	0.94	0.43-1.79	
56 Traffic supervisors	5	0.92	0.30-2.16	1.22	0.40-2.85	
560 Port traffic supervisors	3	4.62	0.95-13.5	6.00	1.24-17.5	*
58 Postal services/couriers	6	0.97	0.36-2.12	0.91	0.33-1.98	
6/7 Industrial and construction work	441	1.19	1.09-1.31	1.08	0.99-1.19	*
612 Furriers	2	8.33	1.01-30.1	8.73	1.06-31.5	*
63 Smelting, metal and foundry work	14	1.36	0.75-2.29	1.29	0.71-2.17	
65 Machine shop/steelworkers	92	1.27	1.03-1.56	1.20	0.96-1.47	*
650 Turners, machinists	23	1.43	0.91-2.14	1.34	0.85-2.00	
651 Fitter-assemblers etc.	14	2.01	1.10-3.37	1.86	1.02-3.12	*
652 Machine and motor repairers	14	0.84	0.46-1.40	0.80	0.44-1.34	
653 Sheetmetalworkers	11	1.67	0.83-2.98	1.59	0.79-2.84	
654 Plumbers	10	1.06	0.51-1.95	1.00	0.48-1.84	
655 Welders and flame cutters	8	1.12	0.48-2.20	1.03	0.44-2.03	
659 Machine shop/steelworkers NOS	9	1.34	0.61-2.55	1.27	0.58-2.40	
66 Electrical work	24	1.10	0.70-1.64	1.03	0.66-1.53	
660 Electricians (indoors)	13	1.10	0.58-1.88	1.02	0.54-1.75	
67 Woodwork	73	0.97	0.76-1.21	0.91	0.71-1.15	

Occupation	Obs.	Crude SIR	Crude 95% CI	Adjusted SIR	Adjusted 95% CI	
671 Timber workers	8	0.85	0.37-1.68	0.81	0.35-1.59	
673 Construction carpenters	54	1.14	0.85-1.48	1.06	0.80-1.39	
675 Bench carpenters	-	-/4.3	0.00-0.85	-/4.3	0.00-0.86	*
68 Painting and lacquering	18	1.30	0.77-2.05	1.25	0.74-1.97	
680 Painters	17	1.32	0.77-2.11	1.27	0.74-2.03	
69 Construction work NOS	73	1.21	0.95-1.52	1.00	0.78-1.25	
690 Bricklayers and tile setters	6	0.78	0.29-1.70	0.73	0.27-1.59	
693 Concrete/cement shutterers	10	1.99	0.95-3.66	1.85	0.89-3.41	
697 Building hands	30	1.23	0.83-1.75	0.95	0.64-1.35	
698 Roadbuilding hands	21	1.29	0.80-1.97	1.01	0.62-1.54	
70 Printing	2	0.41	0.05-1.49	0.39	0.05-1.39	
72 Food industry	4	0.51	0.14-1.31	0.49	0.13-1.24	
73 Chemical process/paper making	18	1.46	0.87-2.31	1.35	0.80-2.13	
735 Paper and board mill workers	5	1.09	0.35-2.55	1.01	0.33-2.35	
75 Industrial work NOS	10	1.24	0.59-2.28	1.19	0.57-2.18	
77 Machinists	30	1.09	0.73-1.55	1.02	0.69-1.46	
772 Construction machinery operator	9	1.00	0.46-1.90	0.98	0.45-1.86	
773 Operators of stationary engine	7	0.99	0.40-2.05	0.92	0.37-1.90	
78 Dock and warehouse work	35	1.59	1.11-2.21	1.30	0.90-1.80	*
780 Dockers	10	1.88	0.90-3.45	1.70	0.82-3.13	
782 Warehousemen	19	1.42	0.85-2.21	1.12	0.68-1.76	
79 Labourers not classified elsewhere	25	1.95	1.26-2.88	1.53	0.99-2.26	*
8 Services	45	1.10	0.80-1.47	1.10	0.80-1.47	
80 Watchmen, security guards	16	0.90	0.51-1.45	0.96	0.55-1.56	
801 Policemen	6	0.83	0.30-1.80	1.01	0.37-2.21	
804 Civilian guards	7	1.29	0.52-2.65	1.15	0.46-2.37	
83 Caretakers and cleaners	24	1.38	0.88-2.05	1.28	0.82-1.91	
830 Caretakers	19	1.22	0.73-1.90	1.14	0.68-1.77	
9 Work not classified elsewhere	11	1.72	0.86-3.08	2.07	1.04-3.71	*
91 Occupation not specified	7	2.72	1.09-5.60	2.56	1.03-5.28	*
ECONOMICALLY INACTIVE PERSONS	254	1.76	1.55-1.98	1.67	1.47-1.88	*

C14. Laryngeal cancer, females

Occupation	Obs.	Crude SIR	Crude 95% CI	Adjusted SIR	Adjusted 95% CI	
WHOLE POPULATION	104	1.10	0.90-1.32	1.12	0.92-1.35	
ECONOMICALLY ACTIVE PERSONS	56	1.00	0.76-1.30	1.00	0.76-1.30	
0 Technical, humanistic, etc. work	4	0.59	0.16-1.50	0.61	0.17-1.57	
1 Administrative and clerical work	8	1.18	0.51-2.33	1.22	0.53-2.41	
2 Sales professions	4	0.74	0.20-1.90	0.72	0.20-1.84	
3 Farming, forestry and fishing	8	0.61	0.26-1.20	0.62	0.27-1.22	
31 Farming, animal husbandry	5	0.52	0.17-1.21	0.52	0.17-1.22	
312 Livestock workers	4	0.48	0.13-1.24	0.49	0.13-1.25	
4 Mining and quarrying	-	-/0.0	0.00-195	-/0.0	0.00-212	
5 Transport and communications	2	1.03	0.13-3.74	1.04	0.13-3.75	
6/7 Industrial and construction work	16	1.60	0.92-2.61	1.60	0.91-2.60	
625 Shoemakers NOS	2	22.3	2.70-80.7	22.4	2.71-80.8	*
65 Machine shop/steelworkers	3	7.84	1.62-22.9	7.85	1.62-22.9	*
659 Machine shop/steelworkers NOS	2	8.54	1.03-30.8	8.65	1.05-31.2	*
670 Round-timber workers	1	43.2	1.09-241	44.0	1.11-245	*
8 Services	14	1.18	0.65-1.98	1.13	0.62-1.90	
815 Hotel reception clerks	1	137	3.47-763	155	3.92-862	*
83 Caretakers and cleaners	3	0.55	0.11-1.62	0.53	0.11-1.55	
831 Cleaners	2	0.41	0.05-1.50	0.39	0.05-1.42	
839 Caretakers/cleaners NOS	1	44.0	1.11-245	43.7	1.11-244	*

Occupation	Obs.	Crude		Adjusted	
		SIR	95% CI	SIR	95% CI
9 Work not classified elsewhere	-	-/0.1	0.00-30.6	-/0.1	0.00-32.4
ECONOMICALLY INACTIVE PERSONS	48	1.25	0.92-1.65	1.32	0.97-1.74

C15. Lung cancer, males

Occupation	Obs.	Crude		Adjusted	
		SIR	95% CI	SIR	95% CI
WHOLE POPULATION	15613	1.10	1.08-1.12	1.09	1.07-1.10 *
ECONOMICALLY ACTIVE PERSONS	12285	1.00	0.98-1.02	1.00	0.98-1.02
0 Technical, humanistic, etc. work	567	0.51	0.47-0.56	0.84	0.77-0.91 *
00 Technical professions	43	0.36	0.26-0.48	0.81	0.59-1.10 *
000 Architects	1	0.13	0.00-0.71	0.29	0.01-1.61 *
001 Civil engineers	12	0.49	0.26-0.86	1.13	0.58-1.97 *
002 Electrical engineers	5	0.31	0.10-0.72	0.70	0.23-1.62 *
003 Teletechnical engineers	2	0.33	0.04-1.20	0.75	0.09-2.72
004 Mechanical engineers	15	0.42	0.23-0.69	0.94	0.53-1.55 *
005 Chemotechnical engineers	4	0.34	0.09-0.88	0.78	0.21-1.99 *
007 Engineers NOS	2	0.27	0.03-0.97	0.61	0.07-2.19 *
008 Surveyors	1	0.13	0.00-0.71	0.28	0.01-1.59 *
01 Technical work	257	0.64	0.56-0.72	0.83	0.73-0.93 *
010 Civil engineering technicians	108	0.71	0.58-0.85	0.92	0.76-1.10 *
011 Power technicians	9	0.28	0.13-0.53	0.36	0.17-0.69 *
012 Teletechnicians	9	0.51	0.23-0.96	0.66	0.30-1.25 *
013 Mechanical technicians	60	0.57	0.44-0.74	0.75	0.57-0.96 *
014 Chemotechnicians	3	0.31	0.06-0.91	0.41	0.08-1.19 *
016 Technicians NOS	30	0.73	0.49-1.04	0.94	0.64-1.35
017 Cartographers	3	0.33	0.07-0.95	0.43	0.09-1.24 *
018 Draughtsmen, survey assistants	20	0.93	0.57-1.44	1.21	0.74-1.87
019 Laboratory assistants	10	0.89	0.42-1.63	1.16	0.56-2.13
02 Chemical/physical/biological work	39	0.54	0.38-0.74	0.92	0.65-1.25 *
020 Chemists	1	0.13	0.00-0.75	0.30	0.01-1.66 *
027 Consultancy, agriculture	11	0.55	0.28-0.99	0.80	0.40-1.44 *
028 Consultancy, forestry	25	0.70	0.45-1.04	1.18	0.76-1.74
03 Medical work and nursing	14	0.26	0.14-0.43	0.42	0.23-0.71 *
030 Medical doctors	6	0.20	0.07-0.44	0.45	0.17-0.99 *
031 Dentists	-	-/5.8	0.00-0.64	-/2.6	0.00-1.43 *
035 Psychiatric nurses	4	0.45	0.12-1.16	0.59	0.16-1.52
039 Medical workers NOS	3	0.36	0.07-1.04	0.32	0.07-0.95 *
04 Health-care related work	15	0.78	0.44-1.29	1.21	0.68-1.99
040 Pharmacists	5	0.63	0.21-1.47	1.40	0.45-3.26
042 Health inspectors	6	1.06	0.39-2.30	1.36	0.50-2.97
05 Teaching	83	0.37	0.29-0.46	0.74	0.59-0.92 *
050 University teachers	5	0.24	0.08-0.57	0.55	0.18-1.28 *
051 Subject teachers	16	0.38	0.22-0.62	0.86	0.49-1.40 *
052 Primary school teachers	26	0.30	0.20-0.44	0.69	0.45-1.00 *
053 Teachers of practical subjects	4	0.32	0.09-0.81	0.56	0.15-1.45 *
054 Vocational teachers	27	0.50	0.33-0.72	0.80	0.52-1.16 *
056 Education officers	2	0.27	0.03-0.99	0.47	0.06-1.70 *
06 Religious professions	3	0.10	0.02-0.30	0.19	0.04-0.55 *
060 Clergy and lay preachers	2	0.07	0.01-0.27	0.14	0.02-0.51 *
07 Legal professions	18	0.51	0.30-0.80	1.04	0.61-1.64 *
070 Barristers and judges	1	0.10	0.00-0.57	0.23	0.01-1.26 *
071 Senior police officials	4	0.57	0.16-1.46	1.25	0.34-3.21
072 Lawyers	8	1.10	0.47-2.16	2.44	1.05-4.80 *
073 Solicitors	1	0.15	0.00-0.85	0.34	0.01-1.90 *
08 Artistic and literary professions	54	0.74	0.55-0.96	1.37	1.03-1.79 *
080 Sculptors, painters, etc.	9	0.97	0.44-1.84	2.15	0.98-4.08
084 Journalists	12	0.49	0.25-0.86	0.99	0.51-1.74 *
086 Performing artists	9	1.56	0.71-2.96	3.18	1.46-6.04 *
087 Musicians	14	0.78	0.42-1.30	1.34	0.74-2.26
09 Humanistic and social work etc.	41	0.58	0.42-0.79	0.99	0.71-1.34 *
090 Auditors	1	0.18	0.00-0.99	0.38	0.01-2.14 *
091 Social workers	15	0.87	0.49-1.44	1.33	0.75-2.20
092 Librarians, museum officials	7	1.04	0.42-2.14	1.87	0.75-3.86
096 PR officers	15	0.56	0.31-0.92	0.87	0.49-1.44 *
099 Humanistic/scientific workers N	1	0.18	0.00-1.00	0.33	0.01-1.81 *

Occupation	Obs.	Crude SIR	95% CI	Adjusted SIR	95% CI	
1 Administrative and clerical work	483	0.64	0.59-0.70	1.11	1.01-1.21	*
10 Public administration	38	0.52	0.37-0.72	1.16	0.82-1.60	
11 Corporate administration	186	0.52	0.45-0.60	1.17	1.01-1.34	*
110 Corporate managers	82	0.49	0.39-0.61	1.09	0.87-1.35	
111 Technical managers	15	0.48	0.27-0.80	1.09	0.61-1.79	
112 Commercial managers	45	0.55	0.40-0.74	1.25	0.91-1.67	
113 Administrative managers	4	0.22	0.06-0.57	0.50	0.14-1.28	
114 Managers of ideal organizations	10	0.61	0.29-1.13	1.37	0.65-2.51	
119 Private sector managers NOS	30	0.72	0.49-1.03	1.63	1.10-2.32	*
12 Clerical work	23	0.72	0.46-1.08	1.05	0.67-1.58	
120 Book-keepers, accountants	18	0.67	0.39-1.05	0.99	0.59-1.57	
13 Stenographers and typists	2	0.35	0.04-1.25	0.45	0.05-1.62	
14/15 Clerical work NOS	234	0.82	0.72-0.93	1.08	0.95-1.22	*
143 Photocopier operators etc.	1	0.20	0.01-1.12	0.26	0.01-1.45	
144 Office clerks	34	0.73	0.51-1.02	0.95	0.65-1.32	
145 Bank clerks	6	0.37	0.14-0.81	0.61	0.22-1.33	*
146 Insurance clerks	6	0.77	0.28-1.67	1.19	0.44-2.60	
147 Social insurance clerks	-	-/4.5	0.00-0.81	-/3.5	0.00-1.06	*
149 Shipping agents	15	1.04	0.58-1.72	1.35	0.76-2.23	
150 Property managers, warehousemen	134	0.92	0.77-1.08	1.19	1.00-1.40	*
151 Bid calculators, orders clerks	11	1.17	0.59-2.10	1.56	0.78-2.79	
159 Clerical workers NOS	26	0.76	0.50-1.11	0.99	0.64-1.44	
2 Sales professions	437	0.77	0.70-0.84	0.91	0.83-1.00	*
20 Wholesale and retail dealers	129	0.74	0.62-0.87	0.97	0.81-1.14	
200 Wholesalers	13	1.73	0.92-2.95	2.60	1.38-4.44	*
201 Retailers	116	0.70	0.58-0.83	0.90	0.75-1.07	
21 Real estate, services, securities	34	0.79	0.55-1.11	1.09	0.75-1.52	
210 Insurance salesmen	22	0.86	0.54-1.30	1.13	0.71-1.71	
211 Real estate/stockbrokers	7	1.03	0.41-2.11	1.33	0.53-2.73	
212 Advertising sales	4	0.46	0.13-1.19	0.79	0.22-2.03	
22 Sales representatives	104	0.92	0.76-1.11	1.21	0.99-1.45	
220 Commercial travellers, etc.	94	0.92	0.74-1.13	1.20	0.97-1.47	
221 Sales agents	10	0.98	0.47-1.80	1.27	0.61-2.33	
23 Sales work	170	0.71	0.61-0.82	0.74	0.63-0.86	*
230 Buyers, office sales staff	27	0.59	0.39-0.86	0.82	0.54-1.19	
231 Shop personnel	100	0.68	0.55-0.82	0.64	0.52-0.77	*
232 Door-to-door salesmen	24	1.41	0.90-2.10	1.79	1.15-2.67	*
233 Service station attendants	15	0.86	0.48-1.41	1.12	0.63-1.84	
239 Sales staff NOS	4	0.34	0.09-0.86	0.33	0.09-0.83	*
3 Farming, forestry and fishing	3305	0.90	0.87-0.93	0.82	0.79-0.85	*
30 Agricultural/forestry management	2501	0.82	0.78-0.85	0.78	0.75-0.81	*
300 Farmers, silviculturists	2355	0.81	0.78-0.84	0.77	0.74-0.80	*
301 Agricultural managers	13	1.12	0.60-1.91	1.46	0.77-2.49	
302 Forestry managers	91	0.86	0.69-1.05	1.11	0.90-1.37	
303 Horticultural managers	11	0.91	0.45-1.62	1.20	0.60-2.16	
304 Livestock breeders	7	1.14	0.46-2.35	1.06	0.43-2.18	
305 Fur-bearing animal breeders	19	1.17	0.70-1.82	1.10	0.66-1.72	
306 Reindeer breeders	5	0.82	0.27-1.90	0.76	0.25-1.78	
31 Farming, animal husbandry	169	0.98	0.84-1.13	0.76	0.65-0.87	*
310 Agricultural workers	120	0.94	0.78-1.11	0.74	0.61-0.87	*
311 Gardeners	26	1.16	0.76-1.70	0.82	0.53-1.20	
312 Livestock workers	15	0.92	0.52-1.52	0.73	0.41-1.21	
33 Fishing	33	1.00	0.69-1.40	0.91	0.63-1.28	
330 Fishermen	31	0.97	0.66-1.38	0.89	0.60-1.26	
34 Forestry work	602	1.54	1.42-1.67	1.07	0.98-1.15	*
4 Mining and quarrying	151	2.23	1.88-2.59	2.10	1.77-2.44	*
40 Mining and quarrying	99	2.34	1.90-2.85	2.21	1.80-2.69	*
41 Deep drilling	13	2.17	1.15-3.70	2.09	1.11-3.57	*
42 Concentration plant work	7	1.46	0.59-3.00	1.35	0.54-2.79	
49 Mining and quarrying NOS	32	2.18	1.49-3.07	2.01	1.37-2.84	*
5 Transport and communications	1068	0.95	0.89-1.01	1.01	0.95-1.07	
50 Ship's officers	47	0.95	0.70-1.27	1.38	1.02-1.84	*
500 Ship's masters and mates	18	0.82	0.49-1.30	1.40	0.83-2.21	
501 Ship pilots	13	1.37	0.73-2.35	1.78	0.95-3.04	
502 Chief engineers in ships	16	0.90	0.51-1.46	1.16	0.66-1.88	
51 Deck and engine-room crew	39	1.36	0.97-1.86	1.25	0.89-1.71	
510 Deck crew	27	1.38	0.91-2.01	1.27	0.84-1.85	

Occupation	Obs.	Crude SIR	95% CI	Adjusted SIR	95% CI	
511 Engine-room crew	12	1.31	0.68-2.29	1.21	0.63-2.12	
53 Engine drivers	34	0.66	0.46-0.92	0.61	0.43-0.86	*
54 Road transport	718	1.07	0.99-1.15	1.13	1.04-1.21	*
540 Motor-vehicle and tram drivers	717	1.07	0.99-1.15	1.13	1.05-1.21	*
55 Transport services	74	0.64	0.50-0.80	0.64	0.50-0.81	*
550 Railway staff	72	0.63	0.49-0.79	0.63	0.49-0.80	*
56 Traffic supervisors	39	0.59	0.42-0.80	0.88	0.62-1.20	*
560 Port traffic supervisors	7	0.88	0.35-1.81	1.26	0.51-2.60	
562 Railway traffic supervisors	19	0.57	0.34-0.89	0.81	0.49-1.27	*
563 Road transport supervisors	11	0.48	0.24-0.86	0.76	0.38-1.36	*
57 Post and telecommunications	18	0.53	0.32-0.84	0.69	0.41-1.10	*
570 Post/telecommunications officials	14	0.52	0.29-0.88	0.68	0.37-1.15	*
573 Telegraphists	2	0.36	0.04-1.29	0.46	0.06-1.67	
58 Postal services/couriers	62	0.84	0.64-1.07	0.78	0.60-1.00	*
580 Postmen	36	0.82	0.58-1.14	0.75	0.53-1.05	
581 Caretakers/messengers	26	0.85	0.56-1.25	0.82	0.53-1.20	
59 Communication work NOS	36	1.25	0.87-1.73	1.16	0.81-1.61	
591 Canal/harbour guards, ferrymen	10	1.82	0.87-3.34	1.69	0.81-3.11	
599 Communication workers NOS	22	1.00	0.63-1.51	0.93	0.58-1.41	
6/7 Industrial and construction work	5705	1.29	1.25-1.32	1.14	1.12-1.17	*
60 Textiles	38	0.93	0.66-1.28	0.88	0.62-1.21	
603 Textile machine setters operato	13	1.03	0.55-1.77	0.96	0.51-1.64	
605 Textile finishers/dyers	12	0.96	0.50-1.68	0.89	0.46-1.56	
61 Cutting/sewing etc.	50	1.19	0.88-1.57	1.23	0.91-1.62	
610 Tailors	14	1.08	0.59-1.82	1.16	0.64-1.95	
614 Upholsterers	11	0.82	0.41-1.47	0.86	0.43-1.55	
616 Garment workers	5	0.94	0.31-2.20	0.94	0.31-2.20	
619 Cutting/sewing workers NOS	6	3.48	1.28-7.57	3.45	1.27-7.51	*
62 Shoes and leather	42	1.18	0.85-1.60	1.24	0.89-1.67	
620 Shoemakers and cobblers	22	1.76	1.10-2.67	2.09	1.31-3.16	*
626 Saddlers, leather sewers, etc.	8	0.85	0.37-1.67	0.91	0.39-1.79	
63 Smelting, metal and foundry work	177	1.42	1.22-1.64	1.36	1.16-1.56	*
630 Smelter furnacemen	24	1.17	0.75-1.73	1.08	0.69-1.60	
632 Hot-rollers	11	2.36	1.18-4.23	2.19	1.09-3.92	*
634 Blacksmiths	64	1.86	1.43-2.38	1.91	1.47-2.44	*
635 Founders	46	1.29	0.94-1.72	1.19	0.87-1.59	
639 Metalworkers NOS	23	1.10	0.70-1.66	1.03	0.66-1.55	
64 Precision mechanical work	37	0.78	0.55-1.07	0.82	0.58-1.13	
640 Precision mechanics	13	0.94	0.50-1.61	0.89	0.47-1.52	
641 Watchmakers	10	0.80	0.38-1.47	0.92	0.44-1.69	
643 Dental technicians	3	0.52	0.11-1.52	0.61	0.13-1.78	
644 Goldsmiths, silversmiths etc.	9	0.80	0.36-1.51	0.84	0.38-1.59	
65 Machine shop/steelworkers	1060	1.25	1.17-1.32	1.18	1.11-1.25	*
650 Turners, machinists	216	1.11	0.97-1.27	1.04	0.91-1.19	
651 Fitter-assemblers etc.	86	1.06	0.85-1.30	0.99	0.79-1.22	
652 Machine and motor repairers	228	1.16	1.02-1.32	1.12	0.98-1.27	*
653 Sheetmetalworkers	112	1.45	1.19-1.73	1.39	1.14-1.66	*
654 Plumbers	173	1.58	1.35-1.82	1.50	1.29-1.74	*
655 Welders and flame cutters	101	1.26	1.02-1.51	1.17	0.95-1.41	*
656 Plate/constructional steel work	26	1.03	0.67-1.51	0.96	0.63-1.41	
657 Metal platers and coaters	7	1.31	0.52-2.69	1.24	0.50-2.55	
659 Machine shop/steelworkers NOS	111	1.37	1.13-1.64	1.30	1.07-1.55	*
66 Electrical work	257	1.01	0.89-1.14	0.95	0.84-1.07	
660 Electricians (indoors)	131	0.95	0.80-1.12	0.90	0.75-1.06	
661 Electric machine operators	21	1.04	0.64-1.58	0.96	0.59-1.47	
662 Electric fitters	6	1.05	0.39-2.29	0.98	0.36-2.13	
663 Electronics and telefitters	7	0.54	0.22-1.11	0.54	0.22-1.11	
664 Telephone installers and repair	45	1.19	0.86-1.59	1.10	0.80-1.47	
665 Linemen	30	1.16	0.78-1.66	1.07	0.73-1.53	
666 Electronic equipment assemblers	10	1.29	0.62-2.38	1.20	0.58-2.21	
669 Electrical workers NOS	7	1.10	0.44-2.27	1.11	0.44-2.28	
67 Woodwork	1117	1.20	1.13-1.27	1.13	1.07-1.20	*
670 Round-timber workers	26	1.26	0.82-1.85	1.18	0.77-1.73	
671 Timber workers	88	0.77	0.62-0.95	0.73	0.59-0.90	*
672 Plywood makers	39	1.28	0.91-1.75	1.19	0.85-1.63	
673 Construction carpenters	801	1.36	1.27-1.46	1.27	1.19-1.36	*
674 Boatbuilders etc.	20	0.91	0.55-1.40	0.91	0.55-1.40	
675 Bench carpenters	46	0.86	0.63-1.14	0.88	0.64-1.17	
676 Cabinetmakers etc.	32	0.95	0.65-1.34	0.93	0.64-1.31	
677 Woodworking machine operators e	45	0.89	0.65-1.19	0.84	0.61-1.13	

Appendix Table C

Occupation	Obs.	Crude SIR	95% CI	Adjusted SIR	95% CI	
678 Wooden surface finishers	7	1.19	0.48-2.45	1.09	0.44-2.25	
679 Woodworkers NOS	13	1.20	0.64-2.06	1.13	0.60-1.94	
68 Painting and lacquering	217	1.30	1.13-1.48	1.26	1.10-1.44	*
680 Painters	210	1.35	1.17-1.54	1.31	1.14-1.50	*
681 Lacquerers	7	0.60	0.24-1.24	0.58	0.23-1.20	
69 Construction work NOS	1224	1.67	1.58-1.77	1.27	1.20-1.35	*
690 Bricklayers and tile setters	142	1.51	1.27-1.77	1.42	1.20-1.66	*
691 Reinforced concreters etc.	6	3.32	1.22-7.23	3.09	1.13-6.72	*
692 Reinforcing iron workers	37	1.70	1.20-2.35	1.57	1.10-2.16	*
693 Concrete/cement shutterers	89	1.48	1.19-1.82	1.39	1.11-1.71	*
694 Asphalt roofers	18	3.50	2.07-5.53	3.25	1.92-5.13	*
695 Insulators	62	3.71	2.85-4.76	3.56	2.73-4.56	*
697 Building hands	495	1.68	1.54-1.84	1.17	1.06-1.27	*
698 Roadbuilding hands	327	1.61	1.44-1.79	1.13	1.01-1.26	*
699 Construction workers NOS	40	1.30	0.93-1.77	1.29	0.92-1.76	
70 Printing	50	0.90	0.67-1.18	0.84	0.62-1.10	
700 Typographers etc.	16	0.73	0.41-1.18	0.67	0.38-1.09	
701 Printers	19	1.16	0.70-1.82	1.08	0.65-1.69	
702 Lithographers	1	0.21	0.01-1.15	0.19	0.00-1.05	
703 Bookbinders	7	0.94	0.38-1.95	0.88	0.35-1.82	
709 Printing workers NOS	7	1.36	0.55-2.79	1.38	0.55-2.84	
71 Glass and ceramic work	33	1.12	0.77-1.58	1.05	0.72-1.48	
710 Glass formers	10	1.10	0.53-2.02	1.02	0.49-1.88	
711 Potters	10	1.10	0.53-2.02	1.04	0.50-1.91	
72 Food industry	87	0.93	0.75-1.15	0.90	0.72-1.10	
720 Grain millers	14	0.89	0.49-1.49	0.88	0.48-1.48	
721 Bakers and pastry chiefs	21	0.99	0.61-1.51	1.00	0.62-1.53	
723 Brewers and beverage producers	4	0.80	0.22-2.05	0.74	0.20-1.90	
724 Food preservation	-	-/4.0	0.00-0.93	-/4.2	0.00-0.87	*
725 Butchers and sausage makers	27	1.13	0.75-1.65	1.06	0.70-1.54	
726 Dairy workers	7	0.60	0.24-1.23	0.56	0.22-1.15	
73 Chemical process/paper making	173	1.19	1.02-1.37	1.10	0.94-1.27	*
731 Cookers (chemical processes)	13	1.33	0.71-2.27	1.23	0.66-2.11	
733 Wood grinders	10	0.96	0.46-1.76	0.89	0.42-1.63	
734 Pulp mill workers	60	1.47	1.12-1.90	1.36	1.04-1.76	*
735 Paper and board mill workers	53	0.99	0.74-1.29	0.91	0.69-1.20	
739 Chemical process workers NOS	31	1.18	0.80-1.68	1.10	0.75-1.56	
75 Industrial work NOS	104	1.08	0.88-1.30	1.05	0.86-1.26	
750 Basket and brush makers	9	1.67	0.76-3.17	2.05	0.94-3.89	
751 Industrial rubber products	14	0.96	0.52-1.61	0.89	0.49-1.50	
752 Plastics	16	0.93	0.53-1.52	0.89	0.51-1.44	
753 Tanners and pelt dressers	3	0.42	0.09-1.23	0.40	0.08-1.16	
756 Stone cutters	20	1.67	1.02-2.58	1.68	1.03-2.60	*
757 Paper products	11	1.25	0.62-2.23	1.15	0.58-2.06	
758 Cast concrete products	14	1.07	0.58-1.79	1.02	0.55-1.70	
759 Industrial workers NOS	14	0.95	0.52-1.60	0.93	0.51-1.56	
76 Packing and labelling	36	0.93	0.65-1.29	0.86	0.60-1.19	
77 Machinists	384	1.20	1.08-1.32	1.13	1.02-1.25	*
770 Crane and hoist operators	23	1.05	0.67-1.58	0.97	0.61-1.45	
771 Forklift operators	50	1.13	0.84-1.49	1.05	0.78-1.38	
772 Construction machinery operator	137	1.35	1.13-1.59	1.33	1.12-1.56	*
773 Operators of stationary engine	95	1.11	0.90-1.36	1.03	0.83-1.26	
774 Greasers	27	1.09	0.72-1.59	1.03	0.68-1.50	
775 Industrial personnel, riggers	52	1.21	0.91-1.59	1.13	0.84-1.48	
78 Dock and warehouse work	339	1.27	1.14-1.41	0.96	0.86-1.07	*
780 Dockers	93	1.44	1.17-1.77	1.29	1.04-1.58	*
781 Freight handlers	51	1.31	0.98-1.72	0.92	0.68-1.20	
782 Warehousemen	195	1.20	1.04-1.37	0.87	0.75-1.00	*
79 Labourers not classified elsewhere	277	1.75	1.55-1.96	1.23	1.09-1.38	*
8 Services	512	1.02	0.93-1.11	1.02	0.93-1.11	
80 Watchmen, security guards	189	0.86	0.75-0.99	0.92	0.80-1.06	*
800 Firemen	9	0.44	0.20-0.83	0.49	0.22-0.93	*
801 Policemen	52	0.58	0.44-0.77	0.76	0.56-0.99	*
802 Customs/border control	14	0.70	0.38-1.17	0.93	0.51-1.55	
803 Prison guards	16	0.90	0.51-1.46	0.88	0.50-1.43	
804 Civilian guards	98	1.38	1.12-1.69	1.17	0.95-1.42	*
81 Housekeeping, domestic work, etc.	11	0.86	0.43-1.54	0.95	0.47-1.70	
810 Housekeepers	4	0.55	0.15-1.41	0.72	0.20-1.83	
82 Waiters	10	1.07	0.51-1.97	1.30	0.63-2.40	
821 Waiters in cafés etc.	5	0.88	0.28-2.05	1.11	0.36-2.60	

Occupation	Obs.	Crude SIR	95% CI	Adjusted SIR	95% CI	
83 Caretakers and cleaners	250	1.17	1.03-1.32	1.08	0.95-1.22	*
830 Caretakers	218	1.13	0.99-1.29	1.06	0.92-1.20	
831 Cleaners	7	1.88	0.76-3.87	1.32	0.53-2.73	
832 Chimney sweeps	23	1.46	0.93-2.19	1.35	0.86-2.03	
87 Photography	5	0.55	0.18-1.28	0.71	0.23-1.66	
89 Services NOS	33	1.40	0.96-1.96	1.28	0.88-1.79	
890 Hotel porters	29	1.47	0.99-2.12	1.37	0.92-1.96	
9 Work not classified elsewhere	57	0.78	0.59-1.02	0.97	0.74-1.26	
90 Military occupations	22	0.53	0.33-0.80	0.86	0.54-1.30	*
900 Officers etc.	7	0.36	0.14-0.74	0.82	0.33-1.68	*
901 Non-commissioned officers	13	0.62	0.33-1.06	0.81	0.43-1.39	
91 Occupation not specified	35	1.12	0.78-1.56	1.06	0.74-1.48	
ECONOMICALLY INACTIVE PERSONS	3328	1.73	1.67-1.78	1.59	1.54-1.65	*

C16. Lung cancer, females

Occupation	Obs.	Crude SIR	95% CI	Adjusted SIR	95% CI	
WHOLE POPULATION	1868	0.98	0.93-1.02	0.99	0.94-1.03	
ECONOMICALLY ACTIVE PERSONS	1105	1.00	0.94-1.06	1.00	0.94-1.06	
0 Technical, humanistic, etc. work	113	0.85	0.70-1.02	0.85	0.70-1.02	
01 Technical work	6	0.96	0.35-2.09	0.87	0.32-1.90	
03 Medical work and nursing	52	0.91	0.68-1.19	0.91	0.68-1.19	
032 Nurses	16	1.01	0.57-1.63	0.93	0.53-1.51	
035 Psychiatric nurses	-	-/4.1	0.00-0.91	-/4.5	0.00-0.82	*
036 Auxiliary nurses	20	0.79	0.48-1.22	0.87	0.53-1.34	
04 Health-care related work	8	1.01	0.43-1.98	1.05	0.46-2.08	
05 Teaching	22	0.55	0.35-0.84	0.57	0.35-0.86	*
050 University teachers	3	5.08	1.05-14.8	5.38	1.11-15.7	*
051 Subject teachers	3	0.33	0.07-0.96	0.35	0.07-1.02	*
052 Primary school teachers	6	0.31	0.11-0.68	0.33	0.12-0.71	*
053 Teachers of practical subjects	4	0.79	0.22-2.03	0.75	0.20-1.92	
08 Artistic and literary professions	11	2.36	1.18-4.22	2.40	1.20-4.30	*
083 Authors	2	9.87	1.19-35.7	8.81	1.07-31.8	*
084 Journalists	7	3.51	1.41-7.24	3.68	1.48-7.59	*
09 Humanistic and social work etc.	9	0.88	0.40-1.67	0.85	0.39-1.60	
091 Social workers	2	0.42	0.05-1.52	0.39	0.05-1.42	
1 Administrative and clerical work	181	1.38	1.18-1.58	1.25	1.07-1.43	*
110 Corporate managers	5	3.35	1.09-7.81	3.14	1.02-7.33	*
12 Clerical work	36	1.17	0.82-1.61	1.04	0.73-1.44	
120 Book-keepers, accountants	11	0.75	0.37-1.34	0.67	0.33-1.20	
121 Office cashiers	11	1.78	0.89-3.18	1.58	0.79-2.83	
123 Shop and restaurant cashiers	12	1.55	0.80-2.71	1.39	0.72-2.43	
129 Book-keeping workers/cashiers N	2	8.61	1.04-31.1	7.45	0.90-26.9	*
13 Stenographers and typists	20	1.73	1.06-2.68	1.57	0.96-2.42	*
130 Private secretaries	12	1.92	0.99-3.35	1.74	0.90-3.04	
131 Typists	8	1.52	0.65-2.99	1.37	0.59-2.69	
14/15 Clerical work NOS	115	1.39	1.15-1.65	1.25	1.03-1.49	*
144 Office clerks	80	1.43	1.14-1.79	1.29	1.02-1.60	*
145 Bank clerks	8	0.87	0.38-1.72	0.81	0.35-1.60	
150 Property managers, warehousemen	7	2.88	1.16-5.93	2.54	1.02-5.22	*
159 Clerical workers NOS	12	1.56	0.80-2.72	1.38	0.71-2.41	
2 Sales professions	107	1.01	0.83-1.21	1.04	0.85-1.24	
20 Wholesale and retail dealers	18	1.08	0.64-1.71	0.94	0.56-1.49	
201 Retailers	18	1.09	0.64-1.72	0.95	0.56-1.50	
23 Sales work	85	0.97	0.78-1.21	1.04	0.83-1.29	
231 Shop personnel	78	0.95	0.75-1.18	1.02	0.81-1.27	
3 Farming, forestry and fishing	131	0.50	0.42-0.59	0.51	0.43-0.60	*
30 Agricultural/forestry management	37	0.52	0.37-0.72	0.54	0.38-0.74	*
300 Farmers, silviculturists	36	0.52	0.37-0.72	0.54	0.38-0.75	*
31 Farming, animal husbandry	92	0.48	0.39-0.59	0.49	0.40-0.60	*
310 Agricultural workers	13	0.68	0.36-1.16	0.69	0.37-1.18	

Occupation	Obs.	Crude		Adjusted	
		SIR	95% CI	SIR	95% CI
311 Gardeners	4	0.56	0.15-1.44	0.53	0.15-1.37
312 Livestock workers	74	0.45	0.35-0.56	0.46	0.36-0.58 *
4 Mining and quarrying	-	-/0.4	0.00-10.4	-/0.3	0.00-11.6
5 Transport and communications	41	1.08	0.77-1.46	1.03	0.74-1.40
55 Transport services	9	2.65	1.21-5.02	2.97	1.36-5.64 *
552 Bus/tram services	7	2.52	1.01-5.20	2.86	1.15-5.89 *
57 Post and telecommunications	19	0.96	0.58-1.50	0.86	0.52-1.34
570 Post/telecommunications officials	4	0.47	0.13-1.20	0.42	0.11-1.08
571 Telephone operators	7	0.97	0.39-2.01	0.87	0.35-1.79
58 Postal services/couriers	11	0.97	0.48-1.73	1.01	0.50-1.81
580 Postmen	6	0.61	0.22-1.32	0.63	0.23-1.37
581 Caretakers/messengers	5	3.35	1.09-7.81	3.62	1.18-8.46 *
6/7 Industrial and construction work	245	1.24	1.09-1.40	1.34	1.18-1.51 *
60 Textiles	17	0.73	0.42-1.17	0.81	0.47-1.29
601 Spinners etc.	4	0.77	0.21-1.97	0.87	0.24-2.23
602 Weavers	7	0.87	0.35-1.80	0.95	0.38-1.96
61 Cutting/sewing etc.	35	0.87	0.61-1.22	0.93	0.65-1.30
611 Dressmakers	7	0.81	0.33-1.67	0.77	0.31-1.58
616 Garment workers	19	0.86	0.52-1.34	0.95	0.57-1.49
62 Shoes and leather	8	1.09	0.47-2.14	1.20	0.52-2.36
65 Machine shop/steelworkers	13	1.72	0.92-2.95	1.92	1.02-3.29 *
650 Turners, machinists	5	3.13	1.02-7.30	3.53	1.15-8.24 *
67 Woodwork	23	1.36	0.86-2.05	1.53	0.97-2.29
672 Plywood makers	11	1.41	0.71-2.53	1.59	0.79-2.84
69 Construction work NOS	23	2.80	1.78-4.21	2.56	1.62-3.84 *
697 Building hands	21	3.08	1.91-4.71	2.79	1.72-4.26 *
70 Printing	12	1.63	0.84-2.85	1.83	0.94-3.19
72 Food industry	23	0.98	0.62-1.47	1.08	0.69-1.63
721 Bakers and pastry chiefs	14	1.29	0.71-2.17	1.41	0.77-2.37
73 Chemical process/paper making	3	0.46	0.09-1.34	0.52	0.11-1.51
75 Industrial work NOS	12	1.03	0.53-1.79	1.14	0.59-1.99
76 Packing and labelling	27	1.49	0.98-2.17	1.67	1.10-2.43 *
77 Machinists	11	2.74	1.37-4.91	2.72	1.36-4.87 *
78 Dock and warehouse work	20	2.26	1.38-3.49	2.15	1.31-3.32 *
780 Dockers	6	5.90	2.17-12.8	6.56	2.41-14.3 *
782 Warehousemen	14	1.89	1.03-3.17	1.77	0.97-2.97 *
8 Services	283	1.21	1.08-1.36	1.16	1.03-1.30 *
804 Civilian guards	3	7.45	1.54-21.8	7.84	1.62-22.9 *
81 Housekeeping, domestic work, etc.	72	0.90	0.70-1.13	0.87	0.68-1.10
810 Housekeepers	12	1.55	0.80-2.70	1.38	0.71-2.40
811 Chefs, cooks etc.	21	1.04	0.64-1.59	1.17	0.73-1.80
812 Kitchen assistants	15	0.69	0.39-1.14	0.63	0.35-1.03
813 Domestic servants	16	0.76	0.43-1.23	0.73	0.42-1.18
814 Communal home-help services	3	0.62	0.13-1.80	0.56	0.12-1.64
82 Waiters	50	2.19	1.62-2.88	2.26	1.67-2.97 *
820 Waiters in restaurants	33	3.13	2.16-4.40	3.41	2.35-4.79 *
821 Waiters in cafés etc.	17	1.38	0.80-2.21	1.36	0.79-2.18
83 Caretakers and cleaners	130	1.21	1.01-1.43	1.13	0.95-1.34 *
830 Caretakers	6	0.53	0.20-1.16	0.60	0.22-1.30
831 Cleaners	122	1.27	1.06-1.51	1.17	0.98-1.39 *
84 Hygiene and beauty services	14	1.33	0.72-2.22	1.23	0.67-2.06
840 Hairdressers and barbers	10	1.21	0.58-2.22	1.11	0.53-2.04
85 Laundry and pressing	12	1.26	0.65-2.19	1.22	0.63-2.13
850 Launderers	11	1.38	0.69-2.46	1.30	0.65-2.33
9 Work not classified elsewhere	4	1.67	0.45-4.28	1.88	0.51-4.81
ECONOMICALLY INACTIVE PERSONS	763	0.94	0.88-1.01	0.97	0.91-1.04

Occupation	Obs.	Crude		Adjusted	
		SIR	95% CI	SIR	95% CI

C17. Breast cancer, males

Occupation	Obs.	SIR	95% CI	SIR	95% CI
WHOLE POPULATION	47	0.95	0.70-1.27	0.95	0.70-1.26
ECONOMICALLY ACTIVE PERSONS	42	1.00	0.72-1.35	1.00	0.72-1.35
0 Technical, humanistic, etc. work	5	1.25	0.41-2.92	0.96	0.31-2.25
1 Administrative and clerical work	4	1.60	0.44-4.09	1.07	0.29-2.74
2 Sales professions	3	1.47	0.30-4.31	1.67	0.34-4.88
3 Farming, forestry and fishing	11	0.91	0.46-1.63	0.97	0.49-1.74
30 Agricultural/forestry management	8	0.81	0.35-1.59	0.87	0.37-1.71
300 Farmers, silviculturists	8	0.85	0.37-1.68	0.91	0.39-1.79
4 Mining and quarrying	-	-/0.2	0.00-16.1	-/0.2	0.00-17.5
5 Transport and communications	2	0.51	0.06-1.85	0.56	0.07-2.04
6/7 Industrial and construction work	14	0.91	0.50-1.53	0.97	0.53-1.63
8 Services	3	1.81	0.37-5.29	1.96	0.40-5.74
9 Work not classified elsewhere	-	-/0.3	0.00-13.1	-/0.3	0.00-11.5
ECONOMICALLY INACTIVE PERSONS	5	0.68	0.22-1.59	0.67	0.22-1.56

C18. Breast cancer, females

Occupation	Obs.	SIR	95% CI	SIR	95% CI	
WHOLE POPULATION	13782	0.96	0.95-0.98	0.96	0.95-0.98	*
ECONOMICALLY ACTIVE PERSONS	8723	1.00	0.98-1.02	1.00	0.98-1.02	
0 Technical, humanistic, etc. work	1676	1.37	1.30-1.43	1.10	1.04-1.15	*
00 Technical professions	11	1.66	0.83-2.96	1.09	0.54-1.95	
000 Architects	7	2.06	0.83-4.25	1.35	0.54-2.77	
01 Technical work	97	1.57	1.27-1.91	1.31	1.06-1.59	*
016 Technicians NOS	6	3.61	1.32-7.85	3.01	1.11-6.56	*
018 Draughtsmen, survey assistants	32	1.81	1.24-2.56	1.52	1.04-2.15	*
019 Laboratory assistants	54	1.37	1.03-1.78	1.14	0.85-1.48	
02 Chemical/physical/biological work	41	1.81	1.30-2.45	1.38	0.99-1.87	*
020 Chemists	5	1.41	0.46-3.28	0.92	0.30-2.14	
027 Consultancy, agriculture	33	1.98	1.37-2.79	1.59	1.09-2.23	*
03 Medical work and nursing	677	1.24	1.15-1.34	1.16	1.08-1.25	*
030 Medical doctors	16	1.27	0.72-2.05	0.84	0.48-1.36	
031 Dentists	29	1.59	1.07-2.29	1.04	0.70-1.50	*
032 Nurses	269	1.66	1.47-1.86	1.38	1.22-1.55	*
033 Doctor's/dentist's receptionist	16	1.35	0.77-2.18	1.44	0.83-2.34	
034 Midwives	32	1.31	0.90-1.85	1.08	0.74-1.52	
035 Psychiatric nurses	40	1.08	0.77-1.47	0.89	0.64-1.21	
036 Auxiliary nurses	215	0.92	0.80-1.05	1.06	0.93-1.21	
037 Technical nursing assistants	5	0.84	0.27-1.95	0.97	0.31-2.26	
038 Institutional children's nurses	51	1.37	1.02-1.80	1.14	0.85-1.51	*
04 Health-care related work	88	1.25	1.01-1.54	0.89	0.72-1.10	*
040 Pharmacists	57	1.33	1.00-1.72	0.87	0.66-1.12	*
041 Physiotherapists	14	1.56	0.85-2.62	1.31	0.72-2.20	
043 Masseurs, etc.	5	0.89	0.29-2.08	0.76	0.25-1.77	
044 Pharmaceutical assistants	10	0.97	0.46-1.78	0.80	0.38-1.47	
05 Teaching	538	1.49	1.37-1.62	1.03	0.94-1.12	*
050 University teachers	8	1.33	0.57-2.61	0.89	0.39-1.76	
051 Subject teachers	154	1.61	1.36-1.87	1.09	0.92-1.27	*
052 Primary school teachers	239	1.47	1.29-1.67	0.97	0.85-1.09	*

Occupation	Obs.	Crude SIR	95% CI	Adjusted SIR	95% CI
053 Teachers of practical subjects	67	1.46	1.13-1.85	1.10	0.85-1.40 *
054 Vocational teachers	38	1.27	0.90-1.74	0.99	0.70-1.36
055 Preschool teachers	24	1.52	0.98-2.27	1.27	0.81-1.89
06 Religious professions	20	1.06	0.65-1.63	0.85	0.52-1.32
060 Clergy and lay preachers	6	0.92	0.34-2.00	0.71	0.26-1.55
061 Deacons and social workers	14	1.15	0.63-1.92	0.95	0.52-1.59
07 Legal professions	3	0.53	0.11-1.55	0.34	0.07-1.01
073 Solicitors	-	-/3.8	0.00-0.96	-/5.9	0.00-0.62 *
08 Artistic and literary professions	70	1.64	1.28-2.08	1.18	0.92-1.49 *
080 Sculptors, painters, etc.	12	3.93	2.03-6.86	2.59	1.34-4.53 *
081 Commercial artists	5	3.10	1.01-7.24	2.62	0.85-6.11 *
084 Journalists	23	1.28	0.81-1.92	0.92	0.58-1.37
085 Industrial designers	11	2.03	1.01-3.64	1.42	0.71-2.53 *
086 Performing artists	8	1.73	0.75-3.41	1.21	0.52-2.38
09 Humanistic and social work etc.	131	1.45	1.21-1.71	1.07	0.90-1.26 *
091 Social workers	65	1.58	1.22-2.01	1.20	0.92-1.52 *
092 Librarians, museum officials	26	0.98	0.64-1.44	0.71	0.46-1.04
096 PR officers	19	2.21	1.33-3.45	1.69	1.02-2.64 *
099 Humanistic/scientific workers N	8	1.62	0.70-3.20	1.14	0.49-2.24
1 Administrative and clerical work	1554	1.31	1.25-1.38	1.07	1.02-1.12 *
10 Public administration	38	1.91	1.35-2.62	1.24	0.88-1.70 *
11 Corporate administration	40	1.46	1.04-1.99	0.93	0.67-1.27 *
110 Corporate managers	14	1.40	0.76-2.34	0.87	0.48-1.47
112 Commercial managers	-	-/3.6	0.00-1.02	-/5.5	0.00-0.67 *
114 Managers of ideal organizations	6	3.20	1.18-6.97	2.06	0.75-4.47 *
119 Private sector managers NOS	13	1.56	0.83-2.66	1.00	0.53-1.71
12 Clerical work	350	1.35	1.21-1.50	1.10	0.99-1.22 *
120 Book-keepers, accountants	159	1.33	1.13-1.55	1.08	0.92-1.25 *
121 Office cashiers	97	1.96	1.59-2.39	1.60	1.30-1.95 *
122 Bank and post office cashiers	28	1.42	0.95-2.06	1.18	0.78-1.71
123 Shop and restaurant cashiers	65	0.94	0.73-1.20	0.78	0.60-0.99 *
13 Stenographers and typists	159	1.41	1.20-1.63	1.17	1.00-1.36 *
130 Private secretaries	86	1.36	1.09-1.68	1.14	0.91-1.41 *
131 Typists	73	1.47	1.15-1.85	1.22	0.95-1.53 *
14/15 Clerical work NOS	967	1.27	1.19-1.35	1.05	0.98-1.11 *
142 Data storage assistants	11	1.06	0.53-1.89	0.91	0.46-1.63
143 Photocopier operators etc.	21	1.13	0.70-1.73	0.94	0.58-1.43
144 Office clerks	627	1.25	1.15-1.35	1.03	0.95-1.11 *
145 Bank clerks	132	1.31	1.09-1.54	1.09	0.91-1.29 *
146 Insurance clerks	34	1.35	0.94-1.89	1.13	0.78-1.58
147 Social insurance clerks	8	0.77	0.33-1.52	0.65	0.28-1.29
148 Travel agents	8	1.57	0.68-3.09	1.32	0.57-2.61
150 Property managers, warehousemen	22	1.27	0.79-1.92	1.02	0.64-1.55
151 Bid calculators, orders clerks	6	1.45	0.53-3.15	1.21	0.44-2.63
159 Clerical workers NOS	86	1.39	1.11-1.71	1.13	0.90-1.40 *
2 Sales professions	964	1.08	1.01-1.15	1.12	1.05-1.19 *
20 Wholesale and retail dealers	135	1.18	0.99-1.38	0.94	0.79-1.11
201 Retailers	134	1.17	0.98-1.38	0.94	0.79-1.11
21 Real estate, services, securities	8	1.58	0.68-3.12	1.25	0.54-2.46
22 Sales representatives	10	0.68	0.33-1.25	0.56	0.27-1.03
220 Commercial travellers, etc.	8	0.59	0.26-1.17	0.49	0.21-0.97 *
23 Sales work	811	1.07	0.99-1.14	1.16	1.08-1.24 *
230 Buyers, office sales staff	24	1.40	0.90-2.08	1.16	0.75-1.73
231 Shop personnel	756	1.05	0.98-1.13	1.16	1.08-1.25 *
232 Door-to-door salesmen	8	0.85	0.37-1.67	0.72	0.31-1.41
239 Sales staff NOS	20	1.48	0.91-2.29	1.65	1.01-2.55 *
3 Farming, forestry and fishing	1285	0.71	0.67-0.74	0.77	0.73-0.81 *
30 Agricultural/forestry management	313	0.74	0.66-0.82	0.83	0.74-0.92 *
300 Farmers, silviculturists	304	0.74	0.66-0.82	0.83	0.74-0.93 *
304 Livestock breeders	4	0.50	0.14-1.27	0.56	0.15-1.45
31 Farming, animal husbandry	972	0.70	0.66-0.74	0.76	0.71-0.81 *
310 Agricultural workers	107	0.78	0.64-0.94	0.82	0.68-0.99 *
311 Gardeners	40	0.81	0.58-1.11	1.00	0.72-1.36
312 Livestock workers	817	0.68	0.64-0.73	0.74	0.69-0.79 *
313 Fur-farm workers	6	1.06	0.39-2.31	1.26	0.46-2.73
4 Mining and quarrying	2	0.80	0.10-2.89	0.92	0.11-3.31

Occupation	Obs.	Crude		Adjusted	
		SIR	95% CI	SIR	95% CI
5 Transport and communications	308	1.03	0.92-1.15	0.95	0.85-1.06
54 Road transport	6	0.51	0.19-1.12	0.46	0.17-0.99 *
540 Motor-vehicle and tram drivers	6	0.53	0.20-1.16	0.47	0.17-1.02
55 Transport services	36	1.36	0.95-1.88	1.54	1.08-2.13 *
552 Bus/tram services	28	1.27	0.84-1.83	1.47	0.97-2.12
56 Traffic supervisors	28	2.42	1.61-3.49	1.90	1.26-2.74 *
562 Railway traffic supervisors	26	2.56	1.67-3.75	2.02	1.32-2.95 *
57 Post and telecommunications	188	1.15	0.99-1.32	0.94	0.81-1.07
570 Post/telecommunications officials	79	1.11	0.88-1.39	0.91	0.72-1.13
571 Telephone operators	65	1.14	0.88-1.45	0.92	0.71-1.18
572 Switchboard operators	33	1.26	0.87-1.77	1.04	0.71-1.46
573 Telegraphists	11	1.17	0.58-2.09	0.95	0.48-1.70
58 Postal services/couriers	49	0.59	0.44-0.78	0.71	0.52-0.93 *
580 Postmen	37	0.51	0.36-0.70	0.61	0.43-0.84 *
581 Caretakers/messengers	12	1.22	0.63-2.13	1.44	0.74-2.51
6/7 Industrial and construction work	1424	0.92	0.87-0.96	1.05	0.99-1.10 *
60 Textiles	152	0.88	0.74-1.02	0.99	0.84-1.15
600 Pre-process yarnworker	10	1.12	0.53-2.05	1.29	0.62-2.38
601 Spinners etc.	32	0.83	0.57-1.17	0.96	0.66-1.36
602 Weavers	41	0.71	0.51-0.96	0.78	0.56-1.06 *
604 Knitters	32	1.50	1.03-2.12	1.71	1.17-2.42 *
605 Textile finishers/dyers	14	0.65	0.35-1.09	0.75	0.41-1.26
606 Textile quality controllers	9	0.68	0.31-1.28	0.78	0.36-1.48
609 Textile workers NOS	13	1.09	0.58-1.87	1.18	0.63-2.02
61 Cutting/sewing etc.	361	1.13	1.02-1.25	1.23	1.10-1.36 *
610 Tailors	7	1.12	0.45-2.30	1.16	0.47-2.39
611 Dressmakers	89	1.48	1.19-1.82	1.33	1.07-1.64 *
612 Furriers	8	1.36	0.59-2.67	1.45	0.63-2.86
613 Milliners	9	0.74	0.34-1.41	0.79	0.36-1.50
614 Upholsterers	9	1.29	0.59-2.45	1.44	0.66-2.73
615 Patternmakers and cutters	35	1.24	0.87-1.73	1.43	1.00-2.00
616 Garment workers	191	1.03	0.89-1.18	1.19	1.02-1.36 *
619 Cutting/sewing workers NOS	13	0.89	0.47-1.52	1.00	0.53-1.71
62 Shoes and leather	68	1.16	0.90-1.47	1.31	1.01-1.65 *
622 Shoe sewers	31	1.37	0.93-1.94	1.58	1.07-2.24 *
625 Shoemakers NOS	17	1.21	0.70-1.93	1.40	0.82-2.25
626 Saddlers, leather sewers, etc.	11	0.90	0.45-1.61	0.95	0.47-1.70
63 Smelting, metal and foundry work	8	0.58	0.25-1.14	0.67	0.29-1.33
639 Metalworkers NOS	3	0.44	0.09-1.29	0.51	0.11-1.49
64 Precision mechanical work	5	0.96	0.31-2.24	1.02	0.33-2.39
65 Machine shop/steelworkers	47	0.78	0.58-1.04	0.90	0.66-1.20
650 Turners, machinists	5	0.41	0.13-0.96	0.48	0.15-1.11 *
659 Machine shop/steelworkers NOS	35	0.95	0.66-1.32	1.10	0.76-1.53
66 Electrical work	34	1.01	0.70-1.41	1.16	0.80-1.62
664 Telephone installers and repair	4	4.35	1.18-11.1	5.02	1.37-12.9 *
666 Electronic equipment assemblers	26	0.93	0.61-1.36	1.07	0.70-1.57
67 Woodwork	102	0.78	0.63-0.94	0.90	0.73-1.08 *
671 Timber workers	21	0.81	0.50-1.24	0.94	0.58-1.44
672 Plywood makers	41	0.66	0.48-0.90	0.77	0.55-1.04 *
677 Woodworking machine operators e	15	0.95	0.53-1.56	1.09	0.61-1.80
678 Wooden surface finishers	7	0.96	0.39-1.98	1.11	0.45-2.29
679 Woodworkers NOS	8	0.70	0.30-1.38	0.81	0.35-1.59
68 Painting and lacquering	9	0.51	0.23-0.97	0.59	0.27-1.12 *
680 Painters	7	0.57	0.23-1.18	0.66	0.27-1.36
681 Lacquerers	2	0.37	0.04-1.34	0.42	0.05-1.53
69 Construction work NOS	51	0.86	0.64-1.13	1.07	0.79-1.40
697 Building hands	39	0.79	0.56-1.08	0.99	0.71-1.36
698 Roadbuilding hands	8	1.16	0.50-2.29	1.45	0.63-2.87
70 Printing	74	1.24	0.98-1.56	1.44	1.13-1.81 *
700 Typographers etc.	7	0.67	0.27-1.38	0.78	0.31-1.60
701 Printers	14	1.26	0.69-2.11	1.46	0.80-2.45
703 Bookbinders	39	1.35	0.96-1.84	1.57	1.11-2.14 *
709 Printing workers NOS	12	1.87	0.97-3.27	2.08	1.07-3.62 *
71 Glass and ceramic work	10	0.43	0.20-0.78	0.49	0.24-0.91 *
710 Glass formers	2	0.39	0.05-1.42	0.46	0.06-1.65
711 Potters	2	0.28	0.03-1.00	0.32	0.04-1.15 *
719 Glass/ceramic workers NOS	3	0.53	0.11-1.55	0.62	0.13-1.80
72 Food industry	147	0.79	0.67-0.92	0.90	0.76-1.05 *
721 Bakers and pastry chiefs	66	0.79	0.61-1.01	0.89	0.69-1.13
722 Chocolate and confectionery mak	12	0.99	0.51-1.73	1.14	0.59-1.99

Occupation	Obs.	Crude SIR	95% CI	Adjusted SIR	95% CI
723 Brewers and beverage producers	8	0.96	0.42-1.89	1.12	0.48-2.20
724 Food preservation	6	0.67	0.24-1.45	0.77	0.28-1.67
725 Butchers and sausage makers	19	1.12	0.67-1.75	1.30	0.78-2.02
726 Dairy workers	25	0.62	0.40-0.91	0.72	0.46-1.06 *
727 Prepared foods	8	0.94	0.40-1.84	1.09	0.47-2.14
73 Chemical process/paper making	37	0.74	0.52-1.02	0.86	0.61-1.19
735 Paper and board mill workers	20	0.72	0.44-1.12	0.84	0.51-1.30
739 Chemical process workers NOS	13	0.83	0.44-1.43	0.97	0.51-1.65
74 Tobacco industry	7	1.14	0.46-2.35	1.32	0.53-2.72
75 Industrial work NOS	82	0.86	0.68-1.07	0.98	0.78-1.22
751 Industrial rubber products	9	0.57	0.26-1.08	0.66	0.30-1.25
752 Plastics	14	0.65	0.35-1.08	0.75	0.41-1.25
753 Tanners and pelt dressers	6	0.87	0.32-1.89	1.01	0.37-2.19
754 Photolab. workers	12	1.72	0.89-3.00	1.88	0.97-3.29
757 Paper products	16	0.90	0.52-1.47	1.05	0.60-1.70
759 Industrial workers NOS	20	0.91	0.56-1.41	1.04	0.64-1.61
76 Packing and labelling	136	0.91	0.76-1.07	1.05	0.88-1.24
77 Machinists	27	0.83	0.55-1.21	1.00	0.66-1.46
770 Crane and hoist operators	7	0.70	0.28-1.44	0.81	0.33-1.67
774 Greasers	17	0.93	0.54-1.49	1.16	0.67-1.85
78 Dock and warehouse work	59	0.88	0.67-1.14	1.08	0.82-1.39
780 Dockers	6	0.88	0.32-1.93	1.04	0.38-2.26
782 Warehousemen	51	0.90	0.67-1.18	1.11	0.83-1.46
79 Labourers not classified elsewhere	8	0.66	0.28-1.30	0.82	0.36-1.62
8 Services	1494	0.87	0.82-0.91	0.99	0.94-1.04 *
80 Watchmen, security guards	10	1.79	0.86-3.28	1.86	0.89-3.41
81 Housekeeping, domestic work, etc.	578	0.98	0.90-1.06	1.10	1.01-1.19 *
810 Housekeepers	71	1.24	0.97-1.56	1.01	0.79-1.27
811 Chefs, cooks etc.	124	0.84	0.70-0.99	0.97	0.81-1.15 *
812 Kitchen assistants	161	0.97	0.82-1.12	1.21	1.03-1.40 *
813 Domestic servants	136	0.98	0.82-1.15	1.19	1.00-1.40 *
814 Communal home-help services	54	1.20	0.90-1.57	1.20	0.90-1.56
818 Hotel/restaurant manageresses	12	1.24	0.64-2.17	1.01	0.52-1.76
819 Housekeeping workers NOS	12	0.64	0.33-1.12	0.63	0.33-1.10
82 Waiters	170	0.87	0.75-1.01	0.91	0.78-1.06
820 Waiters in restaurants	92	1.03	0.83-1.26	1.13	0.91-1.39
821 Waiters in cafés etc.	78	0.74	0.59-0.93	0.74	0.59-0.93 *
83 Caretakers and cleaners	583	0.76	0.70-0.82	0.94	0.86-1.02 *
830 Caretakers	71	0.75	0.58-0.94	0.86	0.67-1.09 *
831 Cleaners	506	0.76	0.69-0.82	0.95	0.87-1.03 *
84 Hygiene and beauty services	93	1.08	0.87-1.33	0.98	0.79-1.20
840 Hairdressers and barbers	77	1.13	0.89-1.41	0.98	0.78-1.23
841 Beauticians	5	1.03	0.33-2.39	0.91	0.30-2.13
843 Sauna attendants etc.	10	0.92	0.44-1.69	1.06	0.51-1.96
85 Laundry and pressing	42	0.61	0.44-0.83	0.70	0.50-0.94 *
850 Launderers	33	0.57	0.40-0.81	0.65	0.45-0.91 *
851 Pressers	9	0.82	0.37-1.55	0.95	0.43-1.80
87 Photography	8	1.57	0.68-3.10	1.28	0.55-2.52
89 Services NOS	9	1.20	0.55-2.29	1.41	0.64-2.67
891 Service workers NOS	9	1.54	0.71-2.93	1.81	0.83-3.44
9 Work not classified elsewhere	16	0.89	0.51-1.45	1.02	0.58-1.66
90 Military occupations	3	4.46	0.92-13.0	5.08	1.05-14.9 *
902 Rank and file	3	4.52	0.93-13.2	5.18	1.07-15.1 *
91 Occupation not specified	13	0.75	0.40-1.29	0.86	0.46-1.47
ECONOMICALLY INACTIVE PERSONS	5059	0.91	0.88-0.93	0.90	0.88-0.93 *

C19. Cervical cancer

	Obs.	Crude SIR	95% CI	Adjusted SIR	95% CI
WHOLE POPULATION	1917	0.98	0.94-1.02	0.98	0.94-1.03
ECONOMICALLY ACTIVE PERSONS	1127	1.00	0.94-1.06	1.00	0.94-1.06
0 Technical, humanistic, etc. work	89	0.62	0.50-0.77	0.83	0.67-1.02 *
01 Technical work	7	1.01	0.41-2.08	1.18	0.48-2.44

Occupation	Obs.	Crude		Adjusted	
		SIR	95% CI	SIR	95% CI
03 Medical work and nursing	44	0.71	0.51-0.95	0.79	0.57-1.06 *
032 Nurses	10	0.56	0.27-1.03	0.67	0.32-1.23
036 Auxiliary nurses	26	0.96	0.63-1.41	0.96	0.63-1.40
04 Health-care related work	5	0.60	0.19-1.39	0.96	0.31-2.25
040 Pharmacists	2	0.39	0.05-1.42	0.84	0.10-3.02
05 Teaching	22	0.51	0.32-0.78	0.88	0.55-1.33 *
051 Subject teachers	4	0.38	0.10-0.96	0.73	0.20-1.87 *
052 Primary school teachers	11	0.55	0.27-0.98	1.04	0.52-1.87 *
053 Teachers of practical subjects	3	0.55	0.11-1.61	0.77	0.16-2.26
08 Artistic and literary professions	5	0.99	0.32-2.32	1.60	0.52-3.73
09 Humanistic and social work etc.	5	0.46	0.15-1.07	0.67	0.22-1.56
091 Social workers	2	0.40	0.05-1.45	0.55	0.07-1.98
1 Administrative and clerical work	145	1.03	0.87-1.21	1.24	1.04-1.45 *
12 Clerical work	33	1.03	0.71-1.45	1.21	0.83-1.70
120 Book-keepers, accountants	13	0.86	0.46-1.48	1.02	0.54-1.74
121 Office cashiers	5	0.79	0.26-1.85	0.93	0.30-2.17
123 Shop and restaurant cashiers	11	1.33	0.66-2.38	1.56	0.78-2.80
13 Stenographers and typists	14	1.09	0.60-1.84	1.27	0.70-2.14
130 Private secretaries	9	1.28	0.58-2.43	1.48	0.68-2.81
131 Typists	5	0.87	0.28-2.03	1.02	0.33-2.38
14/15 Clerical work NOS	92	1.03	0.83-1.26	1.21	0.98-1.49
144 Office clerks	65	1.09	0.84-1.39	1.28	0.99-1.64
145 Bank clerks	5	0.47	0.15-1.10	0.56	0.18-1.31
159 Clerical workers NOS	10	1.27	0.61-2.33	1.49	0.71-2.74
2 Sales professions	85	0.77	0.62-0.95	0.80	0.64-0.99 *
20 Wholesale and retail dealers	8	0.49	0.21-0.96	0.57	0.25-1.13 *
201 Retailers	8	0.49	0.21-0.97	0.57	0.25-1.13 *
23 Sales work	75	0.82	0.64-1.03	0.83	0.66-1.04
231 Shop personnel	73	0.84	0.66-1.06	0.86	0.67-1.08
3 Farming, forestry and fishing	184	0.71	0.61-0.82	0.67	0.58-0.77 *
30 Agricultural/forestry management	59	0.87	0.66-1.12	0.80	0.61-1.03
300 Farmers, silviculturists	58	0.88	0.66-1.13	0.81	0.61-1.04
31 Farming, animal husbandry	125	0.66	0.55-0.78	0.63	0.52-0.74 *
310 Agricultural workers	6	0.32	0.12-0.69	0.31	0.11-0.67 *
311 Gardeners	10	1.44	0.69-2.64	1.14	0.55-2.10
312 Livestock workers	109	0.67	0.55-0.80	0.64	0.53-0.77 *
4 Mining and quarrying	1	2.87	0.07-16.0	2.81	0.07-15.7
5 Transport and communications	38	0.99	0.70-1.37	1.05	0.74-1.44
54 Road transport	5	3.43	1.12-8.01	3.83	1.24-8.93 *
57 Post and telecommunications	16	0.79	0.45-1.29	0.93	0.53-1.51
570 Post/telecommunications officials	7	0.81	0.33-1.67	0.95	0.38-1.97
571 Telephone operators	7	0.97	0.39-2.00	1.14	0.46-2.36
58 Postal services/couriers	10	0.88	0.42-1.63	0.78	0.38-1.44
580 Postmen	9	0.91	0.42-1.74	0.81	0.37-1.53
6/7 Industrial and construction work	265	1.32	1.17-1.49	1.28	1.13-1.44 *
60 Textiles	30	1.29	0.87-1.84	1.28	0.87-1.83
601 Spinners etc.	8	1.55	0.67-3.05	1.52	0.66-3.00
602 Weavers	6	0.76	0.28-1.66	0.77	0.28-1.67
61 Cutting/sewing etc.	53	1.29	0.97-1.69	1.32	0.99-1.72
611 Dressmakers	15	1.76	0.99-2.91	1.96	1.09-3.23 *
616 Garment workers	28	1.22	0.81-1.76	1.21	0.80-1.74
62 Shoes and leather	6	0.80	0.29-1.74	0.80	0.29-1.74
65 Machine shop/steelworkers	8	1.05	0.45-2.06	1.04	0.45-2.05
67 Woodwork	29	1.72	1.15-2.47	1.70	1.14-2.45 *
672 Plywood makers	15	1.91	1.07-3.15	1.89	1.06-3.12 *
679 Woodworkers NOS	5	3.43	1.11-8.00	3.35	1.09-7.81 *
69 Construction work NOS	14	1.74	0.95-2.92	1.31	0.72-2.19
697 Building hands	10	1.50	0.72-2.76	1.11	0.53-2.04
70 Printing	9	1.19	0.54-2.26	1.18	0.54-2.23
72 Food industry	23	0.96	0.61-1.44	0.95	0.60-1.42
721 Bakers and pastry chiefs	10	0.91	0.44-1.67	0.90	0.43-1.65
73 Chemical process/paper making	5	0.76	0.25-1.77	0.75	0.24-1.75
75 Industrial work NOS	18	1.50	0.89-2.37	1.49	0.88-2.36
76 Packing and labelling	28	1.50	1.00-2.17	1.49	0.99-2.15
77 Machinists	9	2.21	1.01-4.20	1.85	0.85-3.51 *

Appendix Table C

Occupation	Obs.	Crude		Adjusted	
		SIR	95% CI	SIR	95% CI
774 Greasers	7	2.94	1.18-6.07	2.20	0.89-4.54 *
78 Dock and warehouse work	13	1.47	0.78-2.51	1.14	0.61-1.95
782 Warehousemen	11	1.48	0.74-2.64	1.12	0.56-2.01
8 Services	318	1.36	1.21-1.51	1.15	1.03-1.28 *
81 Housekeeping, domestic work, etc.	95	1.18	0.96-1.45	1.02	0.83-1.25
810 Housekeepers	7	0.90	0.36-1.86	1.07	0.43-2.20
811 Chefs, cooks etc.	24	1.19	0.76-1.77	1.17	0.75-1.74
812 Kitchen assistants	29	1.32	0.89-1.90	0.97	0.65-1.39
813 Domestic servants	25	1.20	0.77-1.77	0.96	0.62-1.42
814 Communal home-help services	2	0.39	0.05-1.39	0.35	0.04-1.25
818 Hotel/restaurant manageresses	5	3.87	1.26-9.03	4.57	1.48-10.7 *
82 Waiters	43	1.81	1.31-2.44	1.85	1.34-2.49 *
820 Waiters in restaurants	24	2.19	1.41-3.26	2.24	1.44-3.34 *
821 Waiters in cafés etc.	19	1.48	0.89-2.31	1.52	0.91-2.37
83 Caretakers and cleaners	153	1.44	1.22-1.67	1.12	0.95-1.30 *
830 Caretakers	17	1.44	0.84-2.30	1.41	0.82-2.26
831 Cleaners	136	1.44	1.21-1.70	1.10	0.92-1.29 *
84 Hygiene and beauty services	14	1.28	0.70-2.15	1.38	0.75-2.31
840 Hairdressers and barbers	10	1.17	0.56-2.14	1.31	0.63-2.42
85 Laundry and pressing	11	1.17	0.58-2.09	1.00	0.50-1.79
850 Launderers	9	1.15	0.52-2.17	0.95	0.44-1.81
9 Work not classified elsewhere	2	0.83	0.10-2.98	0.82	0.10-2.96
ECONOMICALLY INACTIVE PERSONS	790	0.95	0.89-1.02	0.96	0.90-1.03

C20. Cancer of the corpus uteri

Occupation	Obs.	Crude		Adjusted	
		SIR	95% CI	SIR	95% CI
WHOLE POPULATION	3842	0.99	0.96-1.02	0.99	0.95-1.02
ECONOMICALLY ACTIVE PERSONS	2315	1.00	0.96-1.04	1.00	0.96-1.04
0 Technical, humanistic, etc. work	318	1.10	0.98-1.22	0.98	0.87-1.09
01 Technical work	16	1.16	0.66-1.89	1.01	0.58-1.64
019 Laboratory assistants	11	1.23	0.61-2.19	1.06	0.53-1.90
02 Chemical/physical/biological work	8	1.40	0.60-2.75	1.18	0.51-2.32
026 Biologists	2	15.7	1.90-56.7	14.2	1.72-51.3 *
027 Consultancy, agriculture	6	1.42	0.52-3.08	1.20	0.44-2.60
03 Medical work and nursing	125	0.99	0.82-1.17	0.92	0.77-1.09
031 Dentists	7	1.53	0.61-3.15	1.16	0.47-2.39
032 Nurses	52	1.48	1.11-1.94	1.27	0.95-1.67 *
034 Midwives	4	0.66	0.18-1.69	0.56	0.15-1.45
035 Psychiatric nurses	5	0.55	0.18-1.29	0.47	0.15-1.10
036 Auxiliary nurses	46	0.82	0.60-1.09	0.86	0.63-1.15
038 Institutional children's nurses	4	0.50	0.14-1.28	0.44	0.12-1.12
04 Health-care related work	18	1.04	0.62-1.65	0.90	0.53-1.43
040 Pharmacists	9	0.84	0.38-1.59	0.73	0.33-1.38
05 Teaching	95	1.10	0.89-1.35	0.95	0.77-1.16
051 Subject teachers	28	1.37	0.91-1.98	1.27	0.84-1.83
052 Primary school teachers	34	0.82	0.57-1.15	0.69	0.48-0.97 *
053 Teachers of practical subjects	13	1.19	0.63-2.03	1.01	0.54-1.72
054 Vocational teachers	12	1.63	0.84-2.84	1.39	0.72-2.43
06 Religious professions	8	1.77	0.76-3.49	1.51	0.65-2.98
08 Artistic and literary professions	20	1.99	1.22-3.08	1.70	1.04-2.62 *
084 Journalists	10	2.32	1.11-4.27	2.00	0.96-3.67 *
09 Humanistic and social work etc.	26	1.19	0.78-1.75	1.00	0.65-1.46
091 Social workers	14	1.38	0.76-2.32	1.14	0.62-1.91
092 Librarians, museum officials	6	0.91	0.33-1.98	0.75	0.28-1.64
1 Administrative and clerical work	366	1.29	1.16-1.42	1.09	0.98-1.21 *
10 Public administration	7	1.33	0.54-2.75	1.07	0.43-2.20
11 Corporate administration	8	1.07	0.46-2.10	0.82	0.35-1.61
12 Clerical work	94	1.42	1.15-1.74	1.20	0.97-1.47 *
120 Book-keepers, accountants	42	1.35	0.97-1.82	1.13	0.81-1.53
121 Office cashiers	27	2.07	1.37-3.02	1.75	1.15-2.54 *
122 Bank and post office cashiers	5	1.09	0.35-2.53	0.94	0.30-2.19

Occupation	Obs.	Crude		Adjusted	
		SIR	95% CI	SIR	95% CI
123 Shop and restaurant cashiers	20	1.19	0.73-1.84	1.02	0.62-1.57
13 Stenographers and typists	34	1.34	0.93-1.88	1.16	0.80-1.61
130 Private secretaries	15	1.09	0.61-1.80	0.94	0.53-1.55
131 Typists	19	1.64	0.99-2.56	1.41	0.85-2.20
14/15 Clerical work NOS	223	1.24	1.08-1.40	1.06	0.92-1.20 *
143 Photocopier operators etc.	4	0.91	0.25-2.33	0.78	0.21-2.01
144 Office clerks	136	1.12	0.94-1.32	0.96	0.81-1.13
145 Bank clerks	34	1.64	1.13-2.29	1.44	1.00-2.01 *
146 Insurance clerks	10	1.82	0.87-3.35	1.58	0.76-2.91
150 Property managers, warehousemen	6	1.21	0.45-2.64	1.01	0.37-2.20
159 Clerical workers NOS	24	1.48	0.95-2.20	1.25	0.80-1.85
2 Sales professions	241	1.06	0.93-1.20	1.04	0.91-1.17
20 Wholesale and retail dealers	36	1.07	0.75-1.48	0.88	0.62-1.22
201 Retailers	36	1.08	0.75-1.49	0.89	0.62-1.23
23 Sales work	199	1.05	0.91-1.20	1.07	0.93-1.22
231 Shop personnel	185	1.03	0.89-1.19	1.06	0.91-1.22
3 Farming, forestry and fishing	462	0.87	0.79-0.95	0.92	0.84-1.00 *
30 Agricultural/forestry management	135	1.00	0.84-1.18	1.10	0.92-1.30
300 Farmers, silviculturists	131	1.00	0.84-1.18	1.10	0.92-1.30
31 Farming, animal husbandry	327	0.83	0.74-0.92	0.86	0.77-0.96 *
310 Agricultural workers	32	0.82	0.56-1.16	0.84	0.57-1.19
311 Gardeners	11	0.76	0.38-1.37	0.90	0.45-1.61
312 Livestock workers	282	0.83	0.73-0.93	0.86	0.76-0.97 *
4 Mining and quarrying	-	-/0.7	0.00-5.08	-/0.7	0.00-5.37
5 Transport and communications	71	0.88	0.69-1.11	0.82	0.64-1.04
55 Transport services	5	0.69	0.22-1.61	0.74	0.24-1.74
552 Bus/tram services	4	0.67	0.18-1.72	0.73	0.20-1.87
57 Post and telecommunications	41	0.96	0.69-1.30	0.81	0.58-1.10
570 Post/telecommunications officials	26	1.40	0.91-2.05	1.19	0.78-1.75
571 Telephone operators	11	0.72	0.36-1.29	0.61	0.30-1.09
572 Switchboard operators	3	0.47	0.10-1.36	0.40	0.08-1.16
58 Postal services/couriers	17	0.73	0.42-1.16	0.81	0.47-1.30
580 Postmen	15	0.73	0.41-1.21	0.82	0.46-1.35
6/7 Industrial and construction work	413	0.99	0.90-1.09	1.05	0.95-1.16
60 Textiles	48	1.00	0.73-1.32	1.05	0.77-1.39
601 Spinners etc.	12	1.11	0.58-1.95	1.19	0.62-2.08
602 Weavers	16	0.98	0.56-1.59	1.00	0.57-1.63
604 Knitters	6	1.10	0.40-2.39	1.16	0.43-2.52
605 Textile finishers/dyers	3	0.51	0.10-1.49	0.55	0.11-1.61
61 Cutting/sewing etc.	101	1.20	0.98-1.45	1.22	0.99-1.47
611 Dressmakers	21	1.21	0.75-1.86	1.08	0.67-1.66
615 Patternmakers and cutters	9	1.34	0.61-2.54	1.41	0.64-2.67
616 Garment workers	59	1.25	0.95-1.61	1.32	1.01-1.70 *
62 Shoes and leather	25	1.60	1.04-2.37	1.68	1.09-2.48 *
622 Shoe sewers	11	1.88	0.94-3.37	2.01	1.00-3.59 *
65 Machine shop/steelworkers	15	0.94	0.53-1.55	1.00	0.56-1.65
659 Machine shop/steelworkers NOS	9	0.92	0.42-1.75	0.98	0.45-1.86
66 Electrical work	2	0.25	0.03-0.91	0.26	0.03-0.95 *
666 Electronic equipment assemblers	2	0.31	0.04-1.10	0.32	0.04-1.16
67 Woodwork	39	1.09	0.78-1.49	1.16	0.83-1.59
671 Timber workers	5	0.68	0.22-1.60	0.73	0.24-1.71
672 Plywood makers	17	1.02	0.60-1.64	1.09	0.64-1.75
678 Wooden surface finishers	6	3.04	1.12-6.62	3.24	1.19-7.06 *
69 Construction work NOS	12	0.70	0.36-1.22	0.82	0.42-1.43
697 Building hands	10	0.70	0.34-1.29	0.83	0.40-1.52
70 Printing	17	1.09	0.63-1.75	1.16	0.67-1.85
703 Bookbinders	10	1.31	0.63-2.40	1.39	0.66-2.55
71 Glass and ceramic work	2	0.31	0.04-1.11	0.33	0.04-1.19
72 Food industry	48	0.97	0.71-1.28	1.03	0.76-1.36
721 Bakers and pastry chiefs	25	1.11	0.72-1.64	1.16	0.75-1.72
726 Dairy workers	10	0.99	0.47-1.81	1.05	0.50-1.92
73 Chemical process/paper making	13	0.95	0.51-1.63	1.02	0.54-1.75
735 Paper and board mill workers	8	1.07	0.46-2.10	1.15	0.49-2.26
75 Industrial work NOS	22	0.88	0.55-1.34	0.93	0.58-1.41
752 Plastics	6	1.07	0.39-2.34	1.13	0.42-2.46
759 Industrial workers NOS	3	0.52	0.11-1.53	0.55	0.11-1.62

Appendix Table C

Occupation	Obs.	Crude		Adjusted	
		SIR	95% CI	SIR	95% CI
76 Packing and labelling	33	0.85	0.58-1.19	0.90	0.62-1.26
77 Machinists	11	1.27	0.64-2.28	1.41	0.71-2.53
774 Greasers	7	1.38	0.56-2.85	1.59	0.64-3.27
78 Dock and warehouse work	16	0.87	0.50-1.41	0.99	0.56-1.60
782 Warehousemen	14	0.90	0.49-1.52	1.04	0.57-1.75
8 Services	439	0.92	0.83-1.00	1.01	0.92-1.10
81 Housekeeping, domestic work, etc.	173	1.06	0.91-1.22	1.14	0.98-1.32
810 Housekeepers	21	1.32	0.82-2.02	1.10	0.68-1.68
811 Chefs, cooks etc.	37	0.90	0.63-1.24	0.97	0.68-1.33
812 Kitchen assistants	48	1.05	0.78-1.40	1.23	0.91-1.63
813 Domestic servants	43	1.05	0.76-1.41	1.25	0.90-1.68
814 Communal home-help services	14	1.30	0.71-2.19	1.34	0.73-2.25
819 Housekeeping workers NOS	5	0.92	0.30-2.16	0.88	0.29-2.05
82 Waiters	52	1.06	0.79-1.39	1.05	0.78-1.38
820 Waiters in restaurants	24	1.06	0.68-1.58	1.10	0.71-1.64
821 Waiters in cafés etc.	28	1.05	0.70-1.52	1.01	0.67-1.46
83 Caretakers and cleaners	171	0.78	0.67-0.90	0.92	0.78-1.06 *
830 Caretakers	21	0.88	0.54-1.35	0.94	0.58-1.44
831 Cleaners	149	0.77	0.65-0.89	0.91	0.77-1.07 *
84 Hygiene and beauty services	23	1.05	0.66-1.57	0.94	0.60-1.41
840 Hairdressers and barbers	21	1.21	0.75-1.85	1.05	0.65-1.61
85 Laundry and pressing	14	0.71	0.39-1.19	0.77	0.42-1.29
850 Launderers	12	0.73	0.38-1.27	0.79	0.41-1.38
9 Work not classified elsewhere	5	1.02	0.33-2.38	1.09	0.35-2.54
ECONOMICALLY INACTIVE PERSONS	1527	0.97	0.92-1.01	0.96	0.92-1.01

C21. Ovarian cancer

	Obs.	Crude		Adjusted	
		SIR	95% CI	SIR	95% CI
WHOLE POPULATION	3366	0.94	0.91-0.97	0.94	0.91-0.98 *
ECONOMICALLY ACTIVE PERSONS	2128	1.00	0.96-1.04	1.00	0.96-1.04
0 Technical, humanistic, etc. work	291	1.03	0.92-1.16	0.98	0.87-1.10
01 Technical work	19	1.37	0.82-2.14	1.29	0.78-2.02
019 Laboratory assistants	15	1.68	0.94-2.77	1.58	0.89-2.61
02 Chemical/physical/biological work	7	1.30	0.52-2.67	1.20	0.48-2.47
03 Medical work and nursing	120	0.97	0.80-1.15	0.95	0.79-1.13
032 Nurses	29	0.81	0.54-1.16	0.77	0.51-1.10
034 Midwives	5	0.88	0.29-2.05	0.82	0.27-1.91
035 Psychiatric nurses	9	1.05	0.48-1.99	0.98	0.45-1.86
036 Auxiliary nurses	56	1.04	0.78-1.35	1.06	0.80-1.38
038 Institutional children's nurses	5	0.61	0.20-1.43	0.59	0.19-1.37
04 Health-care related work	10	0.61	0.29-1.11	0.56	0.27-1.03
040 Pharmacists	7	0.69	0.28-1.42	0.63	0.25-1.30
05 Teaching	90	1.08	0.87-1.33	1.00	0.81-1.23
051 Subject teachers	26	1.23	0.81-1.81	1.16	0.76-1.70
052 Primary school teachers	39	1.01	0.72-1.38	0.93	0.66-1.27
053 Teachers of practical subjects	8	0.75	0.33-1.48	0.71	0.30-1.39
054 Vocational teachers	9	1.28	0.59-2.43	1.19	0.54-2.26
08 Artistic and literary professions	11	1.12	0.56-2.00	1.04	0.52-1.87
09 Humanistic and social work etc.	28	1.33	0.88-1.92	1.24	0.82-1.79
091 Social workers	12	1.24	0.64-2.17	1.15	0.60-2.01
092 Librarians, museum officials	10	1.59	0.76-2.92	1.46	0.70-2.68
1 Administrative and clerical work	322	1.17	1.05-1.30	1.09	0.98-1.21 *
10 Public administration	5	1.04	0.34-2.42	0.95	0.31-2.22
11 Corporate administration	10	1.47	0.70-2.70	1.32	0.63-2.43
12 Clerical work	83	1.34	1.07-1.66	1.24	0.99-1.54 *
120 Book-keepers, accountants	42	1.46	1.05-1.97	1.34	0.97-1.81 *
121 Office cashiers	21	1.75	1.08-2.67	1.61	0.99-2.45 *
123 Shop and restaurant cashiers	16	0.99	0.57-1.61	0.93	0.53-1.50
13 Stenographers and typists	24	0.94	0.60-1.40	0.89	0.57-1.32
130 Private secretaries	15	1.06	0.60-1.75	1.01	0.56-1.66
131 Typists	9	0.79	0.36-1.50	0.74	0.34-1.41

Occupation	Obs.	Crude		Adjusted	
		SIR	95% CI	SIR	95% CI
14/15 Clerical work NOS	200	1.14	0.98-1.30	1.06	0.92-1.22
144 Office clerks	132	1.13	0.95-1.33	1.06	0.88-1.24
145 Bank clerks	20	0.92	0.56-1.41	0.88	0.54-1.36
146 Insurance clerks	10	1.79	0.86-3.29	1.69	0.81-3.11
159 Clerical workers NOS	20	1.33	0.81-2.05	1.22	0.75-1.89
2 Sales professions	212	0.99	0.86-1.13	0.99	0.86-1.12
20 Wholesale and retail dealers	32	1.08	0.74-1.52	0.97	0.66-1.37
201 Retailers	31	1.05	0.71-1.49	0.95	0.64-1.34
23 Sales work	177	0.99	0.85-1.14	1.00	0.86-1.15
231 Shop personnel	165	0.98	0.83-1.13	0.99	0.84-1.15
3 Farming, forestry and fishing	391	0.83	0.75-0.92	0.86	0.77-0.94 *
30 Agricultural/forestry management	114	0.99	0.81-1.18	1.03	0.85-1.23
300 Farmers, silviculturists	111	0.99	0.81-1.18	1.03	0.85-1.23
31 Farming, animal husbandry	277	0.79	0.70-0.88	0.80	0.71-0.90 *
310 Agricultural workers	35	1.01	0.70-1.40	1.02	0.71-1.42
311 Gardeners	15	1.19	0.66-1.96	1.27	0.71-2.10
312 Livestock workers	222	0.73	0.64-0.83	0.75	0.65-0.85 *
319 Agricultural workers NOS	3	9.68	2.00-28.3	10.3	2.11-30.0 *
4 Mining and quarrying	-	-/0.6	0.00-5.82	-/0.6	0.00-6.03
5 Transport and communications	92	1.26	1.01-1.54	1.21	0.98-1.49 *
55 Transport services	8	1.22	0.53-2.41	1.25	0.54-2.47
552 Bus/tram services	6	1.11	0.41-2.41	1.14	0.42-2.47
57 Post and telecommunications	49	1.24	0.92-1.64	1.15	0.85-1.52
570 Post/telecommunications officials	20	1.17	0.72-1.81	1.08	0.66-1.67
571 Telephone operators	20	1.44	0.88-2.22	1.32	0.80-2.03
572 Switchboard operators	7	1.14	0.46-2.34	1.06	0.43-2.18
58 Postal services/couriers	29	1.39	0.93-2.00	1.46	0.98-2.09
580 Postmen	27	1.48	0.97-2.15	1.55	1.02-2.25 *
6/7 Industrial and construction work	378	0.99	0.90-1.10	1.02	0.92-1.13
60 Textiles	40	0.92	0.66-1.26	0.95	0.68-1.29
601 Spinners etc.	7	0.73	0.29-1.50	0.75	0.30-1.55
602 Weavers	14	0.96	0.53-1.61	0.97	0.53-1.64
604 Knitters	4	0.78	0.21-2.01	0.80	0.22-2.06
605 Textile finishers/dyers	8	1.49	0.64-2.94	1.55	0.67-3.04
61 Cutting/sewing etc.	80	1.03	0.82-1.28	1.04	0.82-1.29
611 Dressmakers	17	1.10	0.64-1.77	1.04	0.60-1.66
615 Patternmakers and cutters	11	1.69	0.84-3.03	1.73	0.87-3.10
616 Garment workers	43	0.97	0.70-1.31	1.00	0.72-1.35
62 Shoes and leather	12	0.84	0.43-1.46	0.86	0.44-1.50
621 Shoe cutters etc.	4	3.59	0.98-9.20	3.71	1.01-9.50 *
622 Shoe sewers	3	0.55	0.11-1.61	0.57	0.12-1.66
65 Machine shop/steelworkers	16	1.09	0.63-1.78	1.13	0.64-1.83
659 Machine shop/steelworkers NOS	9	1.01	0.46-1.91	1.04	0.47-1.97
66 Electrical work	5	0.65	0.21-1.51	0.66	0.22-1.55
666 Electronic equipment assemblers	4	0.63	0.17-1.61	0.64	0.18-1.65
67 Woodwork	17	0.53	0.31-0.84	0.54	0.32-0.87 *
671 Timber workers	3	0.46	0.10-1.35	0.48	0.10-1.40
672 Plywood makers	8	0.53	0.23-1.04	0.55	0.24-1.08
69 Construction work NOS	14	0.93	0.51-1.56	1.00	0.55-1.68
697 Building hands	12	0.96	0.50-1.68	1.04	0.54-1.82
70 Printing	30	2.08	1.40-2.97	2.15	1.45-3.06 *
700 Typographers etc.	8	3.19	1.38-6.29	3.30	1.42-6.50 *
702 Lithographers	3	5.31	1.09-15.5	5.44	1.12-15.9 *
703 Bookbinders	10	1.42	0.68-2.61	1.47	0.70-2.70
709 Printing workers NOS	5	3.19	1.04-7.45	3.26	1.06-7.62 *
71 Glass and ceramic work	4	0.68	0.19-1.74	0.71	0.19-1.81
72 Food industry	35	0.77	0.54-1.07	0.80	0.55-1.11
721 Bakers and pastry chiefs	16	0.78	0.45-1.27	0.80	0.46-1.30
726 Dairy workers	8	0.84	0.36-1.65	0.86	0.37-1.70
73 Chemical process/paper making	20	1.62	0.99-2.50	1.68	1.03-2.59 *
735 Paper and board mill workers	11	1.61	0.81-2.89	1.67	0.84-3.00
75 Industrial work NOS	28	1.22	0.81-1.76	1.25	0.83-1.80
751 Industrial rubber products	9	2.33	1.06-4.42	2.41	1.10-4.57 *
752 Plastics	7	1.35	0.54-2.79	1.39	0.56-2.86
759 Industrial workers NOS	5	0.94	0.31-2.20	0.97	0.32-2.26
76 Packing and labelling	45	1.25	0.91-1.67	1.29	0.94-1.73

Appendix Table C

Occupation	Obs.	Crude SIR	95% CI	Adjusted SIR	95% CI
77 Machinists	11	1.39	0.70-2.50	1.46	0.73-2.62
78 Dock and warehouse work	18	1.08	0.64-1.71	1.14	0.68-1.80
782 Warehousemen	13	0.93	0.49-1.59	0.98	0.52-1.67
8 Services	439	1.02	0.92-1.12	1.06	0.96-1.16
81 Housekeeping, domestic work, etc.	159	1.08	0.92-1.25	1.11	0.94-1.29
810 Housekeepers	14	0.98	0.54-1.64	0.89	0.49-1.50
811 Chefs, cooks etc.	48	1.30	0.96-1.72	1.35	0.99-1.79
812 Kitchen assistants	42	1.02	0.74-1.38	1.08	0.78-1.45
813 Domestic servants	41	1.13	0.81-1.54	1.19	0.86-1.62
814 Communal home-help services	9	0.87	0.40-1.65	0.89	0.41-1.68
82 Waiters	50	1.08	0.80-1.43	1.08	0.80-1.42
820 Waiters in restaurants	20	0.94	0.57-1.45	0.95	0.58-1.47
821 Waiters in cafés etc.	30	1.21	0.81-1.72	1.18	0.80-1.69
83 Caretakers and cleaners	178	0.91	0.78-1.05	0.98	0.84-1.13
830 Caretakers	25	1.11	0.72-1.63	1.14	0.74-1.69
831 Cleaners	153	0.89	0.76-1.04	0.96	0.82-1.12
84 Hygiene and beauty services	31	1.50	1.02-2.12	1.42	0.97-2.02 *
840 Hairdressers and barbers	27	1.64	1.08-2.39	1.54	1.01-2.24 *
85 Laundry and pressing	15	0.86	0.48-1.42	0.90	0.50-1.48
850 Launderers	11	0.76	0.38-1.35	0.79	0.39-1.41
9 Work not classified elsewhere	3	0.67	0.14-1.97	0.70	0.14-2.03
ECONOMICALLY INACTIVE PERSONS	1238	0.86	0.81-0.91	0.86	0.81-0.91 *

C22. Prostate cancer

Occupation	Obs.	Crude SIR	95% CI	Adjusted SIR	95% CI
WHOLE POPULATION	3270	1.00	0.96-1.03	1.00	0.96-1.03
ECONOMICALLY ACTIVE PERSONS	2757	1.00	0.96-1.04	1.00	0.96-1.04
0 Technical, humanistic, etc. work	271	1.15	1.02-1.29	1.03	0.91-1.15 *
00 Technical professions	32	1.32	0.90-1.86	1.09	0.75-1.54
001 Civil engineers	8	1.69	0.73-3.34	1.39	0.60-2.74
004 Mechanical engineers	7	0.97	0.39-2.00	0.80	0.32-1.65
01 Technical work	99	1.15	0.94-1.40	1.11	0.90-1.36
010 Civil engineering technicians	35	1.06	0.74-1.48	1.03	0.72-1.44
011 Power technicians	6	0.92	0.34-2.00	0.89	0.33-1.93
013 Mechanical technicians	30	1.34	0.90-1.91	1.30	0.87-1.85
016 Technicians NOS	12	1.33	0.69-2.32	1.28	0.66-2.24
02 Chemical/physical/biological work	20	1.26	0.77-1.95	1.11	0.68-1.72
028 Consultancy, forestry	11	1.36	0.68-2.43	1.20	0.60-2.15
03 Medical work and nursing	8	0.69	0.30-1.36	0.60	0.26-1.18
030 Medical doctors	3	0.46	0.09-1.35	0.38	0.08-1.10
04 Health-care related work	8	1.74	0.75-3.44	1.56	0.67-3.08
05 Teaching	50	1.09	0.81-1.44	0.92	0.68-1.22
050 University teachers	6	1.31	0.48-2.84	1.07	0.39-2.32
051 Subject teachers	12	1.39	0.72-2.42	1.13	0.59-1.98
052 Primary school teachers	13	0.78	0.41-1.33	0.65	0.34-1.10
054 Vocational teachers	11	0.96	0.48-1.72	0.87	0.43-1.55
06 Religious professions	9	1.26	0.57-2.38	1.06	0.48-2.00
060 Clergy and lay preachers	8	1.20	0.52-2.37	1.01	0.43-1.98
07 Legal professions	13	1.55	0.83-2.65	1.28	0.68-2.20
08 Artistic and literary professions	18	1.13	0.67-1.79	0.96	0.57-1.52
084 Journalists	5	0.95	0.31-2.22	0.80	0.26-1.86
09 Humanistic and social work etc.	14	0.91	0.50-1.53	0.80	0.44-1.34
096 PR officers	3	0.50	0.10-1.47	0.45	0.09-1.33
1 Administrative and clerical work	212	1.25	1.09-1.42	1.09	0.95-1.25 *
10 Public administration	26	1.54	1.01-2.26	1.26	0.82-1.85 *
11 Corporate administration	100	1.27	1.04-1.53	1.05	0.85-1.26 *
110 Corporate managers	48	1.25	0.92-1.66	1.03	0.76-1.36
111 Technical managers	9	1.39	0.64-2.64	1.15	0.53-2.19
112 Commercial managers	16	0.95	0.54-1.54	0.79	0.45-1.28
119 Private sector managers NOS	18	1.93	1.14-3.04	1.58	0.94-2.50 *
12 Clerical work	13	1.74	0.93-2.98	1.60	0.85-2.74

Occupation	Obs.	Crude		Adjusted	
		SIR	95% CI	SIR	95% CI
120 Book-keepers, accountants	9	1.43	0.65-2.71	1.30	0.60-2.47
121 Office cashiers	4	5.74	1.56-14.7	5.53	1.51-14.2 *
14/15 Clerical work NOS	71	1.08	0.84-1.36	1.04	0.81-1.31
144 Office clerks	9	0.82	0.38-1.56	0.80	0.36-1.51
150 Property managers, warehousemen	43	1.27	0.92-1.70	1.23	0.89-1.65
159 Clerical workers NOS	10	1.26	0.61-2.32	1.22	0.58-2.24
2 Sales professions	131	1.08	0.90-1.27	1.05	0.88-1.24
20 Wholesale and retail dealers	46	1.14	0.84-1.53	1.11	0.81-1.48
201 Retailers	45	1.17	0.85-1.56	1.13	0.83-1.52
21 Real estate, services, securities	14	1.51	0.82-2.53	1.43	0.78-2.40
210 Insurance salesmen	9	1.59	0.73-3.01	1.52	0.70-2.89
22 Sales representatives	24	1.08	0.69-1.60	1.04	0.67-1.55
220 Commercial travellers, etc.	20	1.00	0.61-1.54	0.97	0.59-1.50
23 Sales work	47	0.95	0.70-1.26	0.94	0.69-1.25
230 Buyers, office sales staff	6	0.62	0.23-1.35	0.59	0.22-1.29
231 Shop personnel	30	1.00	0.68-1.43	1.01	0.68-1.44
3 Farming, forestry and fishing	782	0.89	0.83-0.96	0.92	0.86-0.99 *
30 Agricultural/forestry management	692	0.93	0.86-1.00	0.94	0.87-1.01 *
300 Farmers, silviculturists	656	0.92	0.85-1.00	0.94	0.87-1.01 *
302 Forestry managers	21	0.87	0.54-1.33	0.84	0.52-1.29
31 Farming, animal husbandry	35	0.93	0.65-1.29	1.03	0.72-1.43
310 Agricultural workers	22	0.80	0.50-1.20	0.87	0.55-1.32
311 Gardeners	10	1.89	0.91-3.48	2.19	1.05-4.02 *
33 Fishing	7	0.87	0.35-1.79	0.89	0.36-1.82
330 Fishermen	6	0.77	0.28-1.67	0.78	0.29-1.71
34 Forestry work	47	0.57	0.42-0.76	0.66	0.48-0.88 *
4 Mining and quarrying	14	0.95	0.52-1.60	0.97	0.53-1.62
40 Mining and quarrying	11	1.19	0.59-2.12	1.20	0.60-2.14
5 Transport and communications	224	0.95	0.83-1.08	0.94	0.82-1.06
50 Ship's officers	15	1.32	0.74-2.18	1.22	0.68-2.01
500 Ship's masters and mates	9	1.77	0.81-3.35	1.54	0.71-2.93
51 Deck and engine-room crew	5	0.88	0.28-2.04	0.89	0.29-2.08
53 Engine drivers	11	1.13	0.57-2.03	1.13	0.56-2.02
54 Road transport	125	0.91	0.75-1.07	0.90	0.75-1.06
540 Motor-vehicle and tram drivers	125	0.91	0.76-1.08	0.90	0.75-1.07
55 Transport services	20	0.80	0.49-1.24	0.79	0.49-1.23
550 Railway staff	20	0.81	0.49-1.25	0.80	0.49-1.24
56 Traffic supervisors	16	1.05	0.60-1.71	0.96	0.55-1.56
562 Railway traffic supervisors	3	0.39	0.08-1.15	0.36	0.07-1.05
563 Road transport supervisors	11	2.12	1.06-3.80	1.92	0.96-3.43 *
57 Post and telecommunications	8	1.09	0.47-2.15	1.06	0.46-2.09
570 Post/telecommunications officials	7	1.23	0.49-2.53	1.20	0.48-2.47
58 Postal services/couriers	19	1.15	0.69-1.79	1.16	0.70-1.81
580 Postmen	7	0.78	0.32-1.61	0.80	0.32-1.64
581 Caretakers/messengers	12	1.57	0.81-2.74	1.58	0.82-2.76
59 Communication work NOS	5	0.77	0.25-1.79	0.77	0.25-1.81
6/7 Industrial and construction work	975	1.00	0.94-1.06	1.03	0.97-1.10
60 Textiles	18	2.00	1.18-3.16	2.02	1.20-3.19 *
601 Spinners etc.	4	4.44	1.21-11.4	4.47	1.22-11.5 *
61 Cutting/sewing etc.	7	0.72	0.29-1.48	0.71	0.29-1.47
62 Shoes and leather	8	0.94	0.41-1.86	0.94	0.41-1.85
621 Shoe cutters etc.	4	4.57	1.24-11.7	4.64	1.26-11.9 *
63 Smelting, metal and foundry work	33	1.17	0.81-1.65	1.18	0.81-1.66
631 Hardeners, temperers, etc.	3	5.19	1.07-15.2	5.27	1.09-15.4 *
634 Blacksmiths	10	1.17	0.56-2.15	1.17	0.56-2.14
635 Founders	7	0.89	0.36-1.83	0.90	0.36-1.85
64 Precision mechanical work	11	1.09	0.54-1.95	1.08	0.54-1.94
65 Machine shop/steelworkers	171	0.95	0.82-1.10	0.96	0.82-1.11
650 Turners, machinists	36	0.84	0.59-1.17	0.85	0.60-1.18
651 Fitter-assemblers etc.	12	0.71	0.37-1.24	0.72	0.37-1.26
652 Machine and motor repairers	34	0.83	0.58-1.16	0.84	0.58-1.17
653 Sheetmetalworkers	15	0.90	0.50-1.48	0.91	0.51-1.49
654 Plumbers	26	1.17	0.76-1.71	1.18	0.77-1.73
655 Welders and flame cutters	23	1.48	0.94-2.22	1.49	0.95-2.24
656 Plate/constructional steel work	4	0.73	0.20-1.88	0.74	0.20-1.89
659 Machine shop/steelworkers NOS	19	1.06	0.64-1.66	1.07	0.65-1.68

Appendix Table C

Occupation	Obs.	Crude		Adjusted	
		SIR	95% CI	SIR	95% CI
66 Electrical work	48	0.91	0.67-1.21	0.92	0.68-1.22
660 Electricians (indoors)	24	0.86	0.55-1.28	0.87	0.56-1.29
664 Telephone installers and repair	4	0.51	0.14-1.31	0.52	0.14-1.32
665 Linemen	9	1.63	0.74-3.09	1.65	0.75-3.13
67 Woodwork	215	1.01	0.88-1.15	1.02	0.89-1.16
671 Timber workers	28	1.08	0.72-1.56	1.09	0.72-1.57
672 Plywood makers	9	1.38	0.63-2.63	1.40	0.64-2.66
673 Construction carpenters	133	0.98	0.82-1.16	0.99	0.83-1.17
674 Boatbuilders etc.	8	1.54	0.67-3.04	1.54	0.67-3.04
675 Bench carpenters	12	0.96	0.50-1.68	0.96	0.49-1.67
676 Cabinetmakers etc.	6	0.78	0.28-1.69	0.78	0.29-1.69
677 Woodworking machine operators e	13	1.14	0.61-1.95	1.15	0.61-1.97
68 Painting and lacquering	36	0.97	0.68-1.34	0.97	0.68-1.35
680 Painters	32	0.92	0.63-1.30	0.93	0.63-1.31
69 Construction work NOS	161	0.98	0.84-1.14	1.09	0.93-1.26
690 Bricklayers and tile setters	25	1.19	0.77-1.76	1.20	0.78-1.77
693 Concrete/cement shutterers	14	1.09	0.60-1.83	1.10	0.60-1.84
697 Building hands	65	1.01	0.78-1.28	1.17	0.90-1.49
698 Roadbuilding hands	36	0.74	0.52-1.02	0.85	0.60-1.18
699 Construction workers NOS	12	1.76	0.91-3.07	1.76	0.91-3.07
70 Printing	18	1.50	0.89-2.37	1.52	0.90-2.41
71 Glass and ceramic work	10	1.51	0.72-2.77	1.52	0.73-2.80
72 Food industry	12	0.58	0.30-1.02	0.59	0.30-1.03
725 Butchers and sausage makers	2	0.40	0.05-1.44	0.41	0.05-1.46
73 Chemical process/paper making	34	1.08	0.75-1.51	1.09	0.76-1.53
734 Pulp mill workers	8	0.91	0.39-1.79	0.92	0.40-1.81
735 Paper and board mill workers	10	0.87	0.42-1.60	0.89	0.42-1.63
739 Chemical process workers NOS	8	1.43	0.62-2.81	1.44	0.62-2.84
75 Industrial work NOS	23	1.11	0.70-1.66	1.11	0.70-1.67
76 Packing and labelling	6	0.72	0.27-1.58	0.73	0.27-1.59
77 Machinists	71	1.08	0.84-1.36	1.09	0.85-1.37
771 Forklift operators	9	1.04	0.48-1.98	1.05	0.48-2.00
772 Construction machinery operator	19	0.97	0.59-1.52	0.98	0.59-1.52
773 Operators of stationary engine	23	1.19	0.76-1.79	1.21	0.77-1.81
774 Greasers	6	1.15	0.42-2.50	1.17	0.43-2.54
775 Industrial personnel, riggers	8	0.87	0.38-1.72	0.88	0.38-1.74
78 Dock and warehouse work	62	1.03	0.79-1.32	1.14	0.88-1.46
780 Dockers	12	0.85	0.44-1.48	0.87	0.45-1.52
781 Freight handlers	10	1.16	0.56-2.14	1.34	0.64-2.47
782 Warehousemen	39	1.05	0.74-1.43	1.18	0.84-1.62
79 Labourers not classified elsewhere	30	0.80	0.54-1.14	0.92	0.62-1.31
8 Services	127	1.09	0.91-1.29	1.10	0.92-1.30
80 Watchmen, security guards	62	1.22	0.94-1.57	1.22	0.93-1.56
801 Policemen	23	1.12	0.71-1.67	1.07	0.68-1.60
804 Civilian guards	22	1.17	0.74-1.78	1.24	0.78-1.88
83 Caretakers and cleaners	51	1.03	0.77-1.36	1.04	0.78-1.37
830 Caretakers	47	1.05	0.77-1.40	1.07	0.78-1.42
89 Services NOS	7	1.27	0.51-2.62	1.30	0.52-2.67
9 Work not classified elsewhere	21	1.46	0.91-2.24	1.38	0.85-2.11
90 Military occupations	10	1.35	0.65-2.49	1.20	0.58-2.21
91 Occupation not specified	11	1.58	0.79-2.83	1.60	0.80-2.86
ECONOMICALLY INACTIVE PERSONS	513	0.97	0.89-1.06	0.99	0.91-1.08

C23. Kidney cancer, males

	Obs.	Crude		Adjusted	
		SIR	95% CI	SIR	95% CI
WHOLE POPULATION	1864	1.00	0.95-1.04	1.00	0.96-1.05
ECONOMICALLY ACTIVE PERSONS	1658	1.00	0.95-1.05	1.00	0.95-1.05
0 Technical, humanistic, etc. work	197	1.23	1.06-1.41	1.05	0.91-1.20 *
00 Technical professions	25	1.35	0.87-1.99	1.12	0.72-1.65
004 Mechanical engineers	7	1.27	0.51-2.62	1.05	0.42-2.17
01 Technical work	76	1.31	1.03-1.64	1.17	0.93-1.47 *
010 Civil engineering technicians	27	1.27	0.84-1.85	1.14	0.75-1.66

Occupation	Obs.	Crude		Adjusted	
		SIR	95% CI	SIR	95% CI
011 Power technicians	3	0.62	0.13-1.82	0.56	0.12-1.63
013 Mechanical technicians	23	1.52	0.96-2.28	1.37	0.87-2.05
016 Technicians NOS	7	1.19	0.48-2.45	1.07	0.43-2.20
02 Chemical/physical/biological work	13	1.31	0.70-2.23	1.09	0.58-1.86
028 Consultancy, forestry	8	1.73	0.74-3.40	1.42	0.61-2.80
03 Medical work and nursing	10	1.24	0.59-2.28	1.06	0.51-1.95
030 Medical doctors	7	1.58	0.64-3.27	1.28	0.51-2.63
05 Teaching	33	0.96	0.66-1.35	0.80	0.55-1.13
050 University teachers	12	4.02	2.08-7.02	3.18	1.64-5.55 *
051 Subject teachers	5	0.75	0.24-1.76	0.62	0.20-1.45
052 Primary school teachers	4	0.29	0.08-0.75	0.25	0.07-0.63 *
054 Vocational teachers	10	1.27	0.61-2.34	1.09	0.52-2.00
06 Religious professions	6	1.57	0.57-3.41	1.20	0.44-2.62
07 Legal professions	5	1.10	0.36-2.57	0.84	0.27-1.95
08 Artistic and literary professions	14	1.33	0.73-2.24	1.09	0.60-1.83
09 Humanistic and social work etc.	11	1.09	0.54-1.95	0.92	0.46-1.64
1 Administrative and clerical work	120	1.19	0.98-1.41	0.98	0.81-1.16
10 Public administration	9	0.94	0.43-1.79	0.72	0.33-1.37
11 Corporate administration	67	1.38	1.07-1.76	1.09	0.84-1.38 *
110 Corporate managers	38	1.74	1.23-2.39	1.34	0.95-1.84 *
111 Technical managers	3	0.69	0.14-2.00	0.56	0.11-1.62
112 Commercial managers	13	1.09	0.58-1.86	0.88	0.47-1.51
119 Private sector managers NOS	6	1.07	0.39-2.33	0.84	0.31-1.83
14/15 Clerical work NOS	40	1.05	0.75-1.43	0.94	0.67-1.27
144 Office clerks	7	1.13	0.46-2.33	1.02	0.41-2.10
150 Property managers, warehousemen	21	1.12	0.69-1.71	1.00	0.62-1.53
159 Clerical workers NOS	4	0.88	0.24-2.26	0.79	0.22-2.02
2 Sales professions	106	1.30	1.07-1.56	1.21	0.99-1.45 *
20 Wholesale and retail dealers	26	1.16	0.76-1.70	1.03	0.67-1.51
201 Retailers	25	1.17	0.75-1.72	1.04	0.67-1.54
21 Real estate, services, securities	9	1.50	0.69-2.85	1.34	0.61-2.54
210 Insurance salesmen	-	-/3.5	0.00-1.06	-/3.9	0.00-0.95 *
211 Real estate/stockbrokers	6	7.02	2.58-15.3	6.25	2.30-13.6 *
22 Sales representatives	23	1.32	0.84-1.98	1.19	0.75-1.78
220 Commercial travellers, etc.	18	1.12	0.67-1.77	1.01	0.60-1.59
221 Sales agents	5	3.70	1.20-8.63	3.29	1.07-7.68 *
23 Sales work	48	1.35	0.99-1.79	1.31	0.97-1.74
230 Buyers, office sales staff	8	1.22	0.52-2.40	1.08	0.47-2.13
231 Shop personnel	29	1.29	0.87-1.86	1.32	0.88-1.89
3 Farming, forestry and fishing	307	0.67	0.59-0.74	0.71	0.63-0.79 *
30 Agricultural/forestry management	256	0.68	0.60-0.76	0.70	0.61-0.78 *
300 Farmers, silviculturists	241	0.68	0.59-0.76	0.70	0.61-0.79 *
302 Forestry managers	10	0.72	0.35-1.33	0.65	0.31-1.19
31 Farming, animal husbandry	17	0.68	0.40-1.09	0.80	0.47-1.29
310 Agricultural workers	12	0.63	0.33-1.10	0.73	0.38-1.28
34 Forestry work	30	0.55	0.37-0.78	0.73	0.49-1.04 *
4 Mining and quarrying	8	0.85	0.37-1.67	0.87	0.37-1.71
40 Mining and quarrying	5	0.87	0.28-2.03	0.88	0.29-2.07
5 Transport and communications	214	1.33	1.16-1.52	1.28	1.12-1.46 *
50 Ship's officers	14	2.11	1.15-3.54	1.81	0.99-3.04 *
500 Ship's masters and mates	8	2.73	1.18-5.37	2.23	0.96-4.39 *
53 Engine drivers	10	1.38	0.66-2.53	1.39	0.67-2.56
54 Road transport	145	1.46	1.23-1.71	1.41	1.19-1.65 *
540 Motor-vehicle and tram drivers	144	1.45	1.23-1.70	1.40	1.18-1.64 *
55 Transport services	16	1.05	0.60-1.70	1.04	0.59-1.68
550 Railway staff	16	1.07	0.61-1.74	1.06	0.60-1.71
56 Traffic supervisors	8	0.93	0.40-1.82	0.78	0.34-1.54
562 Railway traffic supervisors	1	0.24	0.01-1.32	0.20	0.01-1.11
57 Post and telecommunications	4	0.89	0.24-2.27	0.80	0.22-2.04
58 Postal services/couriers	9	0.89	0.40-1.68	0.91	0.42-1.73
580 Postmen	3	0.46	0.10-1.35	0.48	0.10-1.39
6/7 Industrial and construction work	625	1.03	0.95-1.11	1.10	1.01-1.18 *
60 Textiles	7	1.25	0.50-2.57	1.28	0.51-2.63
61 Cutting/sewing etc.	5	0.92	0.30-2.15	0.90	0.29-2.10
63 Smelting, metal and foundry work	17	1.02	0.59-1.63	1.04	0.60-1.66

Appendix Table C

Occupation	Obs.	Crude SIR	95% CI	Adjusted SIR	95% CI
64 Precision mechanical work	6	0.89	0.33-1.94	0.86	0.32-1.88
65 Machine shop/steelworkers	130	1.06	0.89-1.25	1.08	0.90-1.27
650 Turners, machinists	25	0.95	0.61-1.40	0.97	0.63-1.43
651 Fitter-assemblers etc.	13	1.09	0.58-1.87	1.11	0.59-1.90
652 Machine and motor repairers	33	1.15	0.79-1.62	1.16	0.80-1.63
653 Sheetmetalworkers	18	1.60	0.95-2.53	1.62	0.96-2.56
654 Plumbers	15	0.93	0.52-1.54	0.94	0.53-1.55
655 Welders and flame cutters	14	1.09	0.60-1.83	1.11	0.61-1.86
659 Machine shop/steelworkers NOS	8	0.73	0.31-1.43	0.74	0.32-1.46
66 Electrical work	27	0.72	0.48-1.05	0.73	0.48-1.07
660 Electricians (indoors)	13	0.64	0.34-1.10	0.65	0.35-1.11
664 Telephone installers and repair	4	0.70	0.19-1.80	0.72	0.20-1.84
665 Linemen	-	-/3.7	0.00-1.00	-/3.6	0.00-1.02 *
67 Woodwork	121	1.01	0.84-1.20	1.03	0.86-1.22
670 Round-timber workers	7	2.53	1.02-5.21	2.60	1.05-5.36 *
671 Timber workers	14	0.92	0.50-1.55	0.94	0.51-1.58
673 Construction carpenters	74	0.99	0.78-1.24	1.02	0.80-1.28
675 Bench carpenters	4	0.58	0.16-1.48	0.57	0.16-1.46
677 Woodworking machine operators e	6	0.88	0.32-1.92	0.90	0.33-1.96
68 Painting and lacquering	29	1.26	0.84-1.81	1.27	0.85-1.82
680 Painters	27	1.27	0.84-1.85	1.28	0.84-1.86
69 Construction work NOS	99	1.03	0.83-1.25	1.26	1.02-1.53 *
690 Bricklayers and tile setters	8	0.65	0.28-1.29	0.67	0.29-1.32
693 Concrete/cement shutterers	9	1.09	0.50-2.08	1.11	0.51-2.11
697 Building hands	46	1.17	0.86-1.56	1.59	1.16-2.12 *
698 Roadbuilding hands	12	0.47	0.25-0.83	0.65	0.33-1.13 *
699 Construction workers NOS	9	2.23	1.02-4.23	2.22	1.01-4.21 *
70 Printing	12	1.42	0.73-2.48	1.45	0.75-2.54
72 Food industry	13	0.99	0.53-1.69	1.00	0.53-1.70
73 Chemical process/paper making	25	1.21	0.78-1.79	1.24	0.81-1.84
734 Pulp mill workers	6	1.07	0.39-2.32	1.10	0.40-2.39
735 Paper and board mill workers	12	1.53	0.79-2.68	1.58	0.81-2.75
75 Industrial work NOS	12	0.89	0.46-1.56	0.90	0.46-1.57
76 Packing and labelling	5	0.91	0.30-2.14	0.94	0.31-2.20
77 Machinists	56	1.18	0.89-1.53	1.20	0.90-1.55
771 Forklift operators	7	1.02	0.41-2.09	1.04	0.42-2.14
772 Construction machinery operator	18	1.13	0.67-1.79	1.12	0.66-1.77
773 Operators of stationary engine	16	1.40	0.80-2.27	1.44	0.82-2.34
775 Industrial personnel, riggers	3	0.50	0.10-1.45	0.51	0.11-1.49
78 Dock and warehouse work	34	0.95	0.66-1.33	1.16	0.80-1.62
780 Dockers	8	0.93	0.40-1.84	0.99	0.43-1.94
781 Freight handlers	4	0.74	0.20-1.90	0.98	0.27-2.51
782 Warehousemen	22	1.01	0.63-1.53	1.28	0.80-1.94
79 Labourers not classified elsewhere	18	0.90	0.53-1.42	1.22	0.72-1.93
8 Services	65	0.98	0.76-1.25	0.98	0.76-1.25
80 Watchmen, security guards	28	0.97	0.64-1.40	0.94	0.62-1.35
801 Policemen	14	1.19	0.65-2.00	1.07	0.59-1.80
804 Civilian guards	9	1.10	0.50-2.09	1.25	0.57-2.37
83 Caretakers and cleaners	31	1.12	0.76-1.59	1.16	0.79-1.65
830 Caretakers	28	1.13	0.75-1.64	1.17	0.78-1.69
9 Work not classified elsewhere	16	1.39	0.80-2.26	1.30	0.75-2.12
90 Military occupations	9	1.23	0.56-2.34	1.10	0.50-2.09
ECONOMICALLY INACTIVE PERSONS	206	0.97	0.84-1.11	1.04	0.90-1.18

C24. Kidney cancer, females

Occupation	Obs.	Crude SIR	95% CI	Adjusted SIR	95% CI
WHOLE POPULATION	1269	1.05	0.99-1.10	1.05	0.99-1.11
ECONOMICALLY ACTIVE PERSONS	712	1.00	0.93-1.07	1.00	0.93-1.07
0 Technical, humanistic, etc. work	84	0.97	0.77-1.20	0.93	0.74-1.15
03 Medical work and nursing	36	0.95	0.67-1.32	0.93	0.65-1.28
032 Nurses	11	1.05	0.52-1.87	0.95	0.48-1.70
036 Auxiliary nurses	14	0.84	0.46-1.40	0.87	0.47-1.45

Occupation	Obs.	Crude SIR	95% CI	Adjusted SIR	95% CI
04 Health-care related work	6	1.15	0.42-2.51	1.05	0.39-2.29
05 Teaching	27	1.04	0.69-1.52	1.02	0.67-1.48
051 Subject teachers	7	1.16	0.47-2.39	1.21	0.49-2.49
052 Primary school teachers	13	1.04	0.55-1.78	1.01	0.54-1.72
09 Humanistic and social work etc.	3	0.45	0.09-1.32	0.42	0.09-1.23
1 Administrative and clerical work	93	1.08	0.87-1.33	0.99	0.80-1.21
12 Clerical work	20	1.00	0.61-1.54	0.90	0.55-1.39
120 Book-keepers, accountants	9	0.94	0.43-1.79	0.85	0.39-1.62
123 Shop and restaurant cashiers	6	1.19	0.44-2.58	1.08	0.40-2.35
13 Stenographers and typists	11	1.45	0.72-2.59	1.31	0.66-2.35
14/15 Clerical work NOS	59	1.09	0.83-1.40	0.99	0.76-1.28
144 Office clerks	37	1.01	0.71-1.40	0.93	0.65-1.28
145 Bank clerks	7	1.15	0.46-2.37	1.06	0.43-2.19
159 Clerical workers NOS	8	1.61	0.69-3.17	1.46	0.63-2.87
2 Sales professions	64	0.93	0.71-1.18	0.92	0.71-1.17
20 Wholesale and retail dealers	7	0.66	0.27-1.36	0.59	0.24-1.21
201 Retailers	7	0.67	0.27-1.37	0.59	0.24-1.21
23 Sales work	57	1.00	0.76-1.29	1.01	0.77-1.31
231 Shop personnel	52	0.96	0.72-1.27	0.98	0.73-1.29
3 Farming, forestry and fishing	164	0.98	0.84-1.14	1.01	0.86-1.17
30 Agricultural/forestry management	41	0.94	0.67-1.27	0.98	0.70-1.33
300 Farmers, silviculturists	41	0.96	0.69-1.31	1.01	0.72-1.37
31 Farming, animal husbandry	122	0.99	0.82-1.18	1.01	0.84-1.20
310 Agricultural workers	16	1.31	0.75-2.13	1.32	0.75-2.14
312 Livestock workers	98	0.93	0.75-1.13	0.94	0.77-1.15
4 Mining and quarrying	-	-/0.2	0.00-16.5	-/0.2	0.00-16.9
5 Transport and communications	29	1.18	0.79-1.69	1.14	0.76-1.64
57 Post and telecommunications	16	1.24	0.71-2.01	1.14	0.65-1.85
570 Post/telecommunications officials	7	1.26	0.50-2.59	1.17	0.47-2.41
571 Telephone operators	7	1.50	0.61-3.10	1.38	0.56-2.84
58 Postal services/couriers	5	0.69	0.22-1.60	0.72	0.23-1.68
580 Postmen	3	0.47	0.10-1.38	0.50	0.10-1.45
6/7 Industrial and construction work	119	0.93	0.77-1.11	0.96	0.80-1.14
60 Textiles	15	1.00	0.56-1.66	1.03	0.57-1.69
602 Weavers	7	1.37	0.55-2.83	1.38	0.56-2.84
61 Cutting/sewing etc.	24	0.93	0.60-1.38	0.93	0.60-1.39
611 Dressmakers	4	0.73	0.20-1.88	0.68	0.18-1.73
616 Garment workers	13	0.90	0.48-1.54	0.93	0.50-1.60
67 Woodwork	11	1.01	0.50-1.80	1.04	0.52-1.86
672 Plywood makers	6	1.19	0.44-2.58	1.23	0.45-2.67
69 Construction work NOS	3	0.57	0.12-1.66	0.61	0.13-1.78
72 Food industry	14	0.92	0.50-1.55	0.95	0.52-1.59
721 Bakers and pastry chiefs	4	0.57	0.16-1.47	0.59	0.16-1.51
722 Chocolate and confectionery mak	4	4.08	1.11-10.4	4.21	1.15-10.8 *
75 Industrial work NOS	6	0.79	0.29-1.72	0.81	0.30-1.77
76 Packing and labelling	13	1.10	0.59-1.89	1.14	0.61-1.95
772 Construction machinery operator	1	53.7	1.36-299	47.8	1.21-266 *
78 Dock and warehouse work	4	0.70	0.19-1.80	0.74	0.20-1.90
8 Services	157	1.05	0.90-1.22	1.10	0.93-1.27
81 Housekeeping, domestic work, etc.	48	0.94	0.69-1.25	0.97	0.71-1.28
810 Housekeepers	6	1.21	0.44-2.64	1.08	0.40-2.35
811 Chefs, cooks etc.	14	1.09	0.59-1.82	1.13	0.62-1.90
812 Kitchen assistants	14	1.00	0.55-1.68	1.05	0.58-1.77
813 Domestic servants	10	0.76	0.37-1.40	0.82	0.39-1.50
82 Waiters	14	0.94	0.51-1.57	0.94	0.51-1.57
820 Waiters in restaurants	6	0.87	0.32-1.89	0.89	0.33-1.95
821 Waiters in cafés etc.	8	0.99	0.43-1.96	0.97	0.42-1.91
83 Caretakers and cleaners	77	1.12	0.89-1.41	1.21	0.95-1.51
830 Caretakers	9	1.24	0.57-2.35	1.29	0.59-2.46
831 Cleaners	66	1.08	0.84-1.38	1.17	0.90-1.49
84 Hygiene and beauty services	12	1.76	0.91-3.08	1.66	0.86-2.89
840 Hairdressers and barbers	5	0.93	0.30-2.18	0.86	0.28-2.00
843 Sauna attendants etc.	6	6.02	2.21-13.1	6.29	2.31-13.7 *
85 Laundry and pressing	3	0.49	0.10-1.43	0.51	0.10-1.48

Appendix Table C

Occupation	Obs.	Crude		Adjusted	
		SIR	95% CI	SIR	95% CI
850 Launderers	1	0.20	0.00-1.09	0.20	0.01-1.12
9 Work not classified elsewhere	2	1.31	0.16-4.72	1.36	0.16-4.90
ECONOMICALLY INACTIVE PERSONS	557	1.11	1.02-1.21	1.12	1.03-1.21 *

C25. Cancer of the bladder, ureter and urethra, males

WHOLE POPULATION	2121	1.04	1.00-1.08	1.04	1.00-1.08
ECONOMICALLY ACTIVE PERSONS	1780	1.00	0.95-1.05	1.00	0.95-1.05
0 Technical, humanistic, etc. work	138	0.84	0.70-0.98	0.86	0.72-1.01 *
00 Technical professions	19	1.03	0.62-1.62	1.05	0.63-1.64
004 Mechanical engineers	5	0.91	0.30-2.12	0.93	0.30-2.17
01 Technical work	47	0.78	0.58-1.04	0.82	0.60-1.09
010 Civil engineering technicians	20	0.90	0.55-1.38	0.92	0.56-1.43
013 Mechanical technicians	13	0.83	0.44-1.42	0.87	0.46-1.48
016 Technicians NOS	5	0.82	0.27-1.91	0.85	0.28-1.99
02 Chemical/physical/biological work	9	0.85	0.39-1.62	0.86	0.40-1.64
028 Consultancy, forestry	4	0.79	0.21-2.01	0.79	0.21-2.01
03 Medical work and nursing	11	1.35	0.67-2.41	1.35	0.67-2.41
05 Teaching	24	0.70	0.45-1.04	0.72	0.46-1.08
051 Subject teachers	6	0.92	0.34-2.01	0.95	0.35-2.07
052 Primary school teachers	7	0.52	0.21-1.08	0.55	0.22-1.13
054 Vocational teachers	3	0.37	0.08-1.08	0.38	0.08-1.12
07 Legal professions	5	0.99	0.32-2.32	1.00	0.33-2.34
08 Artistic and literary professions	13	1.19	0.64-2.04	1.22	0.65-2.09
09 Humanistic and social work etc.	7	0.67	0.27-1.38	0.68	0.28-1.41
1 Administrative and clerical work	129	1.18	0.99-1.40	1.20	1.00-1.42 *
10 Public administration	8	0.77	0.33-1.51	0.76	0.33-1.51
11 Corporate administration	68	1.31	1.02-1.66	1.32	1.03-1.67 *
110 Corporate managers	32	1.33	0.91-1.88	1.33	0.91-1.88
112 Commercial managers	14	1.14	0.63-1.92	1.18	0.64-1.97
119 Private sector managers NOS	13	2.16	1.15-3.69	2.13	1.14-3.65 *
12 Clerical work	10	2.20	1.06-4.05	2.23	1.07-4.10 *
120 Book-keepers, accountants	9	2.34	1.07-4.45	2.37	1.08-4.49 *
14/15 Clerical work NOS	41	1.00	0.71-1.35	1.02	0.73-1.39
144 Office clerks	6	0.89	0.33-1.95	0.92	0.34-2.00
150 Property managers, warehousemen	18	0.87	0.52-1.38	0.89	0.53-1.40
2 Sales professions	95	1.13	0.91-1.38	1.15	0.93-1.41
20 Wholesale and retail dealers	31	1.25	0.85-1.78	1.27	0.87-1.81
201 Retailers	31	1.31	0.89-1.86	1.33	0.90-1.89
21 Real estate, services, securities	6	0.95	0.35-2.08	0.98	0.36-2.14
22 Sales representatives	26	1.51	0.99-2.21	1.59	1.04-2.33 *
220 Commercial travellers, etc.	24	1.52	0.98-2.27	1.61	1.03-2.40 *
23 Sales work	32	0.89	0.61-1.26	0.90	0.61-1.26
230 Buyers, office sales staff	5	0.74	0.24-1.72	0.77	0.25-1.80
231 Shop personnel	18	0.81	0.48-1.27	0.80	0.47-1.26
3 Farming, forestry and fishing	430	0.83	0.75-0.91	0.83	0.75-0.91 *
30 Agricultural/forestry management	344	0.80	0.72-0.89	0.81	0.72-0.89 *
300 Farmers, silviculturists	322	0.79	0.71-0.88	0.79	0.71-0.88 *
302 Forestry managers	17	1.12	0.65-1.80	1.15	0.67-1.84
31 Farming, animal husbandry	21	0.82	0.51-1.25	0.79	0.49-1.21
310 Agricultural workers	16	0.83	0.47-1.34	0.80	0.46-1.31
34 Forestry work	63	1.10	0.84-1.40	1.02	0.79-1.31
4 Mining and quarrying	11	1.11	0.55-1.99	1.11	0.55-1.98
40 Mining and quarrying	8	1.31	0.56-2.58	1.31	0.56-2.58
5 Transport and communications	173	1.04	0.89-1.20	1.04	0.89-1.21
50 Ship's officers	5	0.70	0.23-1.64	0.72	0.23-1.69
53 Engine drivers	8	1.04	0.45-2.06	1.05	0.45-2.06
54 Road transport	99	0.98	0.79-1.19	0.98	0.80-1.20
540 Motor-vehicle and tram drivers	98	0.97	0.79-1.18	0.98	0.79-1.19

Occupation	Obs.	Crude SIR	95% CI	Adjusted SIR	95% CI
55 Transport services	22	1.32	0.83-2.00	1.33	0.83-2.01
550 Railway staff	22	1.34	0.84-2.04	1.35	0.85-2.05
56 Traffic supervisors	8	0.84	0.36-1.66	0.85	0.37-1.68
58 Postal services/couriers	12	1.11	0.57-1.94	1.11	0.57-1.93
580 Postmen	5	0.76	0.25-1.77	0.75	0.24-1.75
6/7 Industrial and construction work	712	1.10	1.02-1.19	1.09	1.01-1.17 *
60 Textiles	7	1.18	0.47-2.43	1.18	0.47-2.42
61 Cutting/sewing etc.	6	1.00	0.37-2.18	1.00	0.37-2.18
62 Shoes and leather	5	0.99	0.32-2.31	0.99	0.32-2.31
63 Smelting, metal and foundry work	23	1.28	0.81-1.92	1.28	0.81-1.92
635 Founders	6	1.16	0.42-2.52	1.16	0.43-2.52
64 Precision mechanical work	7	1.00	0.40-2.05	1.00	0.40-2.06
65 Machine shop/steelworkers	145	1.15	0.97-1.34	1.14	0.97-1.34
650 Turners, machinists	27	0.96	0.63-1.39	0.96	0.63-1.39
651 Fitter-assemblers etc.	15	1.23	0.69-2.03	1.22	0.69-2.02
652 Machine and motor repairers	30	1.02	0.69-1.46	1.02	0.69-1.46
653 Sheetmetalworkers	16	1.39	0.80-2.26	1.38	0.79-2.25
654 Plumbers	20	1.22	0.75-1.88	1.21	0.74-1.88
655 Welders and flame cutters	18	1.45	0.86-2.28	1.43	0.85-2.26
656 Plate/constructional steel work	-	-/3.7	0.00-0.99	-/3.7	0.00-0.99 *
659 Machine shop/steelworkers NOS	16	1.36	0.78-2.21	1.36	0.78-2.21
66 Electrical work	39	1.02	0.73-1.40	1.02	0.72-1.39
660 Electricians (indoors)	23	1.11	0.71-1.67	1.10	0.70-1.66
664 Telephone installers and repair	7	1.22	0.49-2.52	1.21	0.49-2.49
67 Woodwork	138	1.04	0.87-1.22	1.05	0.88-1.23
671 Timber workers	15	0.91	0.51-1.50	0.91	0.51-1.51
673 Construction carpenters	86	1.03	0.83-1.28	1.04	0.83-1.28
675 Bench carpenters	8	1.05	0.45-2.06	1.05	0.45-2.08
677 Woodworking machine operators e	5	0.68	0.22-1.60	0.68	0.22-1.60
68 Painting and lacquering	25	1.03	0.66-1.51	1.03	0.66-1.52
680 Painters	21	0.93	0.57-1.42	0.93	0.58-1.42
69 Construction work NOS	130	1.24	1.04-1.46	1.19	1.00-1.41 *
690 Bricklayers and tile setters	18	1.33	0.79-2.11	1.34	0.80-2.12
693 Concrete/cement shutterers	10	1.14	0.55-2.10	1.14	0.55-2.10
697 Building hands	54	1.27	0.96-1.66	1.19	0.90-1.56
698 Roadbuilding hands	38	1.34	0.95-1.84	1.28	0.90-1.75
70 Printing	9	1.07	0.49-2.02	1.06	0.48-2.00
72 Food industry	15	1.09	0.61-1.80	1.09	0.61-1.80
73 Chemical process/paper making	17	0.79	0.46-1.27	0.79	0.46-1.26
734 Pulp mill workers	4	0.67	0.18-1.72	0.67	0.18-1.72
735 Paper and board mill workers	4	0.50	0.14-1.28	0.50	0.14-1.27
75 Industrial work NOS	13	0.92	0.49-1.57	0.92	0.49-1.57
76 Packing and labelling	9	1.58	0.72-3.01	1.58	0.72-3.00
77 Machinists	62	1.29	0.99-1.65	1.28	0.99-1.65
771 Forklift operators	8	1.18	0.51-2.33	1.17	0.50-2.30
772 Construction machinery operator	18	1.15	0.68-1.82	1.16	0.69-1.83
773 Operators of stationary engine	18	1.46	0.86-2.30	1.46	0.86-2.30
775 Industrial personnel, riggers	7	1.11	0.45-2.28	1.11	0.44-2.28
78 Dock and warehouse work	36	0.94	0.66-1.30	0.90	0.63-1.25
780 Dockers	7	0.76	0.30-1.56	0.75	0.30-1.55
781 Freight handlers	3	0.53	0.11-1.54	0.50	0.10-1.46
782 Warehousemen	26	1.11	0.73-1.63	1.06	0.69-1.55
79 Labourers not classified elsewhere	21	0.94	0.58-1.44	0.90	0.55-1.37
8 Services	81	1.13	0.89-1.40	1.14	0.90-1.41
80 Watchmen, security guards	35	1.12	0.78-1.55	1.14	0.79-1.58
801 Policemen	13	1.02	0.55-1.75	1.05	0.56-1.80
804 Civilian guards	15	1.55	0.87-2.56	1.55	0.87-2.56
83 Caretakers and cleaners	36	1.18	0.83-1.64	1.18	0.83-1.64
830 Caretakers	33	1.21	0.83-1.70	1.21	0.84-1.70
9 Work not classified elsewhere	11	0.98	0.49-1.75	1.01	0.50-1.80
90 Military occupations	5	0.74	0.24-1.73	0.78	0.25-1.81
ECONOMICALLY INACTIVE PERSONS	341	1.31	1.18-1.45	1.32	1.18-1.46 *

Appendix Table C

Occupation	Obs.	Crude SIR	95% CI	Adjusted SIR	95% CI

C26. Cancer of the bladder, ureter and urethra, females

Occupation	Obs.	Crude SIR	95% CI	Adjusted SIR	95% CI
WHOLE POPULATION	564	0.94	0.87-1.02	0.92	0.85-1.00
ECONOMICALLY ACTIVE PERSONS	337	1.00	0.90-1.11	1.00	0.90-1.11
0 Technical, humanistic, etc. work	56	1.45	1.10-1.88	1.15	0.87-1.50 *
014 Chemotechnicians	1	53.8	1.36-300	51.6	1.30-287 *
03 Medical work and nursing	22	1.33	0.83-2.01	1.22	0.76-1.85
036 Auxiliary nurses	11	1.49	0.74-2.66	1.40	0.70-2.51
05 Teaching	17	1.46	0.85-2.34	1.00	0.58-1.60
052 Primary school teachers	9	1.56	0.71-2.96	0.97	0.44-1.83
1 Administrative and clerical work	42	1.09	0.78-1.47	1.02	0.74-1.38
12 Clerical work	4	0.43	0.12-1.10	0.41	0.11-1.06
131 Typists	6	3.92	1.44-8.52	3.85	1.41-8.38 *
14/15 Clerical work NOS	29	1.20	0.80-1.72	1.16	0.78-1.67
144 Office clerks	19	1.16	0.70-1.81	1.13	0.68-1.76
2 Sales professions	33	1.04	0.71-1.46	0.98	0.67-1.38
20 Wholesale and retail dealers	7	1.33	0.53-2.73	1.26	0.51-2.60
201 Retailers	7	1.33	0.54-2.75	1.27	0.51-2.62
21 Real estate, services, securities	2	13.2	1.59-47.6	11.9	1.43-42.8 *
23 Sales work	23	0.89	0.56-1.33	0.84	0.53-1.26
231 Shop personnel	21	0.86	0.53-1.31	0.81	0.50-1.24
3 Farming, forestry and fishing	54	0.65	0.49-0.85	0.68	0.51-0.89 *
30 Agricultural/forestry management	16	0.70	0.40-1.13	0.76	0.43-1.23
300 Farmers, silviculturists	16	0.72	0.41-1.16	0.78	0.44-1.26
31 Farming, animal husbandry	38	0.64	0.45-0.87	0.66	0.46-0.90 *
310 Agricultural workers	4	0.66	0.18-1.70	0.67	0.18-1.72
312 Livestock workers	32	0.63	0.43-0.88	0.64	0.44-0.90 *
4 Mining and quarrying	-	-/0.1	0.00-33.5	-/0.1	0.00-32.6
5 Transport and communications	14	1.21	0.66-2.02	1.21	0.66-2.03
550 Railway staff	2	11.7	1.41-42.1	11.5	1.39-41.5 *
57 Post and telecommunications	9	1.50	0.69-2.86	1.47	0.67-2.78
6/7 Industrial and construction work	74	1.23	0.96-1.54	1.21	0.95-1.52
60 Textiles	4	0.55	0.15-1.42	0.53	0.14-1.35
61 Cutting/sewing etc.	20	1.64	1.00-2.53	1.55	0.95-2.40 *
616 Garment workers	10	1.50	0.72-2.76	1.42	0.68-2.61
67 Woodwork	5	0.97	0.31-2.26	0.94	0.30-2.19
72 Food industry	8	1.12	0.48-2.21	1.08	0.46-2.12
729 Food-product workers NOS	2	10.6	1.28-38.2	10.2	1.23-36.8 *
76 Packing and labelling	7	1.29	0.52-2.65	1.22	0.49-2.51
773 Operators of stationary engine	2	28.1	3.39-101	27.3	3.30-98.6 *
78 Dock and warehouse work	7	2.57	1.03-5.29	3.23	1.30-6.65 *
780 Dockers	3	9.32	1.92-27.2	9.42	1.94-27.5 *
8 Services	63	0.87	0.67-1.11	1.04	0.80-1.32
81 Housekeeping, domestic work, etc.	20	0.81	0.49-1.24	0.92	0.56-1.43
811 Chefs, cooks etc.	7	1.12	0.45-2.30	1.09	0.44-2.24
812 Kitchen assistants	8	1.20	0.52-2.36	1.65	0.71-3.25
813 Domestic servants	3	0.45	0.09-1.31	0.58	0.12-1.69
82 Waiters	8	1.17	0.51-2.31	1.13	0.49-2.22
83 Caretakers and cleaners	28	0.83	0.55-1.20	1.10	0.73-1.59
831 Cleaners	22	0.73	0.46-1.11	1.01	0.63-1.53
9 Work not classified elsewhere	1	1.35	0.03-7.55	1.32	0.03-7.35
ECONOMICALLY INACTIVE PERSONS	227	0.87	0.76-0.99	0.83	0.72-0.94 *

Occupation	Obs.	Crude SIR	95% CI	Adjusted SIR	95% CI

C27. Skin melanoma, males

Occupation	Obs.	Crude SIR	95% CI	Adjusted SIR	95% CI	
WHOLE POPULATION	1148	0.99	0.93-1.05	0.99	0.94-1.05	
ECONOMICALLY ACTIVE PERSONS	1060	1.00	0.94-1.06	1.00	0.94-1.06	
0 Technical, humanistic, etc. work	157	1.37	1.17-1.60	1.06	0.90-1.23	*
00 Technical professions	18	1.24	0.73-1.95	0.84	0.50-1.33	
001 Civil engineers	5	1.41	0.46-3.28	0.98	0.32-2.28	
004 Mechanical engineers	7	1.64	0.66-3.39	1.12	0.45-2.32	
01 Technical work	47	1.15	0.85-1.53	1.03	0.76-1.37	
010 Civil engineering technicians	12	0.86	0.44-1.50	0.76	0.40-1.34	
013 Mechanical technicians	16	1.47	0.84-2.39	1.33	0.76-2.15	
02 Chemical/physical/biological work	13	1.98	1.06-3.39	1.48	0.79-2.53	*
025 Veterinary surgeons	3	6.86	1.41-20.0	4.66	0.96-13.6	*
03 Medical work and nursing	7	1.18	0.48-2.44	0.89	0.36-1.83	
05 Teaching	44	1.74	1.27-2.34	1.23	0.89-1.65	*
050 University teachers	7	3.14	1.26-6.46	2.11	0.85-4.34	*
051 Subject teachers	10	1.96	0.94-3.60	1.33	0.64-2.45	
052 Primary school teachers	19	1.89	1.14-2.95	1.28	0.77-1.99	*
054 Vocational teachers	6	1.10	0.40-2.39	0.86	0.31-1.86	
08 Artistic and literary professions	7	0.95	0.38-1.95	0.69	0.28-1.42	
09 Humanistic and social work etc.	16	2.20	1.26-3.57	1.65	0.95-2.68	*
093 Community planning professions	3	5.69	1.17-16.6	3.97	0.82-11.6	*
1 Administrative and clerical work	88	1.38	1.10-1.70	1.01	0.81-1.25	*
10 Public administration	2	0.34	0.04-1.24	0.22	0.03-0.80	*
11 Corporate administration	48	1.56	1.15-2.07	1.02	0.75-1.36	*
110 Corporate managers	22	1.70	1.07-2.58	1.10	0.69-1.66	*
112 Commercial managers	9	1.08	0.49-2.05	0.72	0.33-1.37	
119 Private sector managers NOS	6	1.66	0.61-3.62	1.09	0.40-2.37	
14/15 Clerical work NOS	33	1.35	0.93-1.90	1.20	0.83-1.69	
150 Property managers, warehousemen	15	1.33	0.74-2.19	1.20	0.67-1.98	
2 Sales professions	67	1.18	0.91-1.50	1.10	0.86-1.40	
20 Wholesale and retail dealers	9	0.68	0.31-1.30	0.61	0.28-1.16	
201 Retailers	8	0.64	0.27-1.25	0.57	0.25-1.13	
22 Sales representatives	17	1.28	0.75-2.05	1.14	0.67-1.83	
220 Commercial travellers, etc.	16	1.29	0.74-2.09	1.15	0.66-1.86	
23 Sales work	35	1.33	0.93-1.85	1.33	0.93-1.85	
230 Buyers, office sales staff	7	1.50	0.60-3.09	1.28	0.52-2.64	
231 Shop personnel	25	1.47	0.95-2.16	1.56	1.01-2.31	*
3 Farming, forestry and fishing	224	0.85	0.74-0.96	0.93	0.81-1.06	*
30 Agricultural/forestry management	191	0.92	0.80-1.06	0.97	0.83-1.11	
300 Farmers, silviculturists	179	0.92	0.79-1.06	0.97	0.83-1.12	
302 Forestry managers	8	0.97	0.42-1.90	0.87	0.37-1.71	
31 Farming, animal husbandry	17	0.93	0.54-1.49	1.11	0.65-1.78	
310 Agricultural workers	13	0.91	0.48-1.56	1.05	0.56-1.80	
34 Forestry work	15	0.41	0.23-0.67	0.59	0.33-0.98	*
4 Mining and quarrying	3	0.49	0.10-1.42	0.52	0.11-1.51	
5 Transport and communications	97	0.89	0.72-1.08	0.88	0.71-1.07	
50 Ship's officers	7	1.65	0.66-3.40	1.35	0.54-2.79	
54 Road transport	59	0.84	0.64-1.08	0.84	0.64-1.08	
540 Motor-vehicle and tram drivers	59	0.84	0.64-1.08	0.84	0.64-1.09	
55 Transport services	10	1.09	0.52-2.00	1.13	0.54-2.07	
550 Railway staff	10	1.12	0.54-2.06	1.16	0.56-2.13	
56 Traffic supervisors	2	0.38	0.05-1.39	0.31	0.04-1.10	
58 Postal services/couriers	3	0.45	0.09-1.31	0.48	0.10-1.41	
6/7 Industrial and construction work	371	0.94	0.85-1.04	1.04	0.94-1.15	
63 Smelting, metal and foundry work	7	0.66	0.27-1.36	0.70	0.28-1.45	
65 Machine shop/steelworkers	83	0.97	0.77-1.20	1.03	0.82-1.27	
650 Turners, machinists	18	1.06	0.63-1.67	1.13	0.67-1.79	
651 Fitter-assemblers etc.	5	0.59	0.19-1.37	0.63	0.20-1.47	
652 Machine and motor repairers	11	0.54	0.27-0.96	0.56	0.28-1.01	*

Occupation	Obs.	Crude		Adjusted	
		SIR	95% CI	SIR	95% CI
653 Sheetmetalworkers	13	1.60	0.85-2.74	1.69	0.90-2.89
654 Plumbers	14	1.23	0.67-2.07	1.30	0.71-2.19
655 Welders and flame cutters	10	0.98	0.47-1.80	1.04	0.50-1.92
659 Machine shop/steelworkers NOS	8	1.12	0.48-2.21	1.19	0.51-2.35
66 Electrical work	28	1.05	0.70-1.52	1.12	0.74-1.62
660 Electricians (indoors)	21	1.44	0.89-2.21	1.54	0.95-2.36
67 Woodwork	64	0.90	0.69-1.15	0.96	0.74-1.23
671 Timber workers	11	1.16	0.58-2.08	1.24	0.62-2.22
673 Construction carpenters	35	0.82	0.57-1.14	0.89	0.62-1.23
68 Painting and lacquering	22	1.46	0.92-2.21	1.54	0.96-2.33
680 Painters	20	1.46	0.89-2.26	1.54	0.94-2.37
69 Construction work NOS	44	0.75	0.54-1.00	0.96	0.70-1.29
690 Bricklayers and tile setters	6	0.83	0.30-1.81	0.89	0.33-1.94
693 Concrete/cement shutterers	7	1.34	0.54-2.77	1.44	0.58-2.98
697 Building hands	17	0.69	0.40-1.11	1.01	0.59-1.61
698 Roadbuilding hands	11	0.78	0.39-1.39	1.09	0.55-1.96
70 Printing	7	1.08	0.43-2.22	1.14	0.46-2.36
72 Food industry	10	1.11	0.53-2.05	1.18	0.56-2.16
73 Chemical process/paper making	16	1.13	0.65-1.84	1.22	0.70-1.98
735 Paper and board mill workers	6	1.06	0.39-2.31	1.14	0.42-2.48
75 Industrial work NOS	7	0.77	0.31-1.58	0.81	0.32-1.66
77 Machinists	35	1.03	0.72-1.43	1.09	0.76-1.51
771 Forklift operators	3	0.56	0.12-1.65	0.61	0.12-1.77
772 Construction machinery operator	16	1.32	0.76-2.15	1.35	0.77-2.20
773 Operators of stationary engine	5	0.70	0.23-1.64	0.76	0.25-1.77
78 Dock and warehouse work	18	0.79	0.47-1.25	1.04	0.61-1.64
780 Dockers	6	1.14	0.42-2.48	1.26	0.46-2.75
782 Warehousemen	8	0.57	0.25-1.13	0.79	0.34-1.56
789 Dock/warehouse workers NOS	1	34.3	0.87-191	48.0	1.21-267 *
79 Labourers not classified elsewhere	8	0.69	0.30-1.37	0.99	0.43-1.95
8 Services	45	1.10	0.80-1.47	1.11	0.81-1.49
80 Watchmen, security guards	18	0.98	0.58-1.55	0.95	0.56-1.50
801 Policemen	11	1.49	0.74-2.66	1.35	0.67-2.41
83 Caretakers and cleaners	20	1.23	0.75-1.90	1.33	0.81-2.05
830 Caretakers	19	1.31	0.79-2.05	1.42	0.85-2.21
9 Work not classified elsewhere	8	0.89	0.38-1.75	0.76	0.33-1.50
90 Military occupations	7	1.11	0.45-2.29	0.88	0.35-1.81
ECONOMICALLY INACTIVE PERSONS	88	0.86	0.69-1.06	0.93	0.74-1.14

C28. Skin melanoma, females

Occupation	Obs.	Crude		Adjusted	
		SIR	95% CI	SIR	95% CI
WHOLE POPULATION	1234	0.97	0.92-1.03	0.98	0.93-1.04
ECONOMICALLY ACTIVE PERSONS	781	1.00	0.93-1.07	1.00	0.93-1.07
0 Technical, humanistic, etc. work	138	1.22	1.02-1.43	1.05	0.88-1.23 *
01 Technical work	8	1.35	0.58-2.66	1.15	0.50-2.26
028 Consultancy, forestry	1	44.8	1.13-250	40.1	1.02-224 *
03 Medical work and nursing	59	1.16	0.88-1.50	1.11	0.84-1.43
032 Nurses	20	1.29	0.79-1.99	1.08	0.66-1.68
035 Psychiatric nurses	8	2.38	1.03-4.69	2.02	0.87-3.97 *
036 Auxiliary nurses	20	0.93	0.57-1.43	1.06	0.65-1.63
04 Health-care related work	9	1.38	0.63-2.62	1.12	0.51-2.13
040 Pharmacists	5	1.26	0.41-2.93	1.00	0.32-2.33
05 Teaching	36	1.10	0.77-1.52	0.86	0.60-1.19
051 Subject teachers	3	0.34	0.07-0.99	0.27	0.05-0.78 *
052 Primary school teachers	20	1.39	0.85-2.14	1.05	0.64-1.63
053 Teachers of practical subjects	6	1.43	0.52-3.10	1.17	0.43-2.55
07 Legal professions	3	5.87	1.21-17.2	4.76	0.98-13.9 *
09 Humanistic and social work etc.	11	1.31	0.65-2.34	1.08	0.54-1.93
1 Administrative and clerical work	137	1.24	1.04-1.46	1.04	0.87-1.22 *
12 Clerical work	29	1.23	0.82-1.77	1.02	0.69-1.47
120 Book-keepers, accountants	14	1.30	0.71-2.18	1.08	0.59-1.80

Occupation	Obs.	Crude		Adjusted	
		SIR	95% CI	SIR	95% CI
121 Office cashiers	10	2.25	1.08-4.13	1.85	0.89-3.41 *
123 Shop and restaurant cashiers	3	0.47	0.10-1.37	0.39	0.08-1.15
13 Stenographers and typists	12	1.11	0.57-1.93	0.94	0.48-1.64
130 Private secretaries	7	1.14	0.46-2.34	0.96	0.39-1.98
131 Typists	5	1.07	0.35-2.49	0.90	0.29-2.11
14/15 Clerical work NOS	88	1.23	0.99-1.52	1.04	0.83-1.28
144 Office clerks	55	1.18	0.89-1.54	0.99	0.75-1.29
145 Bank clerks	15	1.52	0.85-2.51	1.30	0.73-2.15
159 Clerical workers NOS	4	0.71	0.19-1.82	0.59	0.16-1.51
2 Sales professions	69	0.85	0.66-1.08	0.88	0.68-1.11
20 Wholesale and retail dealers	8	0.81	0.35-1.59	0.64	0.28-1.26
201 Retailers	8	0.81	0.35-1.60	0.64	0.28-1.27
23 Sales work	61	0.88	0.68-1.13	0.96	0.73-1.23
231 Shop personnel	58	0.89	0.68-1.15	0.98	0.74-1.26
3 Farming, forestry and fishing	144	0.91	0.77-1.07	0.98	0.83-1.15
30 Agricultural/forestry management	26	0.73	0.48-1.07	0.81	0.53-1.19
300 Farmers, silviculturists	26	0.76	0.49-1.11	0.84	0.55-1.23
31 Farming, animal husbandry	118	0.97	0.80-1.15	1.04	0.86-1.23
310 Agricultural workers	15	1.26	0.70-2.08	1.31	0.73-2.16
312 Livestock workers	102	0.97	0.79-1.17	1.04	0.85-1.25
4 Mining and quarrying	-	-/0.2	0.00-17.1	-/0.2	0.00-19.1
5 Transport and communications	38	1.43	1.01-1.96	1.33	0.94-1.83 *
57 Post and telecommunications	25	1.69	1.10-2.50	1.42	0.92-2.10 *
570 Post/telecommunications officials	11	1.72	0.86-3.08	1.46	0.73-2.61
571 Telephone operators	8	1.57	0.68-3.09	1.30	0.56-2.57
58 Postal services/couriers	7	0.97	0.39-2.00	1.12	0.45-2.30
580 Postmen	4	0.63	0.17-1.60	0.72	0.20-1.84
6/7 Industrial and construction work	115	0.83	0.69-0.99	0.93	0.77-1.11 *
60 Textiles	10	0.65	0.31-1.20	0.74	0.35-1.35
602 Weavers	4	0.79	0.22-2.03	0.86	0.24-2.21
61 Cutting/sewing etc.	33	1.15	0.79-1.62	1.24	0.85-1.74
611 Dressmakers	5	0.95	0.31-2.22	0.84	0.27-1.96
612 Furriers	3	5.72	1.18-16.7	6.04	1.24-17.6 *
616 Garment workers	17	1.02	0.59-1.63	1.16	0.68-1.86
62 Shoes and leather	5	0.95	0.31-2.22	1.06	0.35-2.48
65 Machine shop/steelworkers	1	0.19	0.00-1.04	0.21	0.01-1.18
67 Woodwork	11	0.94	0.47-1.69	1.08	0.54-1.93
672 Plywood makers	6	1.09	0.40-2.37	1.25	0.46-2.72
69 Construction work NOS	8	1.54	0.67-3.04	1.74	0.75-3.44
70 Printing	5	0.93	0.30-2.17	1.06	0.34-2.47
72 Food industry	12	0.73	0.38-1.27	0.83	0.43-1.45
721 Bakers and pastry chiefs	7	0.95	0.38-1.96	1.07	0.43-2.21
75 Industrial work NOS	5	0.58	0.19-1.36	0.66	0.21-1.54
76 Packing and labelling	7	0.52	0.21-1.08	0.60	0.24-1.24
78 Dock and warehouse work	6	1.02	0.37-2.21	1.16	0.43-2.52
782 Warehousemen	6	1.20	0.44-2.60	1.37	0.50-2.97
8 Services	140	0.92	0.77-1.08	1.00	0.84-1.17
81 Housekeeping, domestic work, etc.	51	0.98	0.73-1.29	1.05	0.79-1.39
810 Housekeepers	5	0.99	0.32-2.30	0.80	0.26-1.87
811 Chefs, cooks etc.	10	0.77	0.37-1.41	0.89	0.43-1.64
812 Kitchen assistants	19	1.29	0.77-2.01	1.46	0.88-2.29
813 Domestic servants	9	0.75	0.34-1.43	0.87	0.40-1.66
82 Waiters	13	0.73	0.39-1.25	0.76	0.40-1.30
820 Waiters in restaurants	6	0.73	0.27-1.58	0.79	0.29-1.73
821 Waiters in cafés etc.	7	0.73	0.30-1.51	0.73	0.29-1.51
83 Caretakers and cleaners	61	0.91	0.70-1.17	1.04	0.80-1.34
830 Caretakers	7	0.81	0.33-1.67	0.93	0.37-1.92
831 Cleaners	54	0.93	0.70-1.22	1.07	0.80-1.39
84 Hygiene and beauty services	8	1.01	0.43-1.99	0.91	0.39-1.79
840 Hairdressers and barbers	7	1.10	0.44-2.26	0.96	0.39-1.99
85 Laundry and pressing	6	1.00	0.37-2.19	1.09	0.40-2.37
850 Launderers	5	1.00	0.32-2.34	1.07	0.35-2.50
9 Work not classified elsewhere	-	-/1.6	0.00-2.31	-/1.4	0.00-2.65

Appendix Table C

Occupation	Obs.	Crude		Adjusted	
		SIR	95% CI	SIR	95% CI
ECONOMICALLY INACTIVE PERSONS	453	0.93	0.85-1.02	0.95	0.86-1.04

C29. Non-melanoma skin cancer, males

Occupation	Obs.	Crude SIR	95% CI	Adjusted SIR	95% CI	
WHOLE POPULATION	745	1.01	0.94-1.09	1.01	0.94-1.09	
ECONOMICALLY ACTIVE PERSONS	638	1.00	0.92-1.08	1.00	0.92-1.08	
0 Technical, humanistic, etc. work	71	1.19	0.93-1.50	1.15	0.90-1.46	
00 Technical professions	7	1.04	0.42-2.14	0.95	0.38-1.95	
01 Technical work	20	0.92	0.56-1.42	0.97	0.59-1.50	
010 Civil engineering technicians	5	0.63	0.20-1.46	0.66	0.21-1.54	
013 Mechanical technicians	8	1.41	0.61-2.78	1.48	0.64-2.92	
05 Teaching	15	1.19	0.67-1.97	1.08	0.60-1.78	
052 Primary school teachers	9	1.85	0.84-3.51	1.60	0.73-3.04	
093 Community planning professions	2	10.6	1.28-38.2	9.88	1.20-35.7	*
1 Administrative and clerical work	38	0.98	0.69-1.34	0.94	0.67-1.29	
11 Corporate administration	14	0.76	0.42-1.28	0.69	0.38-1.16	
110 Corporate managers	8	0.95	0.41-1.87	0.86	0.37-1.70	
112 Commercial managers	5	1.13	0.37-2.65	1.01	0.33-2.35	
14/15 Clerical work NOS	20	1.35	0.82-2.08	1.42	0.87-2.19	
150 Property managers, warehousemen	10	1.35	0.65-2.48	1.43	0.69-2.63	
2 Sales professions	19	0.62	0.37-0.97	0.65	0.39-1.01	*
20 Wholesale and retail dealers	4	0.46	0.12-1.17	0.48	0.13-1.24	
201 Retailers	4	0.48	0.13-1.22	0.51	0.14-1.30	
22 Sales representatives	5	0.79	0.26-1.84	0.83	0.27-1.94	
220 Commercial travellers, etc.	4	0.69	0.19-1.76	0.72	0.20-1.85	
23 Sales work	9	0.69	0.31-1.30	0.69	0.32-1.32	
231 Shop personnel	4	0.49	0.13-1.25	0.49	0.13-1.24	
3 Farming, forestry and fishing	200	1.08	0.94-1.24	1.09	0.94-1.25	
30 Agricultural/forestry management	172	1.12	0.96-1.30	1.13	0.97-1.31	
300 Farmers, silviculturists	162	1.12	0.95-1.30	1.12	0.95-1.30	
302 Forestry managers	8	1.51	0.65-2.97	1.60	0.69-3.15	
31 Farming, animal husbandry	9	0.94	0.43-1.79	0.95	0.44-1.81	
310 Agricultural workers	8	1.11	0.48-2.18	1.12	0.48-2.21	
34 Forestry work	19	0.92	0.56-1.44	0.94	0.56-1.46	
4 Mining and quarrying	4	1.13	0.31-2.88	1.12	0.30-2.86	
5 Transport and communications	41	0.69	0.50-0.94	0.70	0.50-0.95	*
54 Road transport	25	0.69	0.44-1.01	0.70	0.46-1.04	
540 Motor-vehicle and tram drivers	25	0.69	0.45-1.02	0.71	0.46-1.04	
55 Transport services	3	0.53	0.11-1.54	0.53	0.11-1.54	
550 Railway staff	3	0.54	0.11-1.57	0.54	0.11-1.57	
58 Postal services/couriers	-	-/3.9	0.00-0.95	-/3.9	0.00-0.94	*
6/7 Industrial and construction work	237	1.03	0.90-1.16	1.02	0.90-1.16	
63 Smelting, metal and foundry work	8	1.24	0.54-2.44	1.24	0.53-2.44	
65 Machine shop/steelworkers	58	1.27	0.97-1.65	1.27	0.96-1.64	
650 Turners, machinists	12	1.20	0.62-2.10	1.19	0.61-2.08	
652 Machine and motor repairers	11	1.04	0.52-1.86	1.04	0.52-1.86	
654 Plumbers	6	1.02	0.37-2.22	1.02	0.37-2.22	
659 Machine shop/steelworkers NOS	10	2.38	1.14-4.38	2.37	1.14-4.36	*
66 Electrical work	12	0.88	0.45-1.53	0.87	0.45-1.52	
660 Electricians (indoors)	4	0.54	0.15-1.39	0.54	0.15-1.38	
67 Woodwork	45	0.96	0.70-1.29	0.95	0.70-1.28	
670 Round-timber workers	5	4.68	1.52-10.9	4.64	1.51-10.8	*
671 Timber workers	3	0.51	0.11-1.49	0.51	0.10-1.48	
673 Construction carpenters	27	0.93	0.61-1.35	0.91	0.60-1.33	
68 Painting and lacquering	9	1.01	0.46-1.93	1.02	0.47-1.94	
680 Painters	9	1.10	0.50-2.08	1.10	0.50-2.09	
69 Construction work NOS	28	0.75	0.50-1.09	0.76	0.50-1.10	
697 Building hands	10	0.67	0.32-1.22	0.68	0.32-1.24	
698 Roadbuilding hands	10	0.98	0.47-1.81	1.00	0.48-1.83	

Occupation	Obs.	Crude SIR	95% CI	Adjusted SIR	95% CI
72 Food industry	4	0.79	0.22-2.03	0.80	0.22-2.04
73 Chemical process/paper making	12	1.54	0.80-2.69	1.53	0.79-2.67
75 Industrial work NOS	4	0.79	0.21-2.01	0.79	0.21-2.02
77 Machinists	17	0.97	0.57-1.56	0.97	0.57-1.55
772 Construction machinery operator	11	1.93	0.96-3.45	1.95	0.97-3.48
78 Dock and warehouse work	15	1.09	0.61-1.79	1.09	0.61-1.80
782 Warehousemen	11	1.30	0.65-2.32	1.31	0.65-2.34
79 Labourers not classified elsewhere	9	1.12	0.51-2.12	1.13	0.51-2.14
8 Services	24	0.93	0.60-1.39	0.94	0.60-1.39
80 Watchmen, security guards	14	1.24	0.68-2.08	1.26	0.69-2.11
83 Caretakers and cleaners	8	0.74	0.32-1.46	0.73	0.32-1.44
830 Caretakers	6	0.62	0.23-1.35	0.61	0.22-1.33
9 Work not classified elsewhere	4	0.97	0.27-2.50	0.98	0.27-2.52
ECONOMICALLY INACTIVE PERSONS	107	1.08	0.89-1.30	1.08	0.89-1.30

C30. Non-melanoma skin cancer, females

Occupation	Obs.	Crude SIR	95% CI	Adjusted SIR	95% CI	
WHOLE POPULATION	548	1.01	0.93-1.10	1.00	0.92-1.09	
ECONOMICALLY ACTIVE PERSONS	307	1.00	0.89-1.11	1.00	0.89-1.11	
0 Technical, humanistic, etc. work	45	1.19	0.87-1.60	1.05	0.77-1.40	
03 Medical work and nursing	21	1.29	0.80-1.97	1.24	0.77-1.89	
036 Auxiliary nurses	12	1.69	0.87-2.95	1.61	0.83-2.81	
05 Teaching	12	1.06	0.55-1.86	0.83	0.43-1.45	
052 Primary school teachers	6	1.12	0.41-2.44	0.80	0.30-1.75	
1 Administrative and clerical work	44	1.18	0.86-1.59	1.21	0.88-1.63	
114 Managers of ideal organizations	2	30.5	3.69-110	20.5	2.48-74.1	*
12 Clerical work	7	0.81	0.33-1.68	0.87	0.35-1.80	
14/15 Clerical work NOS	30	1.27	0.86-1.82	1.33	0.90-1.90	
144 Office clerks	20	1.27	0.78-1.96	1.34	0.82-2.07	
2 Sales professions	28	0.95	0.63-1.37	0.94	0.63-1.37	
23 Sales work	20	0.82	0.50-1.27	0.80	0.49-1.23	
231 Shop personnel	20	0.87	0.53-1.35	0.84	0.51-1.30	
3 Farming, forestry and fishing	77	1.06	0.84-1.33	1.07	0.84-1.33	
30 Agricultural/forestry management	17	0.86	0.50-1.38	0.86	0.50-1.38	
300 Farmers, silviculturists	17	0.88	0.52-1.42	0.88	0.52-1.42	
31 Farming, animal husbandry	60	1.14	0.87-1.47	1.15	0.88-1.48	
310 Agricultural workers	3	0.56	0.12-1.65	0.56	0.12-1.65	
312 Livestock workers	55	1.22	0.92-1.59	1.22	0.92-1.59	
4 Mining and quarrying	-	-/0.1	0.00-39.2	-/0.1	0.00-37.3	
5 Transport and communications	9	0.87	0.40-1.65	0.89	0.41-1.70	
57 Post and telecommunications	2	0.37	0.04-1.33	0.39	0.05-1.42	
6/7 Industrial and construction work	47	0.86	0.63-1.15	0.84	0.61-1.11	
60 Textiles	4	0.62	0.17-1.59	0.58	0.16-1.50	
61 Cutting/sewing etc.	13	1.16	0.62-1.98	1.14	0.61-1.94	
616 Garment workers	7	1.13	0.45-2.32	1.06	0.43-2.19	
72 Food industry	5	0.77	0.25-1.80	0.73	0.24-1.69	
76 Packing and labelling	8	1.61	0.70-3.18	1.51	0.65-2.98	
8 Services	55	0.85	0.64-1.11	0.93	0.70-1.22	
81 Housekeeping, domestic work, etc.	21	0.95	0.59-1.45	1.01	0.63-1.55	
811 Chefs, cooks etc.	5	0.89	0.29-2.08	0.82	0.27-1.92	
812 Kitchen assistants	5	0.84	0.27-1.96	0.99	0.32-2.32	
813 Domestic servants	4	0.68	0.18-1.74	0.75	0.20-1.91	
82 Waiters	5	0.79	0.26-1.84	0.79	0.26-1.84	
83 Caretakers and cleaners	25	0.85	0.55-1.25	0.96	0.62-1.42	
831 Cleaners	22	0.84	0.52-1.27	0.97	0.61-1.48	

Appendix Table C

Occupation	Obs.	Crude SIR	95% CI	Adjusted SIR	95% CI	
843 Sauna attendants etc.	3	6.87	1.42-20.1	7.68	1.58-22.5	*
9 Work not classified elsewhere	2	3.01	0.36-10.9	2.79	0.34-10.1	
ECONOMICALLY INACTIVE PERSONS	241	1.03	0.90-1.16	1.00	0.88-1.13	

C31. Basal cell carcinoma of the skin, males

Occupation	Obs.	Crude SIR	95% CI	Adjusted SIR	95% CI	
WHOLE POPULATION	6263	0.99	0.97-1.02	1.00	0.98-1.03	
ECONOMICALLY ACTIVE PERSONS	5577	1.00	0.97-1.03	1.00	0.97-1.03	
0 Technical, humanistic, etc. work	786	1.45	1.35-1.56	1.11	1.04-1.19	*
00 Technical professions	89	1.42	1.14-1.74	0.93	0.75-1.15	*
000 Architects	6	1.46	0.54-3.18	0.95	0.35-2.07	
001 Civil engineers	19	1.37	0.82-2.13	0.90	0.54-1.41	
002 Electrical engineers	14	1.65	0.90-2.77	1.09	0.60-1.83	
003 Teletechnical engineers	2	0.58	0.07-2.09	0.38	0.05-1.37	
004 Mechanical engineers	26	1.40	0.91-2.05	0.92	0.60-1.35	
005 Chemotechnical engineers	11	1.90	0.95-3.39	1.25	0.63-2.24	
007 Engineers NOS	4	1.08	0.30-2.77	0.71	0.19-1.83	
008 Surveyors	5	1.41	0.46-3.29	0.92	0.30-2.14	
01 Technical work	274	1.40	1.24-1.57	1.27	1.12-1.43	*
010 Civil engineering technicians	89	1.25	1.00-1.54	1.13	0.91-1.39	*
011 Power technicians	27	1.67	1.10-2.42	1.51	0.99-2.20	*
012 Teletechnicians	15	1.70	0.95-2.80	1.55	0.87-2.55	
013 Mechanical technicians	74	1.44	1.13-1.81	1.31	1.03-1.65	*
014 Chemotechnicians	13	2.60	1.39-4.45	2.36	1.26-4.04	*
016 Technicians NOS	23	1.16	0.73-1.74	1.05	0.67-1.58	
017 Cartographers	10	2.05	0.98-3.77	1.86	0.89-3.42	
018 Draughtsmen, survey assistants	15	1.40	0.78-2.30	1.27	0.71-2.09	
019 Laboratory assistants	6	1.01	0.37-2.20	0.92	0.34-2.00	
02 Chemical/physical/biological work	39	1.16	0.83-1.59	0.87	0.62-1.19	
020 Chemists	3	0.86	0.18-2.51	0.57	0.12-1.66	
027 Consultancy, agriculture	6	0.63	0.23-1.38	0.53	0.19-1.15	
028 Consultancy, forestry	21	1.34	0.83-2.05	1.02	0.63-1.55	
03 Medical work and nursing	47	1.73	1.27-2.30	1.27	0.94-1.69	*
030 Medical doctors	31	2.07	1.41-2.94	1.36	0.92-1.93	*
035 Psychiatric nurses	3	0.63	0.13-1.83	0.56	0.12-1.65	
037 Technical nursing assistants	3	11.7	2.41-34.2	12.7	2.62-37.1	*
04 Health-care related work	9	1.10	0.51-2.10	0.88	0.40-1.67	
05 Teaching	188	1.63	1.41-1.87	1.12	0.97-1.29	*
050 University teachers	18	1.77	1.05-2.80	1.16	0.69-1.84	*
051 Subject teachers	32	1.44	0.98-2.03	0.94	0.64-1.32	
052 Primary school teachers	85	1.88	1.50-2.32	1.23	0.98-1.52	*
053 Teachers of practical subjects	14	2.20	1.20-3.70	1.61	0.88-2.70	*
054 Vocational teachers	33	1.24	0.86-1.75	0.97	0.67-1.37	
06 Religious professions	15	1.16	0.65-1.91	0.83	0.46-1.36	
060 Clergy and lay preachers	14	1.21	0.66-2.03	0.85	0.46-1.42	
07 Legal professions	25	1.63	1.05-2.40	1.11	0.72-1.63	*
070 Barristers and judges	7	1.71	0.69-3.52	1.12	0.45-2.31	
08 Artistic and literary professions	48	1.36	1.00-1.80	0.98	0.72-1.29	*
080 Sculptors, painters, etc.	8	1.91	0.82-3.76	1.25	0.54-2.47	
083 Authors	4	4.34	1.18-11.1	2.83	0.77-7.25	*
084 Journalists	17	1.46	0.85-2.34	1.01	0.59-1.61	
087 Musicians	8	0.93	0.40-1.84	0.70	0.30-1.38	
09 Humanistic and social work etc.	52	1.52	1.14-2.00	1.14	0.85-1.50	*
091 Social workers	13	1.65	0.88-2.82	1.33	0.71-2.27	
094 Systems analysts, programmers	3	0.84	0.17-2.45	0.58	0.12-1.70	
096 PR officers	24	1.96	1.26-2.92	1.54	0.99-2.30	*
1 Administrative and clerical work	486	1.43	1.30-1.56	1.06	0.96-1.15	*
10 Public administration	41	1.28	0.92-1.73	0.84	0.60-1.14	
11 Corporate administration	260	1.60	1.41-1.80	1.05	0.92-1.18	*
110 Corporate managers	123	1.67	1.39-1.98	1.10	0.91-1.30	*
111 Technical managers	31	2.11	1.43-3.00	1.39	0.94-1.97	*
112 Commercial managers	58	1.45	1.10-1.87	0.95	0.72-1.23	*

Occupation	Obs.	Crude SIR	95% CI	Adjusted SIR	95% CI	
113 Administrative managers	13	1.50	0.80-2.57	0.99	0.53-1.69	
114 Managers of ideal organizations	7	1.00	0.40-2.06	0.66	0.26-1.35	
119 Private sector managers NOS	28	1.47	0.98-2.13	0.97	0.64-1.40	
12 Clerical work	17	1.22	0.71-1.96	1.01	0.59-1.62	
120 Book-keepers, accountants	13	1.10	0.59-1.88	0.90	0.48-1.54	
14/15 Clerical work NOS	163	1.26	1.08-1.47	1.14	0.97-1.32	*
144 Office clerks	35	1.67	1.16-2.33	1.53	1.07-2.13	*
145 Bank clerks	10	1.19	0.57-2.19	0.92	0.44-1.69	
146 Insurance clerks	12	3.24	1.67-5.65	2.57	1.33-4.48	*
149 Shipping agents	3	0.43	0.09-1.27	0.40	0.08-1.16	
150 Property managers, warehousemen	78	1.23	0.97-1.54	1.12	0.89-1.40	
151 Bid calculators, orders clerks	4	0.87	0.24-2.24	0.78	0.21-1.99	
159 Clerical workers NOS	16	1.04	0.60-1.70	0.95	0.55-1.55	
2 Sales professions	287	1.05	0.93-1.17	0.99	0.88-1.11	
20 Wholesale and retail dealers	79	1.05	0.83-1.31	0.95	0.75-1.18	
201 Retailers	77	1.07	0.84-1.33	0.97	0.77-1.22	
21 Real estate, services, securities	30	1.48	1.00-2.12	1.28	0.86-1.83	*
210 Insurance salesmen	18	1.53	0.91-2.42	1.37	0.81-2.17	
212 Advertising sales	8	1.66	0.72-3.27	1.25	0.54-2.47	
22 Sales representatives	64	1.09	0.84-1.40	0.99	0.76-1.27	
220 Commercial travellers, etc.	58	1.08	0.82-1.39	0.98	0.74-1.26	
221 Sales agents	6	1.32	0.48-2.87	1.20	0.44-2.62	
23 Sales work	114	0.95	0.78-1.13	0.96	0.79-1.14	
230 Buyers, office sales staff	26	1.17	0.77-1.72	1.01	0.66-1.49	
231 Shop personnel	65	0.86	0.66-1.10	0.93	0.72-1.19	
232 Door-to-door salesmen	6	0.83	0.31-1.81	0.77	0.28-1.67	
233 Service station attendants	10	1.10	0.53-2.02	1.00	0.48-1.84	
239 Sales staff NOS	7	1.19	0.48-2.45	1.26	0.51-2.60	
3 Farming, forestry and fishing	1323	0.85	0.81-0.90	0.92	0.87-0.97	*
30 Agricultural/forestry management	1128	0.89	0.84-0.94	0.93	0.87-0.98	*
300 Farmers, silviculturists	1055	0.88	0.83-0.93	0.92	0.87-0.98	*
301 Agricultural managers	6	1.15	0.42-2.51	1.05	0.39-2.29	
302 Forestry managers	55	1.18	0.89-1.54	1.07	0.81-1.40	
303 Horticultural managers	4	0.72	0.20-1.85	0.65	0.18-1.66	
305 Fur-bearing animal breeders	5	0.69	0.22-1.62	0.74	0.24-1.73	
31 Farming, animal husbandry	58	0.69	0.52-0.89	0.81	0.62-1.05	*
310 Agricultural workers	41	0.64	0.46-0.87	0.74	0.53-1.01	*
311 Gardeners	9	0.93	0.43-1.76	1.21	0.55-2.29	
312 Livestock workers	7	0.89	0.36-1.84	1.04	0.42-2.14	
33 Fishing	9	0.65	0.30-1.24	0.70	0.32-1.34	
330 Fishermen	7	0.53	0.21-1.09	0.57	0.23-1.18	
34 Forestry work	128	0.70	0.58-0.82	0.92	0.77-1.09	*
4 Mining and quarrying	23	0.73	0.46-1.09	0.78	0.49-1.17	
40 Mining and quarrying	9	0.47	0.21-0.89	0.50	0.23-0.95	*
49 Mining and quarrying NOS	8	1.16	0.50-2.29	1.26	0.54-2.48	
5 Transport and communications	521	0.97	0.89-1.05	0.96	0.88-1.05	
50 Ship's officers	39	1.75	1.24-2.39	1.46	1.03-1.99	*
500 Ship's masters and mates	17	1.72	1.00-2.76	1.29	0.75-2.07	*
502 Chief engineers in ships	14	1.74	0.95-2.92	1.59	0.87-2.67	
51 Deck and engine-room crew	18	1.21	0.72-1.91	1.32	0.78-2.08	
510 Deck crew	17	1.68	0.98-2.69	1.82	1.06-2.92	*
53 Engine drivers	33	1.36	0.94-1.91	1.49	1.02-2.09	*
54 Road transport	273	0.82	0.73-0.92	0.83	0.73-0.93	*
540 Motor-vehicle and tram drivers	273	0.82	0.73-0.92	0.83	0.73-0.93	*
55 Transport services	53	1.03	0.77-1.35	1.07	0.80-1.40	
550 Railway staff	51	1.01	0.75-1.33	1.05	0.78-1.38	
56 Traffic supervisors	32	1.10	0.75-1.55	0.90	0.61-1.26	
562 Railway traffic supervisors	20	1.41	0.86-2.17	1.19	0.72-1.83	
563 Road transport supervisors	4	0.39	0.11-1.00	0.31	0.08-0.78	*
57 Post and telecommunications	18	1.19	0.71-1.88	1.08	0.64-1.70	
570 Post/telecommunications officials	13	1.10	0.59-1.88	0.99	0.53-1.70	
58 Postal services/couriers	40	1.17	0.84-1.59	1.26	0.90-1.71	
580 Postmen	27	1.25	0.82-1.81	1.36	0.90-1.98	
581 Caretakers/messengers	13	1.04	0.55-1.77	1.09	0.58-1.86	
59 Communication work NOS	14	1.10	0.60-1.84	1.18	0.64-1.98	
599 Communication workers NOS	12	1.22	0.63-2.13	1.31	0.68-2.29	

Appendix Table C

Occupation	Obs.	Crude SIR	95% CI	Adjusted SIR	95% CI	
6/7 Industrial and construction work	1886	0.93	0.88-0.97	1.02	0.98-1.07	*
60 Textiles	23	1.22	0.78-1.84	1.31	0.83-1.96	
602 Weavers	6	3.08	1.13-6.71	3.18	1.17-6.91	*
603 Textile machine setters operato	7	1.15	0.46-2.37	1.24	0.50-2.56	
605 Textile finishers/dyers	6	1.05	0.38-2.28	1.13	0.41-2.46	
61 Cutting/sewing etc.	19	1.04	0.63-1.63	1.06	0.64-1.66	
610 Tailors	4	0.79	0.22-2.03	0.80	0.22-2.04	
614 Upholsterers	5	0.82	0.27-1.92	0.83	0.27-1.94	
62 Shoes and leather	13	0.84	0.45-1.44	0.86	0.46-1.46	
620 Shoemakers and cobblers	5	1.01	0.33-2.36	0.97	0.32-2.27	
63 Smelting, metal and foundry work	54	0.96	0.72-1.25	1.02	0.77-1.33	
630 Smelter furnacemen	11	1.12	0.56-2.01	1.21	0.61-2.17	
634 Blacksmiths	13	0.93	0.49-1.58	0.94	0.50-1.61	
635 Founders	19	1.16	0.70-1.82	1.26	0.76-1.97	
639 Metalworkers NOS	9	0.93	0.43-1.77	1.00	0.46-1.90	
64 Precision mechanical work	23	1.02	0.65-1.53	1.03	0.65-1.54	
640 Precision mechanics	8	1.15	0.50-2.26	1.24	0.53-2.43	
641 Watchmakers	8	1.43	0.62-2.82	1.38	0.60-2.72	
644 Goldsmiths, silversmiths etc.	3	0.57	0.12-1.67	0.58	0.12-1.69	
65 Machine shop/steelworkers	397	0.97	0.87-1.06	1.03	0.93-1.14	
650 Turners, machinists	99	1.12	0.91-1.36	1.20	0.98-1.46	
651 Fitter-assemblers etc.	38	0.95	0.67-1.31	1.03	0.73-1.41	
652 Machine and motor repairers	88	0.91	0.73-1.13	0.97	0.78-1.19	
653 Sheetmetalworkers	33	0.87	0.60-1.22	0.93	0.64-1.30	
654 Plumbers	62	1.15	0.89-1.48	1.23	0.94-1.58	
655 Welders and flame cutters	31	0.72	0.49-1.02	0.78	0.53-1.10	
656 Plate/constructional steel work	9	0.75	0.34-1.42	0.81	0.37-1.53	
659 Machine shop/steelworkers NOS	37	1.00	0.70-1.38	1.07	0.75-1.47	
66 Electrical work	134	1.07	0.90-1.26	1.15	0.97-1.36	
660 Electricians (indoors)	69	1.02	0.79-1.29	1.09	0.85-1.38	
661 Electric machine operators	9	0.98	0.45-1.87	1.06	0.49-2.02	
663 Electronics and telefitters	9	1.29	0.59-2.45	1.34	0.61-2.54	
664 Telephone installers and repair	20	1.05	0.64-1.62	1.14	0.70-1.76	
665 Linemen	18	1.45	0.86-2.30	1.58	0.93-2.49	
67 Woodwork	399	0.99	0.89-1.09	1.05	0.95-1.16	
670 Round-timber workers	9	0.97	0.44-1.84	1.04	0.47-1.97	
671 Timber workers	42	0.82	0.59-1.11	0.88	0.63-1.18	
672 Plywood makers	24	1.68	1.08-2.50	1.82	1.16-2.70	*
673 Construction carpenters	244	0.97	0.85-1.10	1.04	0.92-1.18	
674 Boatbuilders etc.	9	0.94	0.43-1.79	0.98	0.45-1.86	
675 Bench carpenters	26	1.12	0.73-1.63	1.14	0.74-1.66	
676 Cabinetmakers etc.	13	0.86	0.46-1.48	0.91	0.48-1.55	
677 Woodworking machine operators e	26	1.14	0.74-1.67	1.21	0.79-1.78	
68 Painting and lacquering	67	0.87	0.67-1.10	0.91	0.71-1.16	
680 Painters	59	0.83	0.63-1.07	0.87	0.66-1.12	
681 Lacquerers	8	1.33	0.58-2.62	1.41	0.61-2.77	
69 Construction work NOS	252	0.78	0.69-0.88	0.95	0.84-1.07	*
690 Bricklayers and tile setters	42	1.02	0.74-1.38	1.10	0.79-1.48	
692 Reinforcing iron workers	10	0.97	0.46-1.78	1.05	0.50-1.93	
693 Concrete/cement shutterers	25	0.91	0.59-1.34	0.98	0.63-1.44	
695 Insulators	5	0.58	0.19-1.35	0.62	0.20-1.44	
697 Building hands	91	0.69	0.56-0.85	0.91	0.73-1.12	*
698 Roadbuilding hands	65	0.77	0.59-0.98	0.99	0.77-1.27	*
699 Construction workers NOS	13	0.96	0.51-1.64	0.99	0.53-1.70	
70 Printing	36	1.26	0.88-1.74	1.35	0.95-1.88	
700 Typographers etc.	15	1.34	0.75-2.21	1.45	0.81-2.39	
701 Printers	9	1.03	0.47-1.95	1.11	0.51-2.11	
71 Glass and ceramic work	20	1.51	0.92-2.34	1.63	0.99-2.51	
72 Food industry	46	1.04	0.76-1.38	1.10	0.81-1.47	
720 Grain millers	10	1.47	0.71-2.71	1.53	0.73-2.81	
721 Bakers and pastry chiefs	11	1.06	0.53-1.89	1.09	0.54-1.95	
725 Butchers and sausage makers	13	1.10	0.58-1.87	1.18	0.63-2.02	
726 Dairy workers	7	1.24	0.50-2.55	1.34	0.54-2.76	
73 Chemical process/paper making	70	1.01	0.79-1.27	1.09	0.85-1.38	
734 Pulp mill workers	13	0.69	0.37-1.18	0.75	0.40-1.27	
735 Paper and board mill workers	34	1.29	0.89-1.80	1.40	0.97-1.95	
739 Chemical process workers NOS	10	0.79	0.38-1.45	0.85	0.41-1.57	
75 Industrial work NOS	35	0.77	0.54-1.07	0.82	0.57-1.13	
751 Industrial rubber products	4	0.57	0.16-1.46	0.62	0.17-1.58	
752 Plastics	9	1.02	0.47-1.94	1.10	0.50-2.08	
756 Stone cutters	4	0.80	0.22-2.04	0.82	0.22-2.10	

Occupation	Obs.	Crude SIR	95% CI	Adjusted SIR	95% CI	
758 Cast concrete products	4	0.63	0.17-1.62	0.68	0.18-1.73	
759 Industrial workers NOS	4	0.60	0.16-1.55	0.63	0.17-1.62	
76 Packing and labelling	18	0.98	0.58-1.55	1.06	0.63-1.68	
77 Machinists	131	0.82	0.69-0.97	0.88	0.74-1.04	*
770 Crane and hoist operators	13	1.12	0.59-1.91	1.22	0.65-2.08	
771 Forklift operators	20	0.86	0.53-1.33	0.94	0.57-1.45	
772 Construction machinery operator	44	0.83	0.60-1.11	0.86	0.63-1.15	
773 Operators of stationary engine	25	0.65	0.42-0.96	0.70	0.45-1.04	*
774 Greasers	11	0.89	0.44-1.59	0.95	0.48-1.70	
775 Industrial personnel, riggers	18	0.89	0.53-1.40	0.96	0.57-1.52	
78 Dock and warehouse work	104	0.87	0.71-1.04	1.06	0.87-1.28	
780 Dockers	24	0.84	0.54-1.25	0.92	0.59-1.37	
781 Freight handlers	15	0.83	0.46-1.37	1.08	0.61-1.79	
782 Warehousemen	65	0.89	0.69-1.13	1.12	0.87-1.43	
79 Labourers not classified elsewhere	45	0.67	0.49-0.90	0.88	0.64-1.18	*
8 Services	226	1.01	0.89-1.15	1.03	0.90-1.17	
80 Watchmen, security guards	96	0.98	0.79-1.19	0.96	0.77-1.17	
800 Firemen	10	0.97	0.46-1.78	0.91	0.44-1.68	
801 Policemen	43	1.07	0.77-1.44	0.97	0.70-1.31	
802 Customs/border control	11	0.97	0.48-1.73	0.87	0.43-1.56	
803 Prison guards	12	1.42	0.73-2.48	1.49	0.77-2.61	
804 Civilian guards	19	0.69	0.41-1.07	0.78	0.47-1.21	
81 Housekeeping, domestic work, etc.	5	0.81	0.26-1.89	0.79	0.26-1.85	
83 Caretakers and cleaners	92	0.99	0.80-1.22	1.07	0.86-1.31	
830 Caretakers	82	0.99	0.79-1.23	1.06	0.85-1.32	
832 Chimney sweeps	8	1.14	0.49-2.25	1.24	0.53-2.44	
87 Photography	4	0.88	0.24-2.25	0.80	0.22-2.04	
89 Services NOS	18	1.75	1.03-2.76	1.90	1.13-3.01	*
890 Hotel porters	14	1.62	0.88-2.72	1.75	0.96-2.93	
9 Work not classified elsewhere	39	1.01	0.72-1.38	0.87	0.62-1.19	
90 Military occupations	29	1.18	0.79-1.70	0.92	0.62-1.32	
900 Officers etc.	18	1.69	1.00-2.67	1.12	0.66-1.76	*
901 Non-commissioned officers	10	0.75	0.36-1.38	0.67	0.32-1.24	
91 Occupation not specified	10	0.71	0.34-1.31	0.76	0.36-1.39	
ECONOMICALLY INACTIVE PERSONS	686	0.96	0.89-1.03	1.01	0.93-1.09	

C32. Basal cell carcinoma of the skin, females

	Obs.	Crude SIR	95% CI	Adjusted SIR	95% CI	
WHOLE POPULATION	7218	1.03	1.00-1.05	1.02	1.00-1.05	*
ECONOMICALLY ACTIVE PERSONS	4128	1.00	0.97-1.03	1.00	0.97-1.03	
0 Technical, humanistic, etc. work	689	1.31	1.22-1.41	1.08	1.00-1.16	*
01 Technical work	29	1.14	0.76-1.64	0.99	0.66-1.43	
018 Draughtsmen, survey assistants	9	1.27	0.58-2.41	1.11	0.51-2.11	
019 Laboratory assistants	20	1.22	0.75-1.89	1.06	0.65-1.64	
02 Chemical/physical/biological work	16	1.55	0.89-2.52	1.24	0.71-2.01	
027 Consultancy, agriculture	11	1.44	0.72-2.57	1.20	0.60-2.15	
03 Medical work and nursing	273	1.19	1.05-1.34	1.13	1.00-1.27	*
030 Medical doctors	13	2.38	1.27-4.07	1.61	0.86-2.75	*
031 Dentists	11	1.29	0.64-2.31	0.89	0.44-1.59	
032 Nurses	96	1.45	1.18-1.77	1.26	1.02-1.53	*
033 Doctor's/dentist's receptionist	3	0.58	0.12-1.68	0.61	0.12-1.77	
034 Midwives	15	1.44	0.81-2.37	1.24	0.69-2.05	
035 Psychiatric nurses	14	0.88	0.48-1.48	0.76	0.42-1.28	
036 Auxiliary nurses	98	0.98	0.80-1.20	1.11	0.90-1.35	
038 Institutional children's nurses	18	1.25	0.74-1.97	1.09	0.65-1.72	
04 Health-care related work	38	1.23	0.87-1.69	0.92	0.65-1.26	
040 Pharmacists	26	1.38	0.90-2.02	0.94	0.61-1.37	
044 Pharmaceutical assistants	2	0.47	0.06-1.69	0.40	0.05-1.46	
05 Teaching	251	1.61	1.42-1.82	1.14	1.01-1.29	*
051 Subject teachers	63	1.66	1.28-2.13	1.13	0.87-1.44	*
052 Primary school teachers	124	1.68	1.40-1.99	1.15	0.96-1.36	*
053 Teachers of practical subjects	27	1.36	0.90-1.98	1.06	0.70-1.54	

Occupation	Obs.	Crude SIR	95% CI	Adjusted SIR	95% CI
054 Vocational teachers	18	1.37	0.81-2.16	1.12	0.66-1.76
055 Preschool teachers	12	1.84	0.95-3.22	1.60	0.83-2.80
06 Religious professions	9	1.09	0.50-2.06	0.91	0.42-1.73
061 Deacons and social workers	7	1.35	0.54-2.78	1.16	0.47-2.40
08 Artistic and literary professions	20	1.08	0.66-1.67	0.80	0.49-1.24
084 Journalists	7	0.90	0.36-1.85	0.66	0.27-1.36
09 Humanistic and social work etc.	48	1.21	0.89-1.60	0.92	0.68-1.22
091 Social workers	24	1.31	0.84-1.95	1.04	0.66-1.54
092 Librarians, museum officials	13	1.08	0.58-1.85	0.82	0.43-1.40
1 Administrative and clerical work	668	1.30	1.20-1.40	1.11	1.02-1.19 *
10 Public administration	14	1.50	0.82-2.51	1.03	0.56-1.72
11 Corporate administration	15	1.13	0.63-1.86	0.78	0.43-1.28
110 Corporate managers	5	0.94	0.31-2.20	0.66	0.21-1.53
119 Private sector managers NOS	3	0.76	0.16-2.23	0.52	0.11-1.53
12 Clerical work	168	1.43	1.22-1.65	1.22	1.04-1.41 *
120 Book-keepers, accountants	76	1.38	1.08-1.72	1.17	0.92-1.47 *
121 Office cashiers	31	1.34	0.91-1.90	1.14	0.78-1.62
122 Bank and post office cashiers	20	2.43	1.49-3.76	2.11	1.29-3.26 *
123 Shop and restaurant cashiers	39	1.29	0.92-1.77	1.12	0.79-1.52
13 Stenographers and typists	51	1.09	0.81-1.43	0.95	0.71-1.25
130 Private secretaries	34	1.31	0.91-1.83	1.15	0.79-1.60
131 Typists	17	0.81	0.47-1.30	0.70	0.41-1.12
14/15 Clerical work NOS	420	1.28	1.16-1.41	1.11	1.00-1.21 *
140 Computer book-keepers	5	3.70	1.20-8.63	3.19	1.04-7.44 *
143 Photocopier operators etc.	10	1.27	0.61-2.33	1.10	0.53-2.02
144 Office clerks	272	1.25	1.10-1.40	1.08	0.95-1.21 *
145 Bank clerks	48	1.23	0.90-1.63	1.07	0.79-1.42
146 Insurance clerks	18	1.75	1.03-2.76	1.52	0.90-2.40 *
150 Property managers, warehousemen	9	1.02	0.47-1.94	0.87	0.40-1.64
159 Clerical workers NOS	43	1.49	1.08-2.00	1.27	0.92-1.71 *
2 Sales professions	365	0.90	0.81-1.00	0.93	0.83-1.02 *
20 Wholesale and retail dealers	48	0.80	0.59-1.07	0.68	0.50-0.90 *
201 Retailers	47	0.79	0.58-1.05	0.67	0.49-0.89 *
22 Sales representatives	8	1.25	0.54-2.46	1.08	0.47-2.12
220 Commercial travellers, etc.	6	1.03	0.38-2.25	0.89	0.33-1.94
23 Sales work	308	0.92	0.82-1.02	0.98	0.87-1.09
230 Buyers, office sales staff	7	0.99	0.40-2.03	0.86	0.34-1.76
231 Shop personnel	288	0.91	0.81-1.02	0.98	0.87-1.10
232 Door-to-door salesmen	8	1.53	0.66-3.01	1.34	0.58-2.63
239 Sales staff NOS	4	0.71	0.19-1.82	0.77	0.21-1.98
3 Farming, forestry and fishing	829	0.88	0.82-0.94	0.94	0.87-1.00 *
30 Agricultural/forestry management	223	0.91	0.79-1.03	0.98	0.86-1.11
300 Farmers, silviculturists	215	0.90	0.78-1.02	0.97	0.85-1.11
31 Farming, animal husbandry	602	0.87	0.80-0.94	0.92	0.84-0.99 *
310 Agricultural workers	59	0.85	0.65-1.09	0.88	0.67-1.13
311 Gardeners	23	0.90	0.57-1.36	1.04	0.66-1.56
312 Livestock workers	520	0.87	0.80-0.95	0.92	0.84-1.00 *
4 Mining and quarrying	2	1.59	0.19-5.74	1.75	0.21-6.33
5 Transport and communications	154	1.09	0.93-1.27	1.03	0.88-1.20
54 Road transport	5	0.95	0.31-2.23	0.87	0.28-2.02
540 Motor-vehicle and tram drivers	5	1.00	0.32-2.33	0.90	0.29-2.09
55 Transport services	12	0.95	0.49-1.66	1.04	0.54-1.82
552 Bus/tram services	11	1.06	0.53-1.89	1.18	0.59-2.11
56 Traffic supervisors	4	0.67	0.18-1.71	0.56	0.15-1.43
562 Railway traffic supervisors	2	0.38	0.05-1.36	0.32	0.04-1.15
57 Post and telecommunications	104	1.40	1.14-1.68	1.19	0.98-1.43 *
570 Post/telecommunications officials	43	1.35	0.98-1.82	1.15	0.83-1.55
571 Telephone operators	35	1.31	0.91-1.82	1.12	0.78-1.55
572 Switchboard operators	18	1.55	0.92-2.45	1.33	0.79-2.11
573 Telegraphists	8	1.87	0.81-3.68	1.61	0.69-3.17
58 Postal services/couriers	28	0.68	0.45-0.98	0.76	0.51-1.11 *
580 Postmen	24	0.67	0.43-0.99	0.75	0.48-1.12 *
581 Caretakers/messengers	4	0.75	0.21-1.93	0.85	0.23-2.17
6/7 Industrial and construction work	661	0.90	0.83-0.97	0.99	0.92-1.07 *
60 Textiles	72	0.84	0.66-1.06	0.92	0.72-1.15

Occupation	Obs.	Crude SIR	95% CI	Adjusted SIR	95% CI	
601 Spinners etc.	18	0.95	0.56-1.50	1.06	0.63-1.67	
602 Weavers	25	0.86	0.56-1.27	0.91	0.59-1.35	
604 Knitters	11	1.12	0.56-2.00	1.24	0.62-2.21	
605 Textile finishers/dyers	8	0.76	0.33-1.50	0.85	0.37-1.67	
606 Textile quality controllers	4	0.63	0.17-1.63	0.71	0.19-1.81	
609 Textile workers NOS	4	0.67	0.18-1.71	0.71	0.19-1.81	
61 Cutting/sewing etc.	145	0.96	0.81-1.13	1.02	0.86-1.19	
611 Dressmakers	24	0.77	0.49-1.14	0.71	0.45-1.05	
613 Milliners	8	1.35	0.58-2.67	1.41	0.61-2.78	
615 Patternmakers and cutters	7	0.58	0.23-1.19	0.65	0.26-1.34	
616 Garment workers	86	1.02	0.81-1.26	1.13	0.90-1.40	
619 Cutting/sewing workers NOS	10	1.39	0.67-2.56	1.51	0.72-2.78	
62 Shoes and leather	21	0.76	0.47-1.17	0.84	0.52-1.28	
622 Shoe sewers	4	0.38	0.10-0.98	0.43	0.12-1.09	*
625 Shoemakers NOS	9	1.36	0.62-2.58	1.52	0.70-2.89	
626 Saddlers, leather sewers, etc.	4	0.70	0.19-1.78	0.73	0.20-1.86	
63 Smelting, metal and foundry work	6	0.94	0.34-2.04	1.05	0.39-2.29	
65 Machine shop/steelworkers	20	0.71	0.43-1.10	0.79	0.48-1.22	
650 Turners, machinists	3	0.51	0.10-1.49	0.56	0.12-1.65	
659 Machine shop/steelworkers NOS	14	0.81	0.45-1.37	0.91	0.50-1.52	
66 Electrical work	12	0.85	0.44-1.48	0.95	0.49-1.66	
666 Electronic equipment assemblers	11	0.95	0.47-1.69	1.07	0.53-1.91	
67 Woodwork	54	0.87	0.65-1.13	0.97	0.73-1.26	
671 Timber workers	9	0.71	0.32-1.34	0.79	0.36-1.50	
672 Plywood makers	26	0.90	0.59-1.31	1.00	0.66-1.47	
677 Woodworking machine operators e	9	1.18	0.54-2.25	1.32	0.60-2.50	
679 Woodworkers NOS	5	0.93	0.30-2.16	1.03	0.33-2.40	
68 Painting and lacquering	6	0.73	0.27-1.60	0.82	0.30-1.78	
680 Painters	5	0.87	0.28-2.03	0.97	0.31-2.26	
69 Construction work NOS	22	0.74	0.47-1.12	0.86	0.54-1.30	
697 Building hands	18	0.73	0.43-1.16	0.85	0.50-1.34	
70 Printing	34	1.24	0.86-1.73	1.38	0.95-1.93	
701 Printers	6	1.12	0.41-2.43	1.25	0.46-2.72	
702 Lithographers	4	3.89	1.06-9.96	4.38	1.19-11.2	*
703 Bookbinders	15	1.11	0.62-1.84	1.25	0.70-2.06	
71 Glass and ceramic work	7	0.61	0.24-1.25	0.68	0.27-1.39	
72 Food industry	83	0.95	0.75-1.17	1.04	0.83-1.30	
721 Bakers and pastry chiefs	33	0.82	0.56-1.15	0.89	0.62-1.25	
722 Chocolate and confectionery mak	14	2.46	1.35-4.13	2.74	1.50-4.59	*
725 Butchers and sausage makers	6	0.74	0.27-1.62	0.83	0.30-1.81	
726 Dairy workers	15	0.84	0.47-1.39	0.94	0.53-1.55	
73 Chemical process/paper making	21	0.87	0.54-1.33	0.97	0.60-1.49	
735 Paper and board mill workers	12	0.91	0.47-1.58	1.01	0.52-1.76	
739 Chemical process workers NOS	7	0.93	0.37-1.92	1.04	0.42-2.14	
75 Industrial work NOS	36	0.82	0.57-1.13	0.91	0.63-1.25	
751 Industrial rubber products	9	1.20	0.55-2.28	1.34	0.61-2.55	
752 Plastics	5	0.51	0.17-1.20	0.57	0.19-1.34	
757 Paper products	9	1.11	0.51-2.10	1.24	0.57-2.35	
759 Industrial workers NOS	8	0.79	0.34-1.55	0.87	0.38-1.72	
76 Packing and labelling	54	0.79	0.59-1.03	0.89	0.67-1.16	
77 Machinists	23	1.54	0.97-2.31	1.75	1.11-2.62	*
774 Greasers	15	1.72	0.96-2.83	1.98	1.11-3.26	*
78 Dock and warehouse work	29	0.89	0.60-1.28	1.02	0.68-1.47	
782 Warehousemen	23	0.84	0.53-1.26	0.97	0.61-1.45	
79 Labourers not classified elsewhere	9	1.37	0.63-2.60	1.59	0.73-3.01	
8 Services	756	0.88	0.82-0.95	0.97	0.90-1.04	*
81 Housekeeping, domestic work, etc.	257	0.88	0.77-0.99	0.95	0.83-1.07	*
810 Housekeepers	25	0.88	0.57-1.30	0.75	0.48-1.10	
811 Chefs, cooks etc.	64	0.86	0.67-1.10	0.96	0.74-1.23	
812 Kitchen assistants	65	0.81	0.62-1.03	0.94	0.72-1.19	
813 Domestic servants	63	0.84	0.64-1.07	0.96	0.74-1.23	
814 Communal, home-help services	23	1.20	0.76-1.80	1.21	0.77-1.82	
818 Hotel/restaurant manageresses	6	1.27	0.46-2.76	1.08	0.40-2.35	
819 Housekeeping workers NOS	9	0.93	0.43-1.77	0.91	0.42-1.73	
82 Waiters	82	0.94	0.75-1.16	0.97	0.77-1.20	
820 Waiters in restaurants	38	0.94	0.67-1.29	1.02	0.72-1.39	
821 Waiters in cafés etc.	44	0.93	0.68-1.25	0.93	0.68-1.25	
83 Caretakers and cleaners	347	0.89	0.80-0.99	1.03	0.92-1.14	*
830 Caretakers	38	0.88	0.63-1.21	0.99	0.70-1.36	
831 Cleaners	304	0.88	0.79-0.99	1.03	0.91-1.14	*

Appendix Table C

Occupation	Obs.	Crude		Adjusted	
		SIR	95% CI	SIR	95% CI
84 Hygiene and beauty services	33	0.82	0.57-1.16	0.76	0.52-1.07
840 Hairdressers and barbers	26	0.82	0.54-1.20	0.74	0.48-1.08
843 Sauna attendants etc.	4	0.70	0.19-1.80	0.77	0.21-1.98
85 Laundry and pressing	24	0.70	0.45-1.03	0.76	0.48-1.12
850 Launderers	18	0.62	0.37-0.99	0.68	0.40-1.07 *
851 Pressers	6	1.07	0.39-2.34	1.19	0.44-2.60
9 Work not classified elsewhere	4	0.45	0.12-1.16	0.50	0.14-1.28
91 Occupation not specified	4	0.46	0.13-1.19	0.51	0.14-1.31
ECONOMICALLY INACTIVE PERSONS	3090	1.06	1.03-1.10	1.06	1.02-1.10 *

C33. Cancer of the brain and nervous system, males

Occupation	Obs.	Crude		Adjusted	
		SIR	95% CI	SIR	95% CI
WHOLE POPULATION	1504	1.00	0.95-1.06	1.01	0.96-1.06
ECONOMICALLY ACTIVE PERSONS	1354	1.00	0.95-1.05	1.00	0.95-1.05
0 Technical, humanistic, etc. work	162	1.14	0.97-1.32	1.05	0.90-1.22
00 Technical professions	26	1.46	0.96-2.14	1.33	0.87-1.95
004 Mechanical engineers	9	1.73	0.79-3.28	1.55	0.71-2.94
01 Technical work	51	1.00	0.74-1.32	0.93	0.69-1.23
010 Civil engineering technicians	23	1.30	0.82-1.94	1.20	0.76-1.80
013 Mechanical technicians	12	0.89	0.46-1.56	0.83	0.43-1.45
016 Technicians NOS	4	0.78	0.21-2.00	0.73	0.20-1.86
02 Chemical/physical/biological work	10	1.21	0.58-2.22	1.11	0.53-2.04
03 Medical work and nursing	13	1.77	0.94-3.03	1.68	0.89-2.87
05 Teaching	30	0.96	0.65-1.37	0.89	0.60-1.27
051 Subject teachers	7	1.11	0.45-2.28	1.04	0.42-2.14
052 Primary school teachers	6	0.48	0.18-1.04	0.45	0.16-0.97 *
054 Vocational teachers	7	1.02	0.41-2.11	0.95	0.38-1.96
08 Artistic and literary professions	15	1.62	0.91-2.67	1.49	0.83-2.45
085 Industrial designers	3	7.43	1.53-21.7	6.79	1.40-19.9 *
09 Humanistic and social work etc.	6	0.67	0.24-1.45	0.61	0.22-1.32
1 Administrative and clerical work	88	1.08	0.87-1.33	0.98	0.79-1.21
10 Public administration	8	1.07	0.46-2.10	0.96	0.42-1.90
11 Corporate administration	41	1.05	0.75-1.42	0.96	0.69-1.30
110 Corporate managers	12	0.72	0.37-1.25	0.65	0.34-1.14
112 Commercial managers	18	1.72	1.02-2.72	1.59	0.94-2.51 *
119 Private sector managers NOS	6	1.31	0.48-2.86	1.21	0.44-2.63
14/15 Clerical work NOS	37	1.19	0.84-1.64	1.09	0.77-1.50
144 Office clerks	8	1.59	0.69-3.13	1.45	0.63-2.85
150 Property managers, warehousemen	12	0.82	0.43-1.44	0.75	0.39-1.30
2 Sales professions	82	1.15	0.92-1.43	1.09	0.87-1.36
20 Wholesale and retail dealers	22	1.28	0.80-1.94	1.16	0.73-1.76
201 Retailers	21	1.28	0.79-1.96	1.16	0.72-1.77
21 Real estate, services, securities	3	0.59	0.12-1.73	0.54	0.11-1.59
22 Sales representatives	23	1.40	0.89-2.11	1.33	0.84-1.99
220 Commercial travellers, etc.	20	1.31	0.80-2.02	1.24	0.76-1.91
23 Sales work	34	1.05	0.72-1.46	1.02	0.71-1.43
230 Buyers, office sales staff	4	0.69	0.19-1.75	0.63	0.17-1.62
231 Shop personnel	25	1.19	0.77-1.76	1.20	0.78-1.77
3 Farming, forestry and fishing	320	0.92	0.83-1.03	0.96	0.85-1.06
30 Agricultural/forestry management	264	0.97	0.85-1.09	0.97	0.86-1.10
300 Farmers, silviculturists	250	0.97	0.86-1.10	0.99	0.87-1.11
302 Forestry managers	9	0.85	0.39-1.60	0.77	0.35-1.45
31 Farming, animal husbandry	13	0.57	0.30-0.98	0.62	0.33-1.07 *
310 Agricultural workers	9	0.51	0.23-0.97	0.55	0.25-1.04 *
34 Forestry work	38	0.81	0.57-1.11	0.95	0.67-1.30
4 Mining and quarrying	6	0.76	0.28-1.66	0.77	0.28-1.68
5 Transport and communications	125	0.91	0.75-1.07	0.88	0.73-1.04
50 Ship's officers	2	0.37	0.04-1.34	0.34	0.04-1.23

Occupation	Obs.	Crude		Adjusted	
		SIR	95% CI	SIR	95% CI
53 Engine drivers	6	1.00	0.37-2.17	1.02	0.37-2.22
54 Road transport	92	1.04	0.84-1.28	1.01	0.81-1.24
540 Motor-vehicle and tram drivers	92	1.04	0.84-1.28	1.01	0.82-1.24
55 Transport services	10	0.85	0.41-1.56	0.84	0.40-1.54
550 Railway staff	10	0.87	0.42-1.60	0.86	0.41-1.58
56 Traffic supervisors	6	0.89	0.33-1.95	0.82	0.30-1.78
58 Postal services/couriers	3	0.35	0.07-1.03	0.36	0.07-1.05
580 Postmen	2	0.34	0.04-1.24	0.35	0.04-1.26
6/7 Industrial and construction work	508	1.01	0.92-1.10	1.04	0.95-1.14
63 Smelting, metal and foundry work	13	0.96	0.51-1.65	0.97	0.52-1.66
64 Precision mechanical work	3	0.52	0.11-1.52	0.51	0.10-1.48
65 Machine shop/steelworkers	113	1.05	0.87-1.25	1.06	0.87-1.26
650 Turners, machinists	26	1.20	0.79-1.76	1.22	0.80-1.79
651 Fitter-assemblers etc.	14	1.32	0.72-2.21	1.33	0.73-2.23
652 Machine and motor repairers	24	0.94	0.60-1.40	0.94	0.60-1.40
653 Sheetmetalworkers	9	0.89	0.41-1.69	0.89	0.41-1.69
654 Plumbers	18	1.26	0.75-1.99	1.26	0.75-1.99
655 Welders and flame cutters	10	0.80	0.38-1.47	0.81	0.39-1.48
659 Machine shop/steelworkers NOS	8	0.88	0.38-1.74	0.89	0.38-1.75
66 Electrical work	29	0.87	0.58-1.25	0.88	0.59-1.26
660 Electricians (indoors)	9	0.49	0.23-0.94	0.50	0.23-0.94 *
664 Telephone installers and repair	9	1.74	0.80-3.30	1.76	0.80-3.33
67 Woodwork	98	1.06	0.86-1.30	1.08	0.88-1.32
671 Timber workers	11	0.91	0.45-1.62	0.92	0.46-1.64
673 Construction carpenters	62	1.11	0.85-1.43	1.14	0.87-1.46
675 Bench carpenters	6	1.12	0.41-2.45	1.10	0.40-2.40
677 Woodworking machine operators e	5	0.90	0.29-2.10	0.91	0.30-2.12
68 Painting and lacquering	24	1.25	0.80-1.86	1.25	0.80-1.86
680 Painters	23	1.31	0.83-1.97	1.31	0.83-1.96
69 Construction work NOS	67	0.88	0.68-1.12	0.99	0.76-1.25
690 Bricklayers and tile setters	6	0.64	0.23-1.38	0.65	0.24-1.41
693 Concrete/cement shutterers	8	1.20	0.52-2.36	1.21	0.52-2.39
697 Building hands	25	0.79	0.51-1.16	0.93	0.60-1.38
698 Roadbuilding hands	18	0.96	0.57-1.52	1.16	0.69-1.83
70 Printing	7	0.88	0.35-1.80	0.88	0.35-1.81
72 Food industry	10	0.88	0.42-1.62	0.88	0.42-1.62
73 Chemical process/paper making	27	1.51	1.00-2.20	1.53	1.01-2.23 *
730 Distillers	2	9.87	1.19-35.7	9.95	1.20-35.9 *
735 Paper and board mill workers	16	2.27	1.30-3.69	2.30	1.31-3.73 *
75 Industrial work NOS	9	0.78	0.36-1.48	0.78	0.36-1.48
755 Musical instrument makers etc.	2	8.59	1.04-31.0	8.42	1.02-30.4 *
77 Machinists	43	1.01	0.73-1.36	1.01	0.73-1.37
771 Forklift operators	9	1.37	0.63-2.61	1.38	0.63-2.63
772 Construction machinery operator	18	1.20	0.71-1.90	1.19	0.71-1.89
773 Operators of stationary engine	5	0.54	0.18-1.27	0.55	0.18-1.29
775 Industrial personnel, riggers	7	1.35	0.54-2.79	1.37	0.55-2.83
78 Dock and warehouse work	36	1.23	0.86-1.71	1.39	0.97-1.92
780 Dockers	8	1.17	0.50-2.30	1.21	0.52-2.38
782 Warehousemen	23	1.29	0.82-1.94	1.49	0.95-2.24
79 Labourers not classified elsewhere	3	0.20	0.04-0.58	0.24	0.05-0.69 *
8 Services	46	0.88	0.64-1.17	0.87	0.64-1.16
80 Watchmen, security guards	29	1.25	0.84-1.80	1.22	0.81-1.75
801 Policemen	14	1.52	0.83-2.56	1.38	0.75-2.31
804 Civilian guards	5	0.88	0.29-2.06	0.96	0.31-2.25
83 Caretakers and cleaners	13	0.61	0.33-1.05	0.63	0.33-1.07
830 Caretakers	13	0.69	0.37-1.18	0.70	0.37-1.20
9 Work not classified elsewhere	17	1.54	0.90-2.46	1.50	0.88-2.41
90 Military occupations	10	1.32	0.63-2.43	1.27	0.61-2.33
ECONOMICALLY INACTIVE PERSONS	150	1.05	0.89-1.23	1.09	0.93-1.28

Appendix Table C

C34. Cancer of the brain and nervous system, females

Occupation	Obs.	Crude SIR	95% CI	Adjusted SIR	95% CI	
WHOLE POPULATION	1943	1.04	1.00-1.09	1.04	0.99-1.08	
ECONOMICALLY ACTIVE PERSONS	1143	1.00	0.94-1.06	1.00	0.94-1.06	
0 Technical, humanistic, etc. work	183	1.14	0.98-1.31	1.05	0.91-1.21	
01 Technical work	5	0.61	0.20-1.43	0.58	0.19-1.35	
019 Laboratory assistants	4	0.77	0.21-1.97	0.72	0.20-1.85	
022 Geologists	1	41.1	1.04-229	41.1	1.04-229	*
03 Medical work and nursing	85	1.19	0.95-1.47	1.15	0.92-1.42	
032 Nurses	31	1.45	0.99-2.06	1.37	0.93-1.95	
035 Psychiatric nurses	4	0.83	0.22-2.11	0.76	0.21-1.96	
036 Auxiliary nurses	40	1.30	0.93-1.78	1.33	0.95-1.81	
038 Institutional children's nurses	2	0.41	0.05-1.49	0.39	0.05-1.42	
04 Health-care related work	8	0.87	0.37-1.71	0.79	0.34-1.56	
040 Pharmacists	6	1.06	0.39-2.30	0.96	0.35-2.08	
05 Teaching	52	1.11	0.83-1.45	0.96	0.72-1.26	
051 Subject teachers	7	0.57	0.23-1.17	0.50	0.20-1.03	
052 Primary school teachers	24	1.13	0.73-1.69	0.95	0.61-1.41	
053 Teachers of practical subjects	8	1.34	0.58-2.63	1.21	0.52-2.39	
08 Artistic and literary professions	7	1.24	0.50-2.56	1.13	0.45-2.33	
09 Humanistic and social work etc.	17	1.43	0.84-2.30	1.29	0.75-2.06	
091 Social workers	13	2.41	1.28-4.13	2.16	1.15-3.69	*
1 Administrative and clerical work	178	1.15	0.98-1.32	1.06	0.91-1.22	
10 Public administration	8	3.06	1.32-6.04	2.57	1.11-5.06	*
12 Clerical work	35	1.03	0.72-1.43	0.95	0.66-1.32	
120 Book-keepers, accountants	14	0.89	0.49-1.50	0.82	0.45-1.37	
121 Office cashiers	7	1.08	0.43-2.22	0.99	0.40-2.03	
123 Shop and restaurant cashiers	10	1.11	0.53-2.03	1.03	0.49-1.89	
13 Stenographers and typists	17	1.14	0.66-1.83	1.07	0.63-1.72	
130 Private secretaries	13	1.55	0.83-2.65	1.47	0.78-2.51	
131 Typists	4	0.61	0.17-1.57	0.58	0.16-1.48	
14/15 Clerical work NOS	115	1.15	0.95-1.37	1.07	0.89-1.28	
144 Office clerks	77	1.17	0.92-1.46	1.09	0.86-1.36	
145 Bank clerks	10	0.75	0.36-1.38	0.72	0.34-1.32	
159 Clerical workers NOS	16	1.96	1.12-3.19	1.80	1.03-2.92	*
2 Sales professions	114	0.97	0.80-1.16	0.96	0.79-1.15	
20 Wholesale and retail dealers	16	1.06	0.61-1.73	0.95	0.54-1.54	
201 Retailers	15	1.00	0.56-1.65	0.89	0.50-1.47	
23 Sales work	95	0.96	0.77-1.17	0.96	0.78-1.17	
231 Shop personnel	89	0.95	0.76-1.17	0.96	0.77-1.18	
3 Farming, forestry and fishing	215	0.90	0.78-1.03	0.93	0.81-1.06	
30 Agricultural/forestry management	49	0.88	0.65-1.17	0.94	0.69-1.24	
300 Farmers, silviculturists	47	0.87	0.64-1.16	0.93	0.68-1.24	
31 Farming, animal husbandry	166	0.91	0.78-1.05	0.93	0.80-1.08	
310 Agricultural workers	11	0.61	0.31-1.10	0.62	0.31-1.11	
311 Gardeners	8	1.24	0.54-2.45	1.42	0.61-2.79	
312 Livestock workers	146	0.93	0.78-1.09	0.95	0.80-1.11	
4 Mining and quarrying	-	-/0.3	0.00-11.4	-/0.3	0.00-11.7	
5 Transport and communications	40	1.02	0.73-1.39	0.99	0.71-1.34	
57 Post and telecommunications	20	0.93	0.57-1.44	0.86	0.52-1.32	
570 Post/telecommunications officials	8	0.86	0.37-1.70	0.79	0.34-1.56	
571 Telephone operators	9	1.20	0.55-2.28	1.10	0.50-2.09	
58 Postal services/couriers	16	1.48	0.84-2.40	1.58	0.90-2.56	
580 Postmen	13	1.36	0.73-2.33	1.46	0.78-2.49	
6/7 Industrial and construction work	193	0.95	0.82-1.09	0.97	0.84-1.11	
60 Textiles	14	0.61	0.34-1.03	0.62	0.34-1.05	
601 Spinners etc.	4	0.79	0.22-2.03	0.81	0.22-2.07	
602 Weavers	7	0.92	0.37-1.90	0.93	0.37-1.91	
61 Cutting/sewing etc.	44	1.05	0.76-1.41	1.05	0.76-1.41	
611 Dressmakers	6	0.76	0.28-1.65	0.71	0.26-1.54	

Occupation	Obs.	Crude		Adjusted	
		SIR	95% CI	SIR	95% CI
616 Garment workers	26	1.07	0.70-1.57	1.09	0.71-1.60
62 Shoes and leather	11	1.43	0.71-2.56	1.45	0.72-2.59
65 Machine shop/steelworkers	7	0.89	0.36-1.83	0.91	0.37-1.88
67 Woodwork	9	0.52	0.24-0.99	0.54	0.24-1.02 *
672 Plywood makers	3	0.37	0.08-1.08	0.38	0.08-1.11
69 Construction work NOS	5	0.64	0.21-1.49	0.72	0.23-1.67
697 Building hands	4	0.62	0.17-1.58	0.69	0.19-1.78
70 Printing	8	1.03	0.44-2.02	1.05	0.45-2.06
72 Food industry	29	1.19	0.80-1.71	1.22	0.82-1.75
721 Bakers and pastry chiefs	8	0.73	0.32-1.45	0.75	0.32-1.47
726 Dairy workers	7	1.32	0.53-2.73	1.36	0.55-2.80
727 Prepared foods	4	3.59	0.98-9.18	3.68	1.00-9.43 *
73 Chemical process/paper making	5	0.77	0.25-1.79	0.79	0.26-1.84
74 Tobacco industry	4	4.93	1.34-12.6	5.04	1.37-12.9 *
742 Cigarette makers	3	11.3	2.33-33.0	11.4	2.35-33.3 *
75 Industrial work NOS	12	0.96	0.50-1.68	0.98	0.51-1.71
76 Packing and labelling	13	0.67	0.35-1.14	0.68	0.36-1.17
78 Dock and warehouse work	11	1.25	0.63-2.25	1.38	0.69-2.47
782 Warehousemen	10	1.35	0.65-2.48	1.50	0.72-2.76
8 Services	219	0.97	0.84-1.10	1.04	0.91-1.18
81 Housekeeping, domestic work, etc.	72	0.93	0.73-1.17	0.99	0.77-1.25
810 Housekeepers	8	1.06	0.46-2.10	0.97	0.42-1.91
811 Chefs, cooks etc.	22	1.13	0.71-1.72	1.15	0.72-1.74
812 Kitchen assistants	18	0.82	0.49-1.30	0.93	0.55-1.46
813 Domestic servants	14	0.77	0.42-1.29	0.90	0.49-1.51
814 Communal home-help services	9	1.53	0.70-2.91	1.57	0.72-2.97
82 Waiters	27	1.06	0.70-1.54	1.05	0.69-1.52
820 Waiters in restaurants	12	1.02	0.52-1.77	1.02	0.53-1.78
821 Waiters in cafés etc.	15	1.09	0.61-1.80	1.07	0.60-1.77
83 Caretakers and cleaners	94	0.94	0.76-1.15	1.06	0.86-1.30
830 Caretakers	10	0.80	0.39-1.48	0.82	0.39-1.51
831 Cleaners	83	0.95	0.76-1.18	1.09	0.87-1.35
84 Hygiene and beauty services	15	1.32	0.74-2.18	1.24	0.69-2.04
840 Hairdressers and barbers	12	1.32	0.68-2.31	1.21	0.63-2.12
85 Laundry and pressing	8	0.89	0.38-1.75	0.94	0.41-1.85
850 Launderers	4	0.53	0.15-1.36	0.57	0.15-1.45
9 Work not classified elsewhere	1	0.42	0.01-2.36	0.43	0.01-2.38
ECONOMICALLY INACTIVE PERSONS	800	1.11	1.03-1.19	1.09	1.02-1.17 *

C35. Non-Hodgkin lymphoma, males

WHOLE POPULATION	941	1.02	0.96-1.09	1.02	0.96-1.09
ECONOMICALLY ACTIVE PERSONS	818	1.00	0.93-1.07	1.00	0.93-1.07
0 Technical, humanistic, etc. work	82	1.01	0.81-1.26	0.96	0.76-1.19
00 Technical professions	7	0.74	0.30-1.52	0.73	0.29-1.50
01 Technical work	31	1.06	0.72-1.51	1.01	0.69-1.43
010 Civil engineering technicians	13	1.24	0.66-2.12	1.19	0.63-2.03
013 Mechanical technicians	7	0.92	0.37-1.89	0.86	0.35-1.78
02 Chemical/physical/biological work	6	1.22	0.45-2.66	1.12	0.41-2.45
05 Teaching	25	1.43	0.93-2.11	1.36	0.88-2.01
052 Primary school teachers	7	1.01	0.41-2.09	0.97	0.39-2.00
054 Vocational teachers	9	2.29	1.05-4.34	2.14	0.98-4.06 *
08 Artistic and literary professions	2	0.38	0.05-1.37	0.35	0.04-1.26
09 Humanistic and social work etc.	5	0.98	0.32-2.28	0.94	0.30-2.18
1 Administrative and clerical work	60	1.21	0.92-1.55	1.10	0.84-1.42
10 Public administration	4	0.86	0.23-2.19	0.74	0.20-1.91
11 Corporate administration	37	1.56	1.10-2.15	1.38	0.97-1.90 *
110 Corporate managers	10	0.95	0.45-1.74	0.81	0.39-1.50
111 Technical managers	6	2.81	1.03-6.11	2.56	0.94-5.58 *
112 Commercial managers	13	2.17	1.16-3.71	2.01	1.07-3.43 *
114 Managers of ideal organizations	4	3.97	1.08-10.2	3.39	0.92-8.69 *
14/15 Clerical work NOS	18	0.95	0.56-1.50	0.91	0.54-1.44

Occupation	Obs.	Crude		Adjusted	
		SIR	95% CI	SIR	95% CI
150 Property managers, warehousemen	9	0.98	0.45-1.85	0.94	0.43-1.79
2 Sales professions	40	0.98	0.70-1.33	0.96	0.69-1.31
20 Wholesale and retail dealers	16	1.47	0.84-2.39	1.42	0.81-2.31
201 Retailers	14	1.34	0.73-2.26	1.30	0.71-2.19
22 Sales representatives	5	0.56	0.18-1.32	0.53	0.17-1.24
220 Commercial travellers, etc.	5	0.61	0.20-1.42	0.57	0.19-1.34
23 Sales work	17	0.94	0.55-1.51	0.95	0.55-1.52
231 Shop personnel	7	0.61	0.25-1.26	0.63	0.25-1.30
3 Farming, forestry and fishing	222	0.99	0.87-1.13	1.00	0.88-1.14
30 Agricultural/forestry management	189	1.04	0.90-1.19	1.06	0.91-1.21
300 Farmers, silviculturists	178	1.04	0.89-1.19	1.06	0.91-1.22
302 Forestry managers	9	1.34	0.61-2.54	1.29	0.59-2.46
31 Farming, animal husbandry	11	0.86	0.43-1.54	0.86	0.43-1.54
310 Agricultural workers	8	0.82	0.35-1.62	0.82	0.35-1.61
34 Forestry work	21	0.77	0.48-1.18	0.76	0.47-1.16
4 Mining and quarrying	4	0.86	0.23-2.20	0.88	0.24-2.26
5 Transport and communications	74	0.93	0.73-1.17	0.93	0.73-1.17
54 Road transport	47	0.94	0.69-1.26	0.95	0.70-1.26
540 Motor-vehicle and tram drivers	47	0.95	0.70-1.26	0.95	0.70-1.27
55 Transport services	11	1.50	0.75-2.68	1.54	0.77-2.76
550 Railway staff	11	1.53	0.76-2.74	1.58	0.79-2.83
58 Postal services/couriers	5	0.99	0.32-2.31	1.02	0.33-2.38
6/7 Industrial and construction work	297	0.99	0.88-1.11	1.01	0.90-1.13
63 Smelting, metal and foundry work	13	1.58	0.84-2.70	1.62	0.86-2.78
65 Machine shop/steelworkers	71	1.16	0.91-1.46	1.19	0.93-1.50
650 Turners, machinists	12	0.93	0.48-1.62	0.96	0.50-1.68
651 Fitter-assemblers etc.	7	1.17	0.47-2.41	1.21	0.48-2.48
652 Machine and motor repairers	18	1.25	0.74-1.98	1.28	0.76-2.03
653 Sheetmetalworkers	6	1.05	0.39-2.29	1.08	0.40-2.35
654 Plumbers	7	0.87	0.35-1.79	0.89	0.36-1.84
655 Welders and flame cutters	11	1.66	0.83-2.98	1.71	0.86-3.07
657 Metal platers and coaters	3	8.15	1.68-23.8	8.38	1.73-24.5 *
659 Machine shop/steelworkers NOS	6	1.11	0.41-2.41	1.14	0.42-2.47
66 Electrical work	19	1.02	0.61-1.59	1.05	0.63-1.63
660 Electricians (indoors)	11	1.08	0.54-1.94	1.11	0.56-1.99
67 Woodwork	43	0.74	0.53-1.00	0.76	0.55-1.03 *
671 Timber workers	6	0.80	0.30-1.75	0.83	0.30-1.80
673 Construction carpenters	30	0.84	0.56-1.19	0.87	0.59-1.24
68 Painting and lacquering	7	0.61	0.25-1.26	0.62	0.25-1.29
680 Painters	6	0.57	0.21-1.24	0.58	0.21-1.27
69 Construction work NOS	47	1.00	0.73-1.33	1.01	0.74-1.34
690 Bricklayers and tile setters	6	1.02	0.37-2.22	1.05	0.39-2.29
697 Building hands	15	0.78	0.44-1.29	0.77	0.43-1.28
698 Roadbuilding hands	20	1.63	0.99-2.52	1.66	1.02-2.57 *
72 Food industry	6	0.90	0.33-1.97	0.92	0.34-2.01
73 Chemical process/paper making	10	0.97	0.46-1.78	1.00	0.48-1.84
75 Industrial work NOS	4	0.60	0.16-1.53	0.61	0.17-1.56
77 Machinists	36	1.51	1.06-2.09	1.54	1.08-2.14 *
772 Construction machinery operator	12	1.48	0.77-2.59	1.50	0.77-2.61
773 Operators of stationary engine	12	2.14	1.11-3.74	2.21	1.14-3.87 *
78 Dock and warehouse work	19	1.07	0.65-1.68	1.08	0.65-1.69
781 Freight handlers	7	2.62	1.05-5.40	2.59	1.04-5.34 *
782 Warehousemen	8	0.74	0.32-1.46	0.74	0.32-1.46
79 Labourers not classified elsewhere	7	0.72	0.29-1.48	0.73	0.30-1.51
8 Services	31	0.95	0.65-1.35	0.96	0.65-1.36
80 Watchmen, security guards	18	1.26	0.74-1.98	1.24	0.74-1.96
801 Policemen	4	0.69	0.19-1.77	0.65	0.18-1.68
804 Civilian guards	9	2.25	1.03-4.27	2.38	1.09-4.52 *
83 Caretakers and cleaners	10	0.74	0.36-1.37	0.77	0.37-1.41
830 Caretakers	8	0.67	0.29-1.31	0.69	0.30-1.36
9 Work not classified elsewhere	8	1.37	0.59-2.69	1.33	0.57-2.61
ECONOMICALLY INACTIVE PERSONS	123	1.19	0.99-1.41	1.20	1.00-1.43 *

Occupation	Obs.	Crude		Adjusted	
		SIR	95% CI	SIR	95% CI

C36. Non-Hodgkin lymphoma, females

Occupation	Obs.	SIR	95% CI	SIR	95% CI	
WHOLE POPULATION	746	1.06	0.99-1.14	1.06	0.98-1.14	
ECONOMICALLY ACTIVE PERSONS	423	1.00	0.91-1.10	1.00	0.91-1.10	
0 Technical, humanistic, etc. work	54	0.99	0.74-1.29	1.01	0.76-1.32	
03 Medical work and nursing	22	0.91	0.57-1.38	0.87	0.55-1.32	
032 Nurses	6	0.85	0.31-1.85	0.82	0.30-1.79	
036 Auxiliary nurses	10	0.95	0.46-1.75	0.89	0.43-1.63	
05 Teaching	15	0.93	0.52-1.53	1.04	0.58-1.71	
052 Primary school teachers	6	0.79	0.29-1.72	0.92	0.34-2.01	
061 Deacons and social workers	3	5.48	1.13-16.0	5.31	1.09-15.5	*
1 Administrative and clerical work	45	0.84	0.61-1.12	0.82	0.60-1.09	
12 Clerical work	11	0.90	0.45-1.62	0.88	0.44-1.58	
120 Book-keepers, accountants	4	0.70	0.19-1.80	0.69	0.19-1.76	
13 Stenographers and typists	3	0.60	0.12-1.76	0.58	0.12-1.70	
14/15 Clerical work NOS	31	0.90	0.61-1.28	0.88	0.60-1.24	
144 Office clerks	12	0.53	0.27-0.92	0.51	0.26-0.89	*
147 Social insurance clerks	3	7.34	1.51-21.5	6.95	1.43-20.3	*
2 Sales professions	37	0.89	0.62-1.22	0.84	0.59-1.16	
20 Wholesale and retail dealers	5	0.84	0.27-1.96	0.84	0.27-1.95	
201 Retailers	5	0.84	0.27-1.97	0.84	0.27-1.96	
23 Sales work	30	0.86	0.58-1.23	0.81	0.54-1.15	
231 Shop personnel	26	0.79	0.52-1.16	0.74	0.48-1.08	
3 Farming, forestry and fishing	98	1.03	0.84-1.26	1.02	0.83-1.25	
30 Agricultural/forestry management	21	0.87	0.54-1.33	0.88	0.54-1.34	
300 Farmers, silviculturists	20	0.85	0.52-1.32	0.86	0.53-1.33	
31 Farming, animal husbandry	76	1.08	0.85-1.35	1.06	0.84-1.33	
310 Agricultural workers	3	0.43	0.09-1.25	0.42	0.09-1.23	
312 Livestock workers	69	1.14	0.88-1.44	1.12	0.87-1.42	
4 Mining and quarrying	-	-/0.1	0.00-28.9	-/0.1	0.00-27.2	
5 Transport and communications	8	0.55	0.24-1.09	0.54	0.23-1.07	
57 Post and telecommunications	3	0.39	0.08-1.14	0.38	0.08-1.11	
6/7 Industrial and construction work	94	1.25	1.01-1.53	1.19	0.96-1.46	*
60 Textiles	16	1.84	1.05-2.99	1.71	0.98-2.78	*
61 Cutting/sewing etc.	14	0.91	0.50-1.53	0.86	0.47-1.44	
616 Garment workers	7	0.80	0.32-1.65	0.75	0.30-1.54	
67 Woodwork	9	1.40	0.64-2.66	1.30	0.60-2.47	
713 Glass and ceramics decorators	2	9.67	1.17-34.9	8.91	1.08-32.2	*
72 Food industry	10	1.11	0.53-2.05	1.04	0.50-1.92	
73 Chemical process/paper making	7	2.85	1.15-5.87	2.64	1.06-5.45	*
76 Packing and labelling	8	1.14	0.49-2.25	1.06	0.46-2.09	
8 Services	86	0.99	0.79-1.22	1.08	0.86-1.33	
81 Housekeeping, domestic work, etc.	25	0.84	0.54-1.24	0.89	0.58-1.32	
811 Chefs, cooks etc.	7	0.93	0.37-1.92	0.87	0.35-1.79	
812 Kitchen assistants	6	0.73	0.27-1.59	0.90	0.33-1.95	
813 Domestic servants	8	1.06	0.46-2.10	1.19	0.51-2.35	
82 Waiters	11	1.20	0.60-2.16	1.15	0.57-2.05	
821 Waiters in cafés etc.	8	1.63	0.71-3.22	1.58	0.68-3.12	
83 Caretakers and cleaners	39	0.99	0.71-1.36	1.15	0.82-1.58	
831 Cleaners	31	0.90	0.61-1.27	1.07	0.73-1.52	
9 Work not classified elsewhere	1	1.10	0.03-6.15	1.03	0.03-5.74	
ECONOMICALLY INACTIVE PERSONS	323	1.16	1.04-1.29	1.15	1.03-1.28	*

C37. Multiple myeloma, males

Occupation	Obs.	Crude SIR	95% CI	Adjusted SIR	95% CI	
WHOLE POPULATION	563	1.00	0.92-1.09	1.00	0.92-1.09	
ECONOMICALLY ACTIVE PERSONS	492	1.00	0.91-1.09	1.00	0.91-1.09	
0 Technical, humanistic, etc. work	55	1.20	0.90-1.56	1.21	0.91-1.58	
00 Technical professions	6	1.17	0.43-2.55	1.51	0.55-3.28	
01 Technical work	31	1.85	1.26-2.63	1.59	1.08-2.26	*
010 Civil engineering technicians	12	1.93	1.00-3.38	1.66	0.86-2.89	
011 Power technicians	5	3.67	1.19-8.57	3.10	1.01-7.24	*
013 Mechanical technicians	5	1.15	0.37-2.69	0.99	0.32-2.32	
05 Teaching	6	0.62	0.23-1.35	0.75	0.28-1.63	
1 Administrative and clerical work	31	1.03	0.70-1.46	1.09	0.74-1.54	
11 Corporate administration	15	1.04	0.58-1.72	1.30	0.72-2.14	
110 Corporate managers	7	1.06	0.43-2.18	1.27	0.51-2.61	
14/15 Clerical work NOS	12	1.05	0.54-1.84	0.93	0.48-1.63	
150 Property managers, warehousemen	7	1.22	0.49-2.52	1.07	0.43-2.20	
2 Sales professions	26	1.11	0.72-1.62	1.01	0.66-1.49	
20 Wholesale and retail dealers	7	1.03	0.41-2.11	0.89	0.36-1.84	
201 Retailers	7	1.07	0.43-2.21	0.93	0.37-1.92	
22 Sales representatives	5	1.04	0.34-2.42	0.89	0.29-2.08	
220 Commercial travellers, etc.	5	1.13	0.37-2.64	0.97	0.31-2.26	
23 Sales work	11	1.09	0.55-1.96	1.07	0.54-1.92	
231 Shop personnel	6	0.96	0.35-2.08	0.99	0.36-2.16	
3 Farming, forestry and fishing	144	1.01	0.86-1.19	1.01	0.85-1.18	
30 Agricultural/forestry management	120	1.02	0.85-1.21	1.01	0.84-1.20	
300 Farmers, silviculturists	112	1.01	0.83-1.20	1.01	0.83-1.20	
31 Farming, animal husbandry	11	1.54	0.77-2.75	1.49	0.75-2.67	
310 Agricultural workers	8	1.49	0.64-2.94	1.45	0.63-2.85	
34 Forestry work	13	0.82	0.43-1.40	0.80	0.43-1.37	
4 Mining and quarrying	3	1.09	0.22-3.17	1.12	0.23-3.28	
5 Transport and communications	47	1.02	0.75-1.35	0.98	0.72-1.30	
54 Road transport	28	0.99	0.66-1.43	0.95	0.63-1.37	
540 Motor-vehicle and tram drivers	27	0.96	0.63-1.39	0.91	0.60-1.33	
6/7 Industrial and construction work	160	0.90	0.76-1.04	0.91	0.78-1.06	
63 Smelting, metal and foundry work	5	1.01	0.33-2.35	1.04	0.34-2.42	
65 Machine shop/steelworkers	28	0.80	0.53-1.15	0.82	0.55-1.19	
650 Turners, machinists	5	0.65	0.21-1.51	0.67	0.22-1.57	
652 Machine and motor repairers	5	0.61	0.20-1.43	0.62	0.20-1.45	
66 Electrical work	13	1.23	0.65-2.10	1.27	0.68-2.17	
660 Electricians (indoors)	6	1.05	0.38-2.28	1.08	0.40-2.35	
67 Woodwork	29	0.80	0.53-1.14	0.83	0.56-1.19	
673 Construction carpenters	21	0.92	0.57-1.41	0.97	0.60-1.48	
68 Painting and lacquering	4	0.59	0.16-1.51	0.60	0.16-1.54	
680 Painters	4	0.64	0.17-1.63	0.65	0.18-1.67	
69 Construction work NOS	19	0.66	0.40-1.03	0.65	0.39-1.01	
697 Building hands	6	0.51	0.19-1.12	0.50	0.18-1.08	
698 Roadbuilding hands	6	0.77	0.28-1.67	0.73	0.27-1.60	
73 Chemical process/paper making	8	1.34	0.58-2.63	1.39	0.60-2.75	
77 Machinists	11	0.82	0.41-1.46	0.84	0.42-1.50	
78 Dock and warehouse work	15	1.41	0.79-2.33	1.40	0.78-2.31	
782 Warehousemen	9	1.39	0.63-2.64	1.36	0.62-2.59	
79 Labourers not classified elsewhere	6	0.98	0.36-2.13	0.95	0.35-2.06	
8 Services	22	1.10	0.69-1.67	1.07	0.67-1.63	
80 Watchmen, security guards	12	1.38	0.71-2.40	1.26	0.65-2.20	
83 Caretakers and cleaners	8	0.95	0.41-1.88	1.00	0.43-1.97	
830 Caretakers	5	0.66	0.22-1.55	0.70	0.23-1.63	
831 Cleaners	2	13.9	1.68-50.2	13.4	1.62-48.5	*
9 Work not classified elsewhere	4	1.27	0.34-3.24	1.31	0.36-3.36	
ECONOMICALLY INACTIVE PERSONS	71	1.02	0.80-1.29	1.02	0.80-1.29	

C38. Multiple myeloma, females

Occupation	Obs.	Crude SIR	95% CI	Adjusted SIR	95% CI
WHOLE POPULATION	532	1.03	0.94-1.12	1.04	0.95-1.13
ECONOMICALLY ACTIVE PERSONS	294	1.00	0.89-1.12	1.00	0.89-1.12
0 Technical, humanistic, etc. work	27	0.78	0.51-1.13	0.91	0.60-1.32
03 Medical work and nursing	12	0.80	0.42-1.40	0.86	0.44-1.50
036 Auxiliary nurses	3	0.45	0.09-1.33	0.46	0.10-1.36
05 Teaching	9	0.86	0.39-1.64	1.12	0.51-2.13
052 Primary school teachers	5	0.98	0.32-2.30	1.45	0.47-3.38
070 Barristers and judges	1	25.7	0.65-143	46.5	1.18-259 *
1 Administrative and clerical work	33	0.96	0.66-1.34	1.01	0.69-1.42
12 Clerical work	7	0.86	0.34-1.77	0.88	0.35-1.81
14/15 Clerical work NOS	21	0.97	0.60-1.48	1.01	0.63-1.54
144 Office clerks	12	0.82	0.42-1.43	0.85	0.44-1.49
2 Sales professions	17	0.61	0.35-0.97	0.61	0.36-0.98 *
23 Sales work	15	0.65	0.37-1.08	0.67	0.37-1.10
231 Shop personnel	15	0.69	0.39-1.14	0.71	0.40-1.17
3 Farming, forestry and fishing	84	1.18	0.94-1.46	1.16	0.93-1.44
30 Agricultural/forestry management	30	1.54	1.04-2.20	1.51	1.02-2.16 *
300 Farmers, silviculturists	29	1.53	1.03-2.20	1.50	1.00-2.15 *
31 Farming, animal husbandry	54	1.05	0.79-1.37	1.04	0.78-1.35
310 Agricultural workers	6	1.16	0.43-2.52	1.15	0.42-2.51
312 Livestock workers	46	1.04	0.76-1.39	1.04	0.76-1.38
4 Mining and quarrying	-	-/0.1	0.00-39.2	-/0.1	0.00-38.7
5 Transport and communications	13	1.29	0.69-2.21	1.32	0.70-2.25
57 Post and telecommunications	8	1.54	0.66-3.02	1.60	0.69-3.16
6/7 Industrial and construction work	52	0.99	0.74-1.30	0.99	0.74-1.30
60 Textiles	4	0.64	0.17-1.64	0.66	0.18-1.70
61 Cutting/sewing etc.	5	0.47	0.15-1.09	0.48	0.16-1.12
616 Garment workers	4	0.68	0.19-1.74	0.70	0.19-1.80
69 Construction work NOS	7	3.20	1.28-6.58	2.65	1.07-5.46 *
697 Building hands	7	3.85	1.55-7.92	3.16	1.27-6.51 *
72 Food industry	5	0.80	0.26-1.87	0.83	0.27-1.93
8 Services	67	1.07	0.83-1.36	0.97	0.75-1.23
81 Housekeeping, domestic work, etc.	21	0.98	0.61-1.50	0.91	0.56-1.39
811 Chefs, cooks etc.	5	0.92	0.30-2.15	0.98	0.32-2.28
812 Kitchen assistants	9	1.55	0.71-2.95	1.30	0.59-2.46
813 Domestic servants	3	0.52	0.11-1.53	0.46	0.10-1.36
82 Waiters	7	1.16	0.47-2.39	1.20	0.48-2.46
83 Caretakers and cleaners	35	1.21	0.84-1.68	1.04	0.73-1.45
830 Caretakers	8	2.69	1.16-5.30	2.79	1.21-5.50 *
831 Cleaners	27	1.05	0.69-1.52	0.88	0.58-1.29
9 Work not classified elsewhere	1	1.56	0.04-8.68	1.66	0.04-9.27
ECONOMICALLY INACTIVE PERSONS	238	1.06	0.93-1.20	1.08	0.95-1.22

C39. Leukaemia, males

Occupation	Obs.	Crude SIR	95% CI	Adjusted SIR	95% CI
WHOLE POPULATION	1163	1.01	0.95-1.06	1.01	0.95-1.07
ECONOMICALLY ACTIVE PERSONS	1014	1.00	0.94-1.06	1.00	0.94-1.06
0 Technical, humanistic, etc. work	88	0.90	0.72-1.10	0.86	0.69-1.07
00 Technical professions	4	0.35	0.10-0.90	0.33	0.09-0.84 *
01 Technical work	32	0.90	0.62-1.27	0.91	0.62-1.29
010 Civil engineering technicians	13	1.01	0.54-1.72	1.01	0.54-1.74
013 Mechanical technicians	10	1.08	0.52-1.98	1.08	0.52-1.99
02 Chemical/physical/biological work	5	0.83	0.27-1.93	0.80	0.26-1.88
03 Medical work and nursing	5	1.01	0.33-2.35	0.94	0.30-2.19
05 Teaching	19	0.91	0.55-1.42	0.85	0.51-1.33
052 Primary school teachers	10	1.22	0.59-2.25	1.13	0.54-2.08
08 Artistic and literary professions	6	0.93	0.34-2.02	0.89	0.33-1.93
09 Humanistic and social work etc.	9	1.45	0.66-2.74	1.37	0.62-2.59
1 Administrative and clerical work	68	1.11	0.86-1.40	1.06	0.82-1.34
10 Public administration	6	1.03	0.38-2.24	0.96	0.35-2.08
11 Corporate administration	31	1.06	0.72-1.50	1.00	0.68-1.42
110 Corporate managers	18	1.37	0.81-2.16	1.29	0.76-2.04
112 Commercial managers	6	0.83	0.30-1.81	0.78	0.29-1.69
14/15 Clerical work NOS	27	1.15	0.76-1.68	1.13	0.75-1.65
150 Property managers, warehousemen	16	1.39	0.79-2.25	1.36	0.78-2.21
2 Sales professions	52	1.04	0.78-1.37	1.04	0.78-1.36
20 Wholesale and retail dealers	13	0.95	0.51-1.63	0.94	0.50-1.60
201 Retailers	11	0.84	0.42-1.51	0.83	0.41-1.48
22 Sales representatives	11	1.03	0.51-1.84	1.06	0.53-1.89
220 Commercial travellers, etc.	11	1.12	0.56-2.00	1.15	0.57-2.06
23 Sales work	24	1.10	0.71-1.64	1.09	0.70-1.62
231 Shop personnel	14	1.02	0.56-1.71	1.00	0.55-1.68
239 Sales staff NOS	4	3.77	1.03-9.65	3.71	1.01-9.49 *
3 Farming, forestry and fishing	270	0.95	0.84-1.07	0.97	0.86-1.09
30 Agricultural/forestry management	222	0.96	0.83-1.09	0.96	0.84-1.09
300 Farmers, silviculturists	213	0.97	0.84-1.10	0.98	0.85-1.11
302 Forestry managers	4	0.48	0.13-1.23	0.48	0.13-1.22
31 Farming, animal husbandry	14	0.89	0.49-1.50	0.96	0.52-1.61
310 Agricultural workers	14	1.17	0.64-1.97	1.25	0.69-2.10
34 Forestry work	31	0.93	0.63-1.32	1.03	0.70-1.46
4 Mining and quarrying	11	1.92	0.96-3.44	1.89	0.94-3.39
5 Transport and communications	110	1.13	0.93-1.36	1.11	0.92-1.33
52 Air traffic	2	10.5	1.27-37.8	9.84	1.19-35.6 *
54 Road transport	70	1.16	0.91-1.47	1.14	0.89-1.45
540 Motor-vehicle and tram drivers	70	1.17	0.91-1.47	1.15	0.90-1.45
55 Transport services	10	1.10	0.53-2.03	1.08	0.52-1.99
550 Railway staff	10	1.12	0.54-2.07	1.10	0.53-2.03
56 Traffic supervisors	7	1.34	0.54-2.75	1.29	0.52-2.65
58 Postal services/couriers	6	0.96	0.35-2.10	0.95	0.35-2.08
6/7 Industrial and construction work	348	0.94	0.84-1.04	0.94	0.85-1.05
63 Smelting, metal and foundry work	7	0.69	0.28-1.41	0.67	0.27-1.39
65 Machine shop/steelworkers	72	0.96	0.75-1.21	0.95	0.74-1.20
650 Turners, machinists	20	1.25	0.76-1.93	1.23	0.75-1.91
651 Fitter-assemblers etc.	5	0.69	0.22-1.61	0.68	0.22-1.58
652 Machine and motor repairers	15	0.86	0.48-1.41	0.85	0.47-1.40
653 Sheetmetalworkers	6	0.86	0.32-1.88	0.85	0.31-1.85
654 Plumbers	11	1.12	0.56-2.01	1.10	0.55-1.97
655 Welders and flame cutters	5	0.64	0.21-1.48	0.62	0.20-1.46
659 Machine shop/steelworkers NOS	9	1.34	0.61-2.54	1.32	0.60-2.51
66 Electrical work	25	1.11	0.72-1.63	1.08	0.70-1.60
660 Electricians (indoors)	12	0.98	0.50-1.71	0.95	0.49-1.67
67 Woodwork	77	1.06	0.83-1.32	1.04	0.82-1.30
671 Timber workers	6	0.65	0.24-1.41	0.64	0.23-1.39
673 Construction carpenters	53	1.17	0.88-1.54	1.16	0.87-1.51

Occupation	Obs.	Crude		Adjusted		
		SIR	95% CI	SIR	95% CI	
68 Painting and lacquering	12	0.85	0.44-1.48	0.83	0.43-1.45	
680 Painters	11	0.84	0.42-1.51	0.83	0.41-1.48	
69 Construction work NOS	53	0.90	0.68-1.18	0.97	0.72-1.27	
690 Bricklayers and tile setters	6	0.81	0.30-1.76	0.79	0.29-1.73	
693 Concrete/cement shutterers	6	1.21	0.44-2.64	1.19	0.44-2.58	
697 Building hands	19	0.79	0.48-1.24	0.89	0.53-1.39	
698 Roadbuilding hands	11	0.71	0.35-1.26	0.80	0.40-1.44	
70 Printing	2	0.38	0.05-1.37	0.37	0.05-1.35	
72 Food industry	5	0.62	0.20-1.44	0.61	0.20-1.41	
73 Chemical process/paper making	15	1.18	0.66-1.95	1.16	0.65-1.92	
75 Industrial work NOS	5	0.61	0.20-1.41	0.60	0.19-1.39	
77 Machinists	27	0.93	0.62-1.36	0.92	0.61-1.34	
772 Construction machinery operator	7	0.72	0.29-1.49	0.72	0.29-1.48	
773 Operators of stationary engine	9	1.29	0.59-2.45	1.27	0.58-2.41	
78 Dock and warehouse work	22	1.00	0.63-1.52	1.06	0.67-1.61	
780 Dockers	3	0.57	0.12-1.67	0.57	0.12-1.66	
781 Freight handlers	8	2.44	1.05-4.80	2.66	1.15-5.25	*
782 Warehousemen	11	0.82	0.41-1.47	0.89	0.44-1.59	
79 Labourers not classified elsewhere	11	0.89	0.44-1.58	1.01	0.51-1.81	
8 Services	54	1.34	1.00-1.74	1.34	1.01-1.75	*
80 Watchmen, security guards	28	1.58	1.05-2.28	1.61	1.07-2.33	*
801 Policemen	17	2.41	1.41-3.87	2.42	1.41-3.88	*
804 Civilian guards	7	1.33	0.54-2.75	1.42	0.57-2.93	
83 Caretakers and cleaners	19	1.13	0.68-1.76	1.11	0.67-1.74	
830 Caretakers	17	1.13	0.66-1.81	1.11	0.65-1.78	
9 Work not classified elsewhere	13	1.86	0.99-3.19	1.85	0.99-3.17	
90 Military occupations	10	2.29	1.10-4.20	2.28	1.09-4.19	*
901 Non-commissioned officers	7	2.94	1.18-6.06	3.14	1.26-6.48	*
ECONOMICALLY INACTIVE PERSONS	149	1.04	0.88-1.22	1.07	0.90-1.24	

C40. Leukaemia, females

Occupation	Obs.	Crude		Adjusted		
		SIR	95% CI	SIR	95% CI	
WHOLE POPULATION	967	1.03	0.97-1.10	1.04	0.97-1.10	
ECONOMICALLY ACTIVE PERSONS	544	1.00	0.92-1.09	1.00	0.92-1.09	
0 Technical, humanistic, etc. work	80	1.16	0.92-1.44	1.20	0.95-1.49	
026 Biologists	1	31.7	0.80-177	39.6	1.00-220	*
03 Medical work and nursing	36	1.19	0.83-1.65	1.16	0.81-1.61	
032 Nurses	5	0.58	0.19-1.35	0.57	0.19-1.33	
036 Auxiliary nurses	16	1.22	0.70-1.98	1.17	0.67-1.89	
038 Institutional children's nurses	6	3.10	1.14-6.76	2.96	1.09-6.44	*
05 Teaching	18	0.87	0.52-1.37	0.99	0.59-1.56	
051 Subject teachers	3	0.58	0.12-1.71	0.79	0.16-2.30	
052 Primary school teachers	10	1.03	0.49-1.90	1.16	0.56-2.13	
06 Religious professions	4	3.68	1.00-9.41	3.63	0.99-9.29	*
09 Humanistic and social work etc.	8	1.53	0.66-3.01	1.59	0.69-3.14	
1 Administrative and clerical work	65	0.96	0.74-1.22	0.93	0.72-1.18	
12 Clerical work	15	0.97	0.54-1.60	0.92	0.52-1.52	
120 Book-keepers, accountants	9	1.24	0.57-2.35	1.17	0.54-2.23	
13 Stenographers and typists	7	1.14	0.46-2.34	1.11	0.45-2.29	
14/15 Clerical work NOS	41	0.95	0.68-1.29	0.92	0.66-1.25	
144 Office clerks	26	0.91	0.59-1.33	0.87	0.57-1.28	
145 Bank clerks	3	0.58	0.12-1.71	0.58	0.12-1.70	
151 Bid calculators, orders clerks	2	8.92	1.08-32.2	8.77	1.06-31.7	*
2 Sales professions	42	0.79	0.57-1.06	0.75	0.54-1.02	
20 Wholesale and retail dealers	3	0.38	0.08-1.11	0.36	0.07-1.04	
201 Retailers	3	0.38	0.08-1.12	0.36	0.07-1.05	
23 Sales work	39	0.88	0.62-1.20	0.85	0.60-1.16	
231 Shop personnel	36	0.86	0.60-1.19	0.83	0.58-1.15	
3 Farming, forestry and fishing	136	1.09	0.92-1.28	1.10	0.92-1.29	

Appendix Table C

Occupation	Obs.	Crude SIR	95% CI	Adjusted SIR	95% CI
30 Agricultural/forestry management	41	1.26	0.91-1.71	1.28	0.92-1.74
300 Farmers, silviculturists	41	1.30	0.93-1.76	1.32	0.95-1.79
31 Farming, animal husbandry	95	1.04	0.84-1.27	1.04	0.84-1.27
310 Agricultural workers	14	1.53	0.83-2.56	1.52	0.83-2.56
312 Livestock workers	80	1.02	0.81-1.27	1.02	0.81-1.27
4 Mining and quarrying	-	-/0.2	0.00-22.4	-/0.2	0.00-22.9
5 Transport and communications	24	1.30	0.83-1.93	1.26	0.81-1.87
57 Post and telecommunications	15	1.54	0.86-2.53	1.45	0.81-2.39
58 Postal services/couriers	8	1.47	0.63-2.89	1.50	0.65-2.96
6/7 Industrial and construction work	86	0.89	0.71-1.10	0.88	0.70-1.09
60 Textiles	8	0.71	0.31-1.40	0.71	0.30-1.39
61 Cutting/sewing etc.	13	0.66	0.35-1.12	0.64	0.34-1.09
616 Garment workers	8	0.72	0.31-1.41	0.70	0.30-1.37
67 Woodwork	6	0.73	0.27-1.60	0.73	0.27-1.59
674 Boatbuilders etc.	1	44.5	1.13-248	44.0	1.11-245 *
72 Food industry	10	0.86	0.41-1.59	0.85	0.41-1.57
721 Bakers and pastry chiefs	3	0.56	0.12-1.65	0.56	0.11-1.63
75 Industrial work NOS	9	1.55	0.71-2.95	1.53	0.70-2.90
76 Packing and labelling	18	2.00	1.18-3.15	1.97	1.17-3.12 *
8 Services	111	0.99	0.81-1.18	1.01	0.83-1.21
81 Housekeeping, domestic work, etc.	41	1.06	0.76-1.44	1.09	0.78-1.47
811 Chefs, cooks etc.	15	1.54	0.86-2.55	1.53	0.86-2.52
812 Kitchen assistants	10	0.95	0.45-1.74	1.02	0.49-1.87
813 Domestic servants	7	0.71	0.28-1.46	0.74	0.30-1.52
82 Waiters	9	0.78	0.36-1.48	0.75	0.34-1.43
820 Waiters in restaurants	4	0.75	0.20-1.93	0.72	0.20-1.85
821 Waiters in cafés etc.	5	0.81	0.26-1.88	0.78	0.25-1.81
83 Caretakers and cleaners	49	0.96	0.71-1.26	1.00	0.74-1.32
830 Caretakers	7	1.23	0.49-2.53	1.19	0.48-2.45
831 Cleaners	42	0.93	0.67-1.25	0.98	0.71-1.32
84 Hygiene and beauty services	7	1.33	0.54-2.74	1.27	0.51-2.62
9 Work not classified elsewhere	-	-/1.2	0.00-3.17	-/1.2	0.00-3.11
ECONOMICALLY INACTIVE PERSONS	423	1.08	0.98-1.18	1.09	0.99-1.20

C41. Cancer of all sites, males

Occupation	Obs.	Crude SIR	95% CI	Adjusted SIR	95% CI
WHOLE POPULATION	47178	1.05	1.04-1.06	1.04	1.04-1.05 *
ECONOMICALLY ACTIVE PERSONS	39226	1.00	0.99-1.01	1.00	0.99-1.01
0 Technical, humanistic, etc. work	3099	0.85	0.82-0.88	0.96	0.92-0.99 *
00 Technical professions	325	0.79	0.70-0.88	0.94	0.84-1.04 *
000 Architects	27	1.00	0.66-1.46	1.20	0.79-1.74
001 Civil engineers	74	0.84	0.66-1.05	0.99	0.78-1.24
002 Electrical engineers	43	0.77	0.56-1.04	0.93	0.67-1.25
003 Teletechnical engineers	15	0.68	0.38-1.12	0.80	0.45-1.32
004 Mechanical engineers	96	0.78	0.63-0.95	0.93	0.76-1.14 *
005 Chemotechnical engineers	31	0.80	0.54-1.13	0.95	0.65-1.35
006 Mining engineers	7	0.88	0.36-1.82	1.05	0.42-2.16
007 Engineers NOS	24	0.97	0.62-1.44	1.15	0.74-1.72
008 Surveyors	8	0.32	0.14-0.63	0.38	0.16-0.75 *
01 Technical work	1195	0.90	0.85-0.95	0.97	0.92-1.03 *
010 Civil engineering technicians	470	0.96	0.87-1.04	1.03	0.94-1.13
011 Power technicians	77	0.71	0.56-0.89	0.77	0.61-0.96 *
012 Teletechnicians	49	0.82	0.61-1.09	0.88	0.65-1.17
013 Mechanical technicians	312	0.90	0.80-1.00	0.97	0.87-1.08
014 Chemotechnicians	27	0.82	0.54-1.19	0.89	0.58-1.29
015 Mining technicians	15	1.19	0.66-1.96	1.28	0.71-2.10
016 Technicians NOS	116	0.85	0.71-1.02	0.92	0.76-1.10
017 Cartographers	26	0.82	0.53-1.20	0.88	0.58-1.29
018 Draughtsmen, survey assistants	67	0.93	0.72-1.18	1.00	0.78-1.28

Occupation	Obs.	Crude SIR	95% CI	Adjusted SIR	95% CI	
019 Laboratory assistants	36	0.92	0.64-1.27	0.99	0.69-1.37	
02 Chemical/physical/biological work	191	0.82	0.71-0.94	0.94	0.81-1.08	*
020 Chemists	13	0.54	0.29-0.92	0.65	0.34-1.11	*
022 Geologists	4	0.53	0.14-1.36	0.64	0.17-1.64	
025 Veterinary surgeons	15	1.15	0.64-1.89	1.37	0.76-2.25	
027 Consultancy, agriculture	54	0.83	0.62-1.08	0.92	0.69-1.20	
028 Consultancy, forestry	97	0.87	0.71-1.06	1.00	0.81-1.21	
03 Medical work and nursing	132	0.72	0.60-0.85	0.81	0.68-0.96	*
030 Medical doctors	73	0.72	0.57-0.91	0.86	0.67-1.08	*
031 Dentists	12	0.61	0.31-1.06	0.71	0.37-1.24	
035 Psychiatric nurses	19	0.62	0.37-0.97	0.67	0.40-1.05	*
039 Medical workers NOS	22	0.82	0.51-1.24	0.79	0.50-1.20	
04 Health-care related work	61	1.03	0.79-1.32	1.15	0.88-1.48	
040 Pharmacists	27	1.13	0.75-1.65	1.35	0.89-1.97	
041 Physiotherapists	1	0.14	0.00-0.80	0.16	0.00-0.87	*
042 Health inspectors	18	1.03	0.61-1.63	1.12	0.66-1.76	
043 Masseurs, etc.	13	1.27	0.67-2.17	1.35	0.72-2.30	
05 Teaching	587	0.77	0.71-0.83	0.90	0.83-0.98	*
050 University teachers	62	0.90	0.69-1.15	1.06	0.81-1.36	
051 Subject teachers	128	0.87	0.73-1.03	1.04	0.87-1.22	
052 Primary school teachers	191	0.64	0.56-0.74	0.77	0.67-0.89	*
053 Teachers of practical subjects	44	1.03	0.75-1.39	1.19	0.86-1.59	
054 Vocational teachers	134	0.75	0.63-0.88	0.85	0.71-1.00	*
056 Education officers	22	0.90	0.56-1.36	1.03	0.65-1.56	
059 Teaching workers NOS	6	1.11	0.41-2.43	1.26	0.46-2.73	
06 Religious professions	60	0.64	0.49-0.83	0.74	0.56-0.95	*
060 Clergy and lay preachers	55	0.65	0.49-0.85	0.75	0.57-0.98	*
061 Deacons and social workers	5	0.57	0.18-1.32	0.63	0.20-1.46	
07 Legal professions	91	0.82	0.66-1.01	0.97	0.78-1.19	
070 Barristers and judges	17	0.57	0.33-0.90	0.67	0.39-1.08	*
071 Senior police officials	16	0.75	0.43-1.21	0.89	0.51-1.45	
072 Lawyers	27	1.19	0.79-1.74	1.43	0.94-2.08	
073 Solicitors	12	0.55	0.28-0.95	0.65	0.34-1.14	*
079 Juridical workers NOS	19	1.27	0.76-1.98	1.39	0.83-2.16	
08 Artistic and literary professions	253	1.05	0.92-1.18	1.21	1.06-1.36	*
080 Sculptors, painters, etc.	35	1.18	0.82-1.65	1.42	0.99-1.97	
081 Commercial artists	20	1.19	0.73-1.84	1.29	0.79-2.00	
082 Window dressers, etc.	7	1.13	0.45-2.33	1.21	0.49-2.50	
083 Authors	6	0.93	0.34-2.02	1.10	0.40-2.39	
084 Journalists	77	0.97	0.76-1.21	1.14	0.90-1.42	
085 Industrial designers	13	1.25	0.66-2.13	1.44	0.77-2.47	
086 Performing artists	24	1.27	0.81-1.89	1.50	0.96-2.23	
087 Musicians	55	0.92	0.70-1.20	1.05	0.79-1.37	
088 Film and radio producers	13	1.44	0.77-2.46	1.71	0.91-2.92	
089 Art-related workers NOS	3	0.55	0.11-1.61	0.60	0.12-1.75	
09 Humanistic and social work etc.	204	0.88	0.76-1.00	0.99	0.86-1.14	*
090 Auditors	7	0.39	0.16-0.81	0.46	0.19-0.95	*
091 Social workers	51	0.93	0.69-1.22	1.04	0.77-1.36	
092 Librarians, museum officials	20	0.93	0.57-1.44	1.07	0.65-1.65	
093 Community planning professions	10	0.89	0.43-1.64	1.03	0.50-1.90	
094 Systems analysts, programmers	21	1.04	0.64-1.59	1.18	0.73-1.81	
096 PR officers	79	0.92	0.73-1.15	1.04	0.82-1.30	
099 Humanistic/scientific workers N	15	0.84	0.47-1.39	0.97	0.54-1.60	
1 Administrative and clerical work	2236	0.93	0.90-0.97	1.07	1.03-1.12	*
10 Public administration	194	0.85	0.73-0.97	1.01	0.87-1.16	*
11 Corporate administration	1023	0.90	0.85-0.96	1.08	1.02-1.15	*
110 Corporate managers	483	0.92	0.84-1.01	1.11	1.01-1.21	*
111 Technical managers	73	0.73	0.57-0.92	0.88	0.69-1.10	*
112 Commercial managers	247	0.91	0.80-1.03	1.10	0.97-1.24	
113 Administrative managers	44	0.75	0.54-1.00	0.90	0.65-1.20	
114 Managers of ideal organizations	44	0.87	0.63-1.17	1.05	0.76-1.40	
119 Private sector managers NOS	132	1.00	0.83-1.17	1.19	1.00-1.40	
12 Clerical work	107	1.07	0.88-1.28	1.19	0.97-1.42	
120 Book-keepers, accountants	88	1.04	0.83-1.28	1.16	0.93-1.42	
121 Office cashiers	12	1.28	0.66-2.24	1.39	0.72-2.42	
13 Stenographers and typists	16	0.86	0.49-1.40	0.93	0.53-1.51	
130 Private secretaries	13	1.02	0.54-1.74	1.10	0.59-1.88	
131 Typists	3	0.51	0.11-1.50	0.55	0.11-1.62	
14/15 Clerical work NOS	896	0.98	0.92-1.05	1.07	1.00-1.14	
141 Computer operators	5	0.84	0.27-1.97	0.91	0.29-2.12	

Appendix Table C

Occupation	Obs.	Crude SIR	95% CI	Adjusted SIR	95% CI
143 Photocopier operators etc.	12	0.75	0.39-1.31	0.81	0.42-1.41
144 Office clerks	131	0.88	0.74-1.04	0.95	0.80-1.12
145 Bank clerks	46	0.83	0.61-1.11	0.94	0.69-1.25
146 Insurance clerks	24	0.94	0.60-1.39	1.05	0.67-1.56
147 Social insurance clerks	9	0.64	0.29-1.22	0.69	0.32-1.32
149 Shipping agents	51	1.07	0.80-1.41	1.16	0.86-1.53
150 Property managers, warehousemen	469	1.03	0.94-1.12	1.11	1.01-1.22 *
151 Bid calculators, orders clerks	31	1.00	0.68-1.42	1.09	0.74-1.55
159 Clerical workers NOS	114	1.05	0.87-1.25	1.13	0.93-1.35
2 Sales professions	1770	0.95	0.90-0.99	1.00	0.95-1.04 *
20 Wholesale and retail dealers	520	0.96	0.88-1.04	1.04	0.95-1.13
200 Wholesalers	26	1.10	0.72-1.62	1.23	0.81-1.81
201 Retailers	494	0.95	0.87-1.04	1.03	0.94-1.12
21 Real estate, services, securities	123	0.89	0.74-1.05	0.97	0.81-1.15
210 Insurance salesmen	64	0.78	0.60-1.00	0.85	0.65-1.09
211 Real estate/stockbrokers	30	1.42	0.96-2.03	1.54	1.04-2.19 *
212 Advertising sales	25	0.81	0.53-1.20	0.93	0.60-1.37
219 Real estate etc. workers NOS	4	0.72	0.20-1.85	0.78	0.21-2.00
22 Sales representatives	384	1.00	0.90-1.10	1.08	0.97-1.19
220 Commercial travellers, etc.	347	0.98	0.88-1.09	1.06	0.95-1.18
221 Sales agents	37	1.14	0.81-1.58	1.24	0.87-1.71
23 Sales work	743	0.92	0.86-0.99	0.93	0.87-1.00 *
230 Buyers, office sales staff	138	0.92	0.77-1.08	1.00	0.84-1.18
231 Shop personnel	457	0.91	0.83-1.00	0.89	0.81-0.97 *
232 Door-to-door salesmen	68	1.29	1.00-1.63	1.39	1.08-1.76 *
233 Service station attendants	48	0.80	0.59-1.06	0.87	0.64-1.15
239 Sales staff NOS	32	0.81	0.55-1.14	0.80	0.55-1.13
3 Farming, forestry and fishing	10334	0.91	0.89-0.93	0.89	0.87-0.90 *
30 Agricultural/forestry management	8290	0.88	0.86-0.90	0.87	0.85-0.89 *
300 Farmers, silviculturists	7814	0.88	0.86-0.90	0.86	0.85-0.88 *
301 Agricultural managers	38	1.03	0.73-1.41	1.11	0.79-1.53
302 Forestry managers	305	0.92	0.82-1.03	1.00	0.89-1.11
303 Horticultural managers	42	1.08	0.78-1.46	1.18	0.85-1.59
304 Livestock breeders	20	1.06	0.65-1.63	1.03	0.63-1.59
305 Fur-bearing animal breeders	56	1.09	0.83-1.42	1.07	0.81-1.39
306 Reindeer breeders	15	0.77	0.43-1.27	0.75	0.42-1.24
31 Farming, animal husbandry	541	0.94	0.86-1.02	0.86	0.79-0.94 *
310 Agricultural workers	404	0.93	0.84-1.02	0.86	0.78-0.95 *
311 Gardeners	67	0.96	0.74-1.21	0.85	0.66-1.08
312 Livestock workers	52	0.96	0.72-1.26	0.89	0.67-1.17
313 Fur-farm workers	11	1.01	0.51-1.81	0.89	0.45-1.60
314 Reindeer herders	7	1.16	0.47-2.40	1.03	0.41-2.12
33 Fishing	94	0.92	0.75-1.13	0.90	0.72-1.10
330 Fishermen	87	0.89	0.71-1.09	0.86	0.69-1.06
34 Forestry work	1407	1.11	1.05-1.17	0.98	0.93-1.03 *
4 Mining and quarrying	327	1.49	1.34-1.66	1.46	1.31-1.63 *
40 Mining and quarrying	222	1.64	1.44-1.87	1.61	1.41-1.83 *
41 Deep drilling	26	1.26	0.82-1.84	1.24	0.81-1.82
42 Concentration plant work	17	1.09	0.64-1.75	1.06	0.62-1.70
49 Mining and quarrying NOS	62	1.30	1.00-1.67	1.27	0.97-1.62
5 Transport and communications	3666	1.00	0.97-1.03	1.02	0.98-1.05
50 Ship's officers	161	1.02	0.87-1.19	1.13	0.96-1.31
500 Ship's masters and mates	73	1.04	0.82-1.31	1.19	0.93-1.49
501 Ship pilots	30	0.98	0.66-1.40	1.06	0.72-1.52
502 Chief engineers in ships	58	1.02	0.77-1.32	1.10	0.84-1.42
51 Deck and engine-room crew	112	1.14	0.94-1.36	1.11	0.91-1.32
510 Deck crew	71	1.06	0.83-1.34	1.03	0.80-1.30
511 Engine-room crew	41	1.31	0.94-1.77	1.27	0.91-1.73
52 Air traffic	6	0.93	0.34-2.02	1.08	0.40-2.34
53 Engine drivers	146	0.89	0.75-1.04	0.87	0.73-1.01
54 Road transport	2360	1.05	1.01-1.10	1.07	1.03-1.11 *
540 Motor-vehicle and tram drivers	2354	1.06	1.01-1.10	1.07	1.03-1.12 *
541 Draymen	5	0.99	0.32-2.31	0.96	0.31-2.24
55 Transport services	321	0.89	0.79-0.99	0.89	0.79-0.99 *
550 Railway staff	316	0.89	0.79-0.99	0.89	0.79-0.99 *
551 Flight operations officers	4	0.78	0.21-2.01	0.81	0.22-2.07
56 Traffic supervisors	162	0.78	0.67-0.91	0.87	0.74-1.01 *

Occupation	Obs.	Crude		Adjusted	
		SIR	95% CI	SIR	95% CI
560 Port traffic supervisors	27	1.07	0.71-1.56	1.19	0.78-1.73
561 Air traffic supervisors	7	1.02	0.41-2.11	1.20	0.48-2.47
562 Railway traffic supervisors	69	0.67	0.52-0.85	0.74	0.58-0.94 *
563 Road transport supervisors	59	0.82	0.62-1.05	0.92	0.70-1.19
57 Post and telecommunications	85	0.80	0.64-0.99	0.87	0.69-1.07 *
570 Post/telecommunications officials	68	0.82	0.63-1.03	0.89	0.69-1.12
573 Telegraphists	13	0.71	0.38-1.22	0.77	0.41-1.31
58 Postal services/couriers	222	0.93	0.81-1.05	0.91	0.79-1.03
580 Postmen	127	0.87	0.73-1.03	0.84	0.70-1.00 *
581 Caretakers/messengers	95	1.02	0.82-1.24	1.00	0.81-1.23
59 Communication work NOS	91	1.00	0.81-1.23	0.98	0.79-1.20
591 Canal/harbour guards, ferrymen	15	0.88	0.49-1.45	0.86	0.48-1.42
599 Communication workers NOS	68	0.98	0.76-1.24	0.95	0.74-1.21
6/7 Industrial and construction work	15857	1.11	1.10-1.13	1.07	1.06-1.09 *
60 Textiles	135	1.03	0.86-1.21	1.01	0.84-1.18
600 Pre-process yarnworker	7	1.02	0.41-2.10	0.99	0.40-2.05
601 Spinners etc.	17	1.34	0.78-2.14	1.31	0.76-2.10
602 Weavers	10	0.72	0.35-1.33	0.72	0.35-1.33
603 Textile machine setters operato	43	1.03	0.75-1.39	1.01	0.73-1.35
604 Knitters	9	2.34	1.07-4.45	2.31	1.06-4.39 *
605 Textile finishers/dyers	35	0.87	0.61-1.22	0.85	0.59-1.18
609 Textile workers NOS	11	1.08	0.54-1.93	1.06	0.53-1.90
61 Cutting/sewing etc.	131	1.00	0.83-1.17	1.01	0.84-1.19
610 Tailors	41	1.06	0.76-1.43	1.08	0.77-1.46
612 Furriers	14	1.54	0.84-2.59	1.57	0.86-2.63
614 Upholsterers	35	0.82	0.57-1.14	0.83	0.58-1.16
615 Patternmakers and cutters	11	0.75	0.38-1.35	0.73	0.37-1.31
616 Garment workers	14	0.84	0.46-1.42	0.84	0.46-1.41
619 Cutting/sewing workers NOS	11	2.03	1.01-3.63	2.02	1.01-3.62 *
62 Shoes and leather	119	1.07	0.88-1.27	1.08	0.90-1.28
620 Shoemakers and cobblers	43	1.14	0.82-1.53	1.20	0.87-1.62
621 Shoe cutters etc.	16	1.29	0.74-2.10	1.26	0.72-2.05
623 Lasters	11	1.26	0.63-2.25	1.23	0.61-2.19
624 Sole fitters etc.	6	0.75	0.27-1.63	0.73	0.27-1.59
625 Shoemakers NOS	11	0.85	0.43-1.53	0.84	0.42-1.49
626 Saddlers, leather sewers, etc.	29	0.98	0.66-1.41	1.01	0.68-1.45
63 Smelting, metal and foundry work	477	1.20	1.10-1.31	1.18	1.08-1.29 *
630 Smelter furnacemen	68	1.01	0.78-1.28	0.98	0.76-1.25
631 Hardeners, temperers, etc.	10	1.24	0.59-2.27	1.21	0.58-2.22
632 Hot-rollers	22	1.42	0.89-2.15	1.38	0.87-2.09
633 Cold-rollers	6	0.91	0.33-1.98	0.88	0.32-1.92
634 Blacksmiths	151	1.44	1.22-1.68	1.46	1.23-1.70 *
635 Founders	130	1.14	0.95-1.34	1.11	0.93-1.31
636 Wire and tube drawers	18	1.40	0.83-2.21	1.36	0.81-2.15
639 Metalworkers NOS	72	1.07	0.84-1.35	1.05	0.82-1.32
64 Precision mechanical work	136	0.88	0.74-1.03	0.89	0.75-1.05
640 Precision mechanics	49	1.06	0.78-1.40	1.03	0.76-1.37
641 Watchmakers	29	0.73	0.49-1.05	0.77	0.51-1.10
642 Opticians	6	0.67	0.25-1.46	0.69	0.25-1.50
643 Dental technicians	14	0.75	0.41-1.25	0.78	0.43-1.31
644 Goldsmiths, silversmiths etc.	35	0.96	0.67-1.34	0.98	0.68-1.36
65 Machine shop/steelworkers	3095	1.11	1.07-1.14	1.08	1.05-1.12 *
650 Turners, machinists	614	0.99	0.91-1.07	0.97	0.89-1.05
651 Fitter-assemblers etc.	277	1.03	0.91-1.15	1.00	0.89-1.12
652 Machine and motor repairers	676	1.04	0.96-1.12	1.03	0.95-1.10
653 Sheetmetalworkers	325	1.26	1.13-1.40	1.24	1.11-1.38 *
654 Plumbers	459	1.27	1.15-1.37	1.24	1.13-1.36 *
655 Welders and flame cutters	335	1.19	1.07-1.33	1.17	1.04-1.29 *
656 Plate/constructional steel work	80	0.97	0.77-1.21	0.95	0.75-1.18
657 Metal platers and coaters	30	1.74	1.17-2.48	1.70	1.15-2.43 *
659 Machine shop/steelworkers NOS	299	1.16	1.03-1.29	1.13	1.01-1.27 *
66 Electrical work	843	1.00	0.93-1.07	0.98	0.91-1.04
660 Electricians (indoors)	461	1.01	0.92-1.10	0.99	0.90-1.08
661 Electric machine operators	64	1.00	0.77-1.27	0.97	0.75-1.24
662 Electric fitters	17	0.90	0.53-1.45	0.88	0.51-1.41
663 Electronics and telefitters	46	1.01	0.74-1.35	1.01	0.74-1.35
664 Telephone installers and repair	128	1.00	0.84-1.18	0.98	0.81-1.15
665 Linemen	85	1.00	0.80-1.24	0.98	0.78-1.21
666 Electronic equipment assemblers	20	0.78	0.48-1.21	0.76	0.47-1.18
669 Electrical workers NOS	22	1.04	0.65-1.57	1.04	0.65-1.57

Occupation	Obs.	Crude SIR	95% CI	Adjusted SIR	95% CI
67 Woodwork	3092	1.07	1.03-1.11	1.05	1.01-1.08 *
670 Round-timber workers	86	1.31	1.05-1.62	1.28	1.03-1.58 *
671 Timber workers	344	0.95	0.85-1.05	0.93	0.84-1.03
672 Plywood makers	120	1.22	1.01-1.44	1.18	0.98-1.40 *
673 Construction carpenters	2028	1.12	1.07-1.17	1.09	1.05-1.14 *
674 Boatbuilders etc.	65	0.95	0.73-1.21	0.95	0.73-1.21
675 Bench carpenters	146	0.87	0.74-1.02	0.88	0.74-1.03
676 Cabinetmakers etc.	106	0.99	0.81-1.19	0.98	0.81-1.18
677 Woodworking machine operators e	150	0.93	0.79-1.08	0.91	0.77-1.06
678 Wooden surface finishers	17	0.92	0.54-1.47	0.89	0.52-1.43
679 Woodworkers NOS	30	0.87	0.59-1.24	0.85	0.57-1.22
68 Painting and lacquering	626	1.16	1.07-1.25	1.15	1.06-1.24 *
680 Painters	589	1.18	1.09-1.28	1.17	1.07-1.26 *
681 Lacquerers	37	0.93	0.65-1.28	0.92	0.65-1.27
69 Construction work NOS	2858	1.24	1.20-1.29	1.13	1.09-1.17 *
690 Bricklayers and tile setters	333	1.14	1.02-1.26	1.11	1.00-1.23 *
691 Reinforced concreters etc.	7	1.07	0.43-2.21	1.05	0.42-2.15
692 Reinforcing iron workers	88	1.25	1.00-1.54	1.21	0.97-1.49
693 Concrete/cement shutterers	225	1.17	1.03-1.33	1.15	1.00-1.30 *
694 Asphalt roofers	36	2.12	1.49-2.94	2.07	1.45-2.86 *
695 Insulators	107	1.88	1.54-2.25	1.85	1.52-2.22 *
696 Glaziers	17	1.25	0.73-2.00	1.24	0.72-1.99
697 Building hands	1172	1.26	1.19-1.33	1.11	1.05-1.17 *
698 Roadbuilding hands	749	1.20	1.11-1.29	1.06	0.99-1.14 *
699 Construction workers NOS	124	1.29	1.07-1.53	1.28	1.07-1.52 *
70 Printing	195	1.02	0.88-1.17	1.00	0.86-1.14
700 Typographers etc.	73	0.97	0.76-1.22	0.95	0.74-1.19
701 Printers	69	1.20	0.93-1.52	1.17	0.91-1.48
702 Lithographers	15	0.86	0.48-1.41	0.83	0.47-1.37
703 Bookbinders	19	0.78	0.47-1.23	0.77	0.46-1.20
709 Printing workers NOS	19	1.12	0.67-1.75	1.13	0.68-1.76
71 Glass and ceramic work	103	1.10	0.90-1.33	1.08	0.88-1.30
710 Glass formers	36	1.22	0.85-1.69	1.19	0.83-1.64
711 Potters	25	0.87	0.57-1.29	0.86	0.55-1.26
712 Kiln operators	13	0.92	0.49-1.57	0.90	0.48-1.53
713 Glass and ceramics decorators	15	2.01	1.13-3.32	1.97	1.10-3.24 *
719 Glass/ceramic workers NOS	11	1.04	0.52-1.85	1.02	0.51-1.82
72 Food industry	279	0.91	0.81-1.02	0.90	0.80-1.01
720 Grain millers	44	0.90	0.65-1.20	0.89	0.65-1.20
721 Bakers and pastry chiefs	63	0.88	0.68-1.13	0.89	0.68-1.13
722 Chocolate and confectionery mak	7	0.82	0.33-1.68	0.80	0.32-1.65
723 Brewers and beverage producers	16	1.00	0.57-1.62	0.97	0.56-1.58
724 Food preservation	10	0.77	0.37-1.42	0.76	0.36-1.39
725 Butchers and sausage makers	82	1.02	0.82-1.27	1.00	0.80-1.24
726 Dairy workers	31	0.81	0.55-1.14	0.78	0.53-1.11
728 Sugar processers	13	0.90	0.48-1.54	0.87	0.47-1.49
729 Food-product workers NOS	12	0.91	0.47-1.60	0.89	0.46-1.55
73 Chemical process/paper making	521	1.09	1.00-1.19	1.06	0.97-1.16 *
730 Distillers	8	1.44	0.62-2.84	1.40	0.60-2.76
731 Cookers (chemical processes)	33	1.06	0.73-1.49	1.03	0.71-1.45
732 Crushers and calender operators	14	1.31	0.72-2.20	1.28	0.70-2.14
733 Wood grinders	36	1.09	0.76-1.51	1.06	0.74-1.47
734 Pulp mill workers	148	1.13	0.95-1.32	1.10	0.93-1.28
735 Paper and board mill workers	180	1.01	0.86-1.16	0.98	0.84-1.13
739 Chemical process workers NOS	102	1.18	0.96-1.42	1.15	0.94-1.38
74 Tobacco industry	10	2.01	0.96-3.70	1.96	0.94-3.60
75 Industrial work NOS	307	0.98	0.87-1.09	0.97	0.86-1.08
750 Basket and brush makers	23	1.39	0.88-2.09	1.48	0.94-2.23
751 Industrial rubber products	53	1.10	0.82-1.44	1.07	0.80-1.40
752 Plastics	62	1.07	0.82-1.37	1.05	0.80-1.34
753 Tanners and pelt dressers	12	0.54	0.28-0.94	0.53	0.27-0.92 *
755 Musical instrument makers etc.	8	1.33	0.57-2.61	1.33	0.57-2.62
756 Stone cutters	44	1.19	0.86-1.60	1.19	0.87-1.60
757 Paper products	23	0.77	0.49-1.15	0.75	0.47-1.12
758 Cast concrete products	43	1.00	0.72-1.35	0.98	0.71-1.32
759 Industrial workers NOS	38	0.81	0.57-1.11	0.80	0.57-1.10
76 Packing and labelling	140	1.11	0.93-1.30	1.08	0.91-1.27
77 Machinists	1189	1.11	1.05-1.17	1.09	1.03-1.15 *
770 Crane and hoist operators	84	1.11	0.88-1.37	1.08	0.86-1.33
771 Forklift operators	163	1.07	0.92-1.24	1.04	0.89-1.21
772 Construction machinery operator	405	1.16	1.05-1.28	1.16	1.05-1.27 *

Occupation	Obs.	Crude SIR	95% CI	Adjusted SIR	95% CI	
773 Operators of stationary engine	297	1.09	0.97-1.22	1.07	0.95-1.19	
774 Greasers	94	1.13	0.91-1.38	1.11	0.89-1.35	
775 Industrial personnel, riggers	146	1.05	0.88-1.22	1.02	0.86-1.19	
78 Dock and warehouse work	972	1.14	1.07-1.22	1.04	0.98-1.11	*
780 Dockers	237	1.17	1.02-1.32	1.12	0.98-1.27	*
781 Freight handlers	159	1.26	1.07-1.47	1.12	0.95-1.30	*
782 Warehousemen	574	1.11	1.02-1.20	0.99	0.91-1.08	*
79 Labourers not classified elsewhere	629	1.28	1.18-1.38	1.13	1.05-1.22	*
8 Services	1665	1.05	1.00-1.10	1.05	1.00-1.10	
80 Watchmen, security guards	714	1.03	0.95-1.11	1.05	0.98-1.13	
800 Firemen	53	0.77	0.58-1.01	0.80	0.60-1.04	
801 Policemen	272	0.97	0.86-1.09	1.04	0.92-1.17	
802 Customs/border control	55	0.77	0.58-1.00	0.83	0.63-1.08	*
803 Prison guards	67	1.16	0.90-1.47	1.15	0.89-1.46	
804 Civilian guards	266	1.24	1.10-1.39	1.17	1.04-1.32	*
81 Housekeeping, domestic work, etc.	40	0.95	0.68-1.29	0.98	0.70-1.33	
810 Housekeepers	22	0.94	0.59-1.42	1.02	0.64-1.54	
811 Chefs, cooks etc.	8	1.12	0.48-2.21	1.09	0.47-2.16	
815 Hotel reception clerks	6	1.09	0.40-2.37	1.06	0.39-2.32	
82 Waiters	26	0.85	0.55-1.24	0.90	0.58-1.31	
820 Waiters in restaurants	14	1.08	0.59-1.82	1.12	0.61-1.88	
821 Waiters in cafés etc.	12	0.67	0.35-1.18	0.72	0.37-1.27	
83 Caretakers and cleaners	727	1.09	1.01-1.17	1.06	0.98-1.14	*
830 Caretakers	647	1.08	1.00-1.17	1.05	0.97-1.14	
831 Cleaners	17	1.47	0.85-2.35	1.30	0.76-2.08	
832 Chimney sweeps	56	1.13	0.86-1.47	1.10	0.83-1.43	
839 Caretakers/cleaners NOS	7	0.80	0.32-1.65	0.84	0.34-1.73	
84 Hygiene and beauty services	19	1.38	0.83-2.15	1.45	0.87-2.27	
840 Hairdressers and barbers	14	1.49	0.81-2.50	1.58	0.86-2.65	
85 Laundry and pressing	12	0.85	0.44-1.48	0.87	0.45-1.52	
850 Launderers	12	0.91	0.47-1.60	0.95	0.49-1.65	
86 Sports	4	0.54	0.15-1.39	0.59	0.16-1.50	
87 Photography	24	0.78	0.50-1.17	0.85	0.54-1.26	
88 Undertakers	11	0.89	0.45-1.60	0.85	0.43-1.53	
89 Services NOS	88	1.19	0.95-1.46	1.15	0.92-1.42	
890 Hotel porters	82	1.33	1.06-1.65	1.29	1.03-1.61	*
891 Service workers NOS	6	0.49	0.18-1.06	0.46	0.17-1.01	
9 Work not classified elsewhere	272	1.08	0.95-1.21	1.15	1.01-1.29	*
90 Military occupations	147	0.96	0.81-1.13	1.08	0.92-1.27	
900 Officers etc.	63	0.92	0.71-1.18	1.09	0.84-1.40	
901 Non-commissioned officers	76	0.95	0.75-1.19	1.03	0.81-1.28	
91 Occupation not specified	125	1.25	1.04-1.48	1.23	1.02-1.46	*
ECONOMICALLY INACTIVE PERSONS	7952	1.38	1.35-1.41	1.34	1.31-1.37	*

C42. Cancer of all sites, females

	Obs.	Crude SIR	95% CI	Adjusted SIR	95% CI	
WHOLE POPULATION	46853	1.00	0.99-1.00	1.00	0.99-1.01	
ECONOMICALLY ACTIVE PERSONS	27918	1.00	0.99-1.01	1.00	0.99-1.01	
0 Technical, humanistic, etc. work	4155	1.13	1.10-1.17	1.03	1.00-1.07	*
00 Technical professions	27	1.33	0.88-1.93	1.13	0.75-1.65	
000 Architects	14	1.33	0.73-2.24	1.13	0.62-1.89	
01 Technical work	232	1.29	1.13-1.46	1.17	1.02-1.32	*
016 Technicians NOS	8	1.65	0.71-3.24	1.50	0.65-2.96	
018 Draughtsmen, survey assistants	67	1.32	1.03-1.68	1.21	0.94-1.54	*
019 Laboratory assistants	147	1.27	1.07-1.48	1.15	0.97-1.35	*
02 Chemical/physical/biological work	103	1.46	1.19-1.75	1.29	1.05-1.55	*
020 Chemists	11	1.00	0.50-1.79	0.86	0.43-1.53	
027 Consultancy, agriculture	80	1.53	1.21-1.91	1.37	1.08-1.70	*
03 Medical work and nursing	1758	1.09	1.04-1.14	1.06	1.01-1.11	*
030 Medical doctors	48	1.26	0.93-1.68	1.07	0.79-1.42	
031 Dentists	69	1.19	0.93-1.51	1.00	0.78-1.26	
032 Nurses	609	1.30	1.20-1.41	1.18	1.09-1.28	*

Occupation	Obs.	Crude SIR	95% CI	Adjusted SIR	95% CI
033 Doctor's/dentist's receptionist	39	1.08	0.77-1.48	1.12	0.80-1.53
034 Midwives	67	0.92	0.71-1.16	0.82	0.64-1.04
035 Psychiatric nurses	118	1.06	0.88-1.26	0.96	0.79-1.14
036 Auxiliary nurses	669	0.96	0.89-1.03	1.02	0.95-1.10
037 Technical nursing assistants	19	1.07	0.65-1.68	1.15	0.69-1.79
038 Institutional children's nurses	113	1.08	0.89-1.28	0.98	0.81-1.17
039 Medical workers NOS	7	1.11	0.45-2.29	1.12	0.45-2.30
04 Health-care related work	224	1.05	0.91-1.19	0.91	0.80-1.04
040 Pharmacists	140	1.07	0.90-1.25	0.91	0.77-1.07
041 Physiotherapists	29	1.14	0.76-1.63	1.04	0.70-1.49
042 Health inspectors	4	0.86	0.23-2.21	0.77	0.21-1.98
043 Masseurs, etc.	19	0.98	0.59-1.53	0.89	0.54-1.39
044 Pharmaceutical assistants	31	1.02	0.69-1.45	0.92	0.63-1.31
05 Teaching	1231	1.13	1.07-1.20	0.98	0.92-1.03 *
050 University teachers	29	1.66	1.11-2.38	1.42	0.95-2.04 *
051 Subject teachers	304	1.11	0.99-1.24	0.95	0.85-1.06
052 Primary school teachers	553	1.10	1.01-1.19	0.93	0.86-1.01 *
053 Teachers of practical subjects	162	1.17	1.00-1.36	1.03	0.88-1.20
054 Vocational teachers	112	1.22	1.01-1.46	1.09	0.90-1.30 *
055 Preschool teachers	51	1.11	0.82-1.45	1.00	0.75-1.32
056 Education officers	8	1.52	0.66-3.00	1.36	0.59-2.69
059 Teaching workers NOS	12	1.13	0.58-1.97	0.97	0.50-1.70
06 Religious professions	68	1.19	0.92-1.50	1.06	0.83-1.35
060 Clergy and lay preachers	24	1.18	0.75-1.75	1.04	0.67-1.55
061 Deacons and social workers	44	1.21	0.88-1.63	1.10	0.80-1.47
07 Legal professions	22	1.16	0.73-1.75	0.97	0.61-1.46
073 Solicitors	13	1.01	0.54-1.73	0.84	0.45-1.44
08 Artistic and literary professions	180	1.40	1.20-1.61	1.22	1.05-1.41 *
080 Sculptors, painters, etc.	24	2.46	1.58-3.67	2.09	1.34-3.11 *
081 Commercial artists	8	1.64	0.71-3.23	1.48	0.64-2.92
082 Window dressers, etc.	7	1.13	0.45-2.32	1.05	0.42-2.16
083 Authors	7	1.48	0.59-3.05	1.22	0.49-2.51
084 Journalists	70	1.29	1.00-1.63	1.12	0.88-1.42 *
085 Industrial designers	26	1.64	1.07-2.40	1.42	0.93-2.08 *
086 Performing artists	20	1.47	0.90-2.27	1.28	0.78-1.97
087 Musicians	9	0.97	0.44-1.84	0.84	0.38-1.59
088 Film and radio producers	3	0.65	0.13-1.91	0.57	0.12-1.66
089 Art-related workers NOS	6	1.14	0.42-2.49	1.03	0.38-2.24
09 Humanistic and social work etc.	310	1.12	1.00-1.25	0.98	0.88-1.10 *
090 Auditors	4	0.56	0.15-1.43	0.47	0.13-1.21
091 Social workers	159	1.26	1.07-1.46	1.11	0.94-1.29 *
092 Librarians, museum officials	77	0.93	0.74-1.17	0.81	0.64-1.01
093 Community planning professions	6	1.30	0.48-2.84	1.13	0.41-2.46
094 Systems analysts, programmers	4	0.72	0.20-1.86	0.67	0.18-1.72
095 Psychologists	8	0.94	0.40-1.85	0.82	0.35-1.61
096 PR officers	35	1.36	0.95-1.89	1.20	0.84-1.68
099 Humanistic/scientific workers N	17	1.11	0.65-1.78	0.95	0.56-1.53
1 Administrative and clerical work	4209	1.18	1.14-1.21	1.06	1.03-1.09 *
10 Public administration	87	1.37	1.10-1.69	1.16	0.93-1.43 *
11 Corporate administration	112	1.25	1.03-1.50	1.05	0.86-1.25 *
110 Corporate managers	48	1.38	1.02-1.83	1.14	0.84-1.51 *
112 Commercial managers	5	0.45	0.15-1.06	0.39	0.13-0.90 *
113 Administrative managers	10	1.16	0.56-2.14	0.98	0.47-1.80
114 Managers of ideal organizations	11	1.85	0.92-3.31	1.55	0.77-2.77
119 Private sector managers NOS	32	1.20	0.82-1.70	1.01	0.69-1.43
12 Clerical work	943	1.17	1.09-1.24	1.05	0.98-1.11 *
120 Book-keepers, accountants	428	1.14	1.03-1.25	1.01	0.92-1.11 *
121 Office cashiers	223	1.42	1.24-1.61	1.27	1.11-1.44 *
122 Bank and post office cashiers	64	1.10	0.85-1.41	1.00	0.77-1.28
123 Shop and restaurant cashiers	224	1.07	0.93-1.21	0.96	0.84-1.09
129 Book-keeping workers/cashiers N	4	0.74	0.20-1.89	0.65	0.18-1.68
13 Stenographers and typists	402	1.21	1.10-1.33	1.10	1.00-1.21 *
130 Private secretaries	220	1.20	1.04-1.36	1.09	0.95-1.24 *
131 Typists	182	1.23	1.06-1.42	1.11	0.96-1.28 *
14/15 Clerical work NOS	2665	1.16	1.12-1.21	1.05	1.01-1.09 *
140 Computer book-keepers	11	1.20	0.60-2.14	1.07	0.54-1.92
141 Computer operators	6	0.87	0.32-1.90	0.81	0.30-1.76
142 Data storage assistants	18	0.67	0.40-1.06	0.63	0.37-0.99 *
143 Photocopier operators etc.	60	1.08	0.83-1.39	0.98	0.75-1.26
144 Office clerks	1729	1.14	1.09-1.19	1.03	0.98-1.08 *

Occupation	Obs.	Crude SIR	95% CI	Adjusted SIR	95% CI
145 Bank clerks	315	1.11	0.99-1.24	1.02	0.91-1.13
146 Insurance clerks	93	1.28	1.03-1.56	1.16	0.94-1.42 *
147 Social insurance clerks	32	1.14	0.78-1.60	1.05	0.71-1.48
148 Travel agents	16	1.10	0.63-1.79	1.01	0.58-1.63
149 Shipping agents	11	1.29	0.64-2.30	1.17	0.58-2.09
150 Property managers, warehousemen	85	1.46	1.17-1.81	1.30	1.04-1.60 *
151 Bid calculators, orders clerks	16	1.32	0.76-2.15	1.21	0.69-1.96
159 Clerical workers NOS	273	1.39	1.23-1.56	1.24	1.10-1.39 *
2 Sales professions	2761	0.99	0.96-1.03	1.00	0.97-1.04
20 Wholesale and retail dealers	404	1.03	0.93-1.13	0.91	0.82-1.00
200 Wholesalers	6	2.77	1.02-6.04	2.35	0.86-5.12 *
201 Retailers	398	1.02	0.92-1.12	0.90	0.82-0.99 *
21 Real estate, services, securities	14	0.94	0.51-1.57	0.84	0.46-1.41
212 Advertising sales	10	1.18	0.56-2.17	1.06	0.51-1.95
22 Sales representatives	44	0.99	0.72-1.33	0.89	0.65-1.19
220 Commercial travellers, etc.	38	0.94	0.66-1.29	0.85	0.60-1.16
23 Sales work	2299	0.99	0.95-1.03	1.03	0.98-1.07
230 Buyers, office sales staff	64	1.27	0.98-1.63	1.16	0.89-1.48
231 Shop personnel	2142	0.98	0.93-1.02	1.02	0.98-1.06
232 Door-to-door salesmen	41	1.22	0.87-1.65	1.11	0.79-1.50
233 Service station attendants	7	0.96	0.39-1.98	0.87	0.35-1.80
239 Sales staff NOS	45	1.13	0.82-1.51	1.18	0.86-1.58
3 Farming, forestry and fishing	5166	0.83	0.81-0.86	0.86	0.84-0.89 *
30 Agricultural/forestry management	1385	0.89	0.84-0.94	0.93	0.88-0.98 *
300 Farmers, silviculturists	1349	0.89	0.84-0.94	0.94	0.89-0.99 *
303 Horticultural managers	10	1.21	0.58-2.23	1.09	0.52-2.00
304 Livestock breeders	21	0.72	0.45-1.10	0.76	0.47-1.17
305 Fur-bearing animal breeders	5	0.86	0.28-2.00	0.90	0.29-2.11
31 Farming, animal husbandry	3773	0.82	0.79-0.84	0.84	0.82-0.87 *
310 Agricultural workers	419	0.91	0.83-1.00	0.93	0.84-1.02
311 Gardeners	145	0.87	0.73-1.01	0.93	0.79-1.09
312 Livestock workers	3183	0.80	0.77-0.83	0.83	0.80-0.86 *
313 Fur-farm workers	17	0.93	0.54-1.49	1.00	0.58-1.60
319 Agricultural workers NOS	9	2.21	1.01-4.19	2.37	1.08-4.50 *
33 Fishing	3	0.35	0.07-1.02	0.38	0.08-1.10
330 Fishermen	3	0.39	0.08-1.13	0.42	0.09-1.22
34 Forestry work	5	0.53	0.17-1.23	0.56	0.18-1.32
4 Mining and quarrying	4	0.48	0.13-1.22	0.51	0.14-1.30
5 Transport and communications	1003	1.05	0.99-1.12	1.01	0.94-1.07
54 Road transport	41	1.13	0.81-1.54	1.06	0.76-1.43
540 Motor-vehicle and tram drivers	37	1.07	0.75-1.47	0.99	0.70-1.37
55 Transport services	99	1.16	0.94-1.41	1.24	1.01-1.51 *
550 Railway staff	17	1.45	0.84-2.32	1.52	0.89-2.44
552 Bus/tram services	77	1.09	0.86-1.37	1.18	0.93-1.47
56 Traffic supervisors	59	1.48	1.13-1.91	1.30	0.99-1.68 *
562 Railway traffic supervisors	51	1.45	1.08-1.91	1.27	0.95-1.67 *
57 Post and telecommunications	560	1.10	1.01-1.19	0.98	0.90-1.06 *
570 Post/telecommunications officials	243	1.10	0.97-1.25	0.99	0.87-1.11
571 Telephone operators	192	1.06	0.91-1.21	0.94	0.82-1.08
572 Switchboard operators	97	1.21	0.98-1.47	1.09	0.88-1.33
573 Telegraphists	28	0.95	0.63-1.38	0.85	0.57-1.23
58 Postal services/couriers	242	0.88	0.77-0.99	0.95	0.83-1.07 *
580 Postmen	197	0.82	0.71-0.94	0.88	0.76-1.01 *
581 Caretakers/messengers	45	1.31	0.95-1.75	1.41	1.03-1.88 *
59 Communication work NOS	2	0.36	0.04-1.31	0.39	0.05-1.40
6/7 Industrial and construction work	4953	1.00	0.97-1.02	1.06	1.03-1.09 *
60 Textiles	525	0.92	0.84-1.00	0.97	0.89-1.06 *
600 Pre-process yarnworker	34	1.10	0.76-1.53	1.18	0.82-1.66
601 Spinners etc.	129	1.02	0.85-1.20	1.09	0.91-1.29
602 Weavers	162	0.84	0.72-0.98	0.88	0.75-1.02 *
604 Knitters	70	1.05	0.82-1.32	1.11	0.87-1.41
605 Textile finishers/dyers	51	0.72	0.54-0.95	0.78	0.58-1.03 *
606 Textile quality controllers	30	0.70	0.47-1.00	0.76	0.51-1.08
609 Textile workers NOS	47	1.19	0.87-1.58	1.23	0.90-1.64
61 Cutting/sewing etc.	1094	1.07	1.01-1.14	1.11	1.05-1.18 *
610 Tailors	23	1.05	0.67-1.58	1.07	0.68-1.60

Occupation	Obs.	Crude		Adjusted	
		SIR	95% CI	SIR	95% CI
611 Dressmakers	240	1.17	1.03-1.33	1.10	0.97-1.25 *
612 Furriers	26	1.34	0.88-1.96	1.38	0.90-2.02
613 Milliners	35	0.88	0.62-1.23	0.91	0.63-1.26
614 Upholsterers	24	1.10	0.71-1.64	1.16	0.74-1.72
615 Patternmakers and cutters	103	1.22	1.00-1.47	1.30	1.06-1.56 *
616 Garment workers	598	1.03	0.95-1.12	1.10	1.02-1.19 *
619 Cutting/sewing workers NOS	45	0.94	0.68-1.25	0.99	0.72-1.33
62 Shoes and leather	219	1.17	1.02-1.33	1.24	1.08-1.41 *
620 Shoemakers and cobblers	5	1.04	0.34-2.43	0.96	0.31-2.25
621 Shoe cutters etc.	15	1.04	0.58-1.71	1.12	0.62-1.84
622 Shoe sewers	95	1.33	1.08-1.63	1.43	1.15-1.74 *
623 Lasters	6	1.17	0.43-2.54	1.25	0.46-2.73
624 Sole fitters etc.	7	0.97	0.39-2.00	1.05	0.42-2.15
625 Shoemakers NOS	41	0.91	0.66-1.24	0.98	0.70-1.33
626 Saddlers, leather sewers, etc.	50	1.28	0.95-1.69	1.31	0.98-1.73
63 Smelting, metal and foundry work	36	0.82	0.58-1.14	0.88	0.62-1.22
635 Founders	15	1.10	0.62-1.82	1.19	0.66-1.95
639 Metalworkers NOS	12	0.56	0.29-0.98	0.60	0.31-1.05 *
64 Precision mechanical work	16	0.97	0.56-1.58	1.00	0.57-1.63
644 Goldsmiths, silversmiths etc.	4	0.79	0.22-2.03	0.83	0.23-2.13
65 Machine shop/steelworkers	190	0.99	0.86-1.14	1.06	0.92-1.22
650 Turners, machinists	40	1.01	0.72-1.38	1.09	0.78-1.48
655 Welders and flame cutters	12	1.32	0.68-2.31	1.42	0.73-2.48
657 Metal platers and coaters	17	1.20	0.70-1.92	1.28	0.75-2.06
659 Machine shop/steelworkers NOS	114	0.98	0.80-1.16	1.04	0.86-1.24
66 Electrical work	91	0.91	0.74-1.12	0.97	0.78-1.19
660 Electricians (indoors)	7	1.39	0.56-2.87	1.48	0.60-3.06
664 Telephone installers and repair	7	2.45	0.99-5.05	2.63	1.06-5.42 *
666 Electronic equipment assemblers	69	0.84	0.65-1.06	0.89	0.70-1.13
669 Electrical workers NOS	5	0.71	0.23-1.65	0.72	0.23-1.68
67 Woodwork	375	0.89	0.80-0.98	0.95	0.86-1.05 *
670 Round-timber workers	9	0.82	0.37-1.55	0.87	0.40-1.66
671 Timber workers	65	0.76	0.59-0.97	0.82	0.63-1.05 *
672 Plywood makers	172	0.87	0.75-1.01	0.94	0.80-1.08
676 Cabinetmakers etc.	12	1.01	0.52-1.77	1.07	0.55-1.87
677 Woodworking machine operators e	52	1.01	0.76-1.33	1.09	0.81-1.42
678 Wooden surface finishers	27	1.16	0.77-1.69	1.24	0.82-1.81
679 Woodworkers NOS	33	0.90	0.62-1.27	0.96	0.66-1.35
68 Painting and lacquering	47	0.84	0.62-1.12	0.90	0.66-1.20
680 Painters	29	0.74	0.50-1.07	0.79	0.53-1.14
681 Lacquerers	18	1.08	0.64-1.70	1.14	0.68-1.81
69 Construction work NOS	213	1.08	0.94-1.23	1.16	1.01-1.32 *
697 Building hands	174	1.06	0.91-1.23	1.14	0.98-1.32
698 Roadbuilding hands	25	1.08	0.70-1.59	1.16	0.75-1.71
70 Printing	232	1.23	1.08-1.40	1.32	1.16-1.49 *
700 Typographers etc.	36	1.11	0.78-1.54	1.19	0.83-1.65
701 Printers	44	1.22	0.88-1.63	1.31	0.95-1.75
702 Lithographers	9	1.22	0.56-2.32	1.31	0.60-2.48
703 Bookbinders	115	1.25	1.03-1.49	1.34	1.11-1.60 *
709 Printing workers NOS	28	1.37	0.91-1.98	1.44	0.96-2.08
71 Glass and ceramic work	54	0.70	0.53-0.91	0.75	0.57-0.98 *
710 Glass formers	6	0.37	0.13-0.80	0.40	0.15-0.86 *
711 Potters	15	0.62	0.35-1.02	0.66	0.37-1.10
713 Glass and ceramics decorators	19	1.37	0.83-2.15	1.48	0.89-2.31
719 Glass/ceramic workers NOS	12	0.65	0.34-1.14	0.70	0.36-1.23
72 Food industry	511	0.86	0.79-0.94	0.92	0.84-1.00 *
721 Bakers and pastry chiefs	224	0.83	0.72-0.94	0.88	0.77-1.00 *
722 Chocolate and confectionery mak	41	1.06	0.76-1.44	1.14	0.82-1.55
723 Brewers and beverage producers	25	0.95	0.62-1.41	1.02	0.66-1.51
724 Food preservation	29	0.96	0.64-1.38	1.03	0.69-1.48
725 Butchers and sausage makers	52	0.95	0.71-1.25	1.02	0.76-1.34
726 Dairy workers	100	0.81	0.66-0.98	0.87	0.70-1.04 *
727 Prepared foods	24	0.87	0.56-1.30	0.94	0.60-1.40
728 Sugar processors	2	0.40	0.05-1.46	0.43	0.05-1.57
729 Food-product workers NOS	12	0.79	0.41-1.37	0.84	0.44-1.47
73 Chemical process/paper making	158	0.98	0.83-1.13	1.05	0.89-1.22
734 Pulp mill workers	13	0.94	0.50-1.61	1.01	0.54-1.74
735 Paper and board mill workers	87	0.97	0.78-1.20	1.05	0.84-1.29
739 Chemical process workers NOS	54	1.07	0.80-1.39	1.15	0.86-1.50
74 Tobacco industry	23	1.13	0.72-1.70	1.22	0.77-1.82
740 Preprocess tobacco treatment	6	0.88	0.32-1.91	0.94	0.35-2.06

Occupation	Obs.	Crude		Adjusted	
		SIR	95% CI	SIR	95% CI
742 Cigarette makers	8	1.21	0.52-2.39	1.30	0.56-2.56
75 Industrial work NOS	295	0.98	0.87-1.10	1.04	0.93-1.17
750 Basket and brush makers	14	1.39	0.76-2.34	1.38	0.76-2.32
751 Industrial rubber products	47	0.93	0.68-1.24	1.00	0.73-1.33
752 Plastics	69	1.03	0.80-1.30	1.10	0.85-1.39
753 Tanners and pelt dressers	18	0.80	0.48-1.27	0.86	0.51-1.36
754 Photolab. workers	26	1.24	0.81-1.82	1.29	0.85-1.90
757 Paper products	48	0.86	0.64-1.14	0.93	0.68-1.23
759 Industrial workers NOS	72	1.04	0.81-1.31	1.11	0.87-1.39
76 Packing and labelling	485	1.04	0.95-1.13	1.11	1.01-1.21 *
77 Machinists	117	1.14	0.94-1.36	1.22	1.01-1.46 *
770 Crane and hoist operators	33	1.09	0.75-1.53	1.17	0.81-1.64
771 Forklift operators	8	1.17	0.51-2.31	1.25	0.54-2.46
773 Operators of stationary engine	5	0.91	0.29-2.11	0.97	0.32-2.27
774 Greasers	69	1.17	0.91-1.48	1.25	0.98-1.59
78 Dock and warehouse work	240	1.10	0.97-1.24	1.18	1.03-1.33 *
780 Dockers	28	1.19	0.79-1.73	1.29	0.86-1.86
781 Freight handlers	9	0.88	0.40-1.67	0.91	0.42-1.74
782 Warehousemen	202	1.10	0.95-1.26	1.18	1.02-1.35 *
79 Labourers not classified elsewhere	32	0.75	0.51-1.06	0.81	0.55-1.14
8 Services	5617	0.99	0.96-1.01	1.03	1.00-1.06 *
80 Watchmen, security guards	32	1.69	1.16-2.39	1.72	1.18-2.43 *
804 Civilian guards	17	1.82	1.06-2.92	1.95	1.14-3.13 *
81 Housekeeping, domestic work, etc.	1941	1.00	0.95-1.04	1.03	0.99-1.08
810 Housekeepers	202	1.07	0.93-1.22	0.95	0.82-1.09
811 Chefs, cooks etc.	486	0.99	0.91-1.08	1.06	0.97-1.16
812 Kitchen assistants	540	1.00	0.92-1.09	1.07	0.98-1.16
813 Domestic servants	460	0.94	0.86-1.03	1.01	0.92-1.10
814 Communal home-help services	140	1.04	0.88-1.23	1.04	0.87-1.21
816 Pursers, stewardesses	14	1.54	0.84-2.58	1.43	0.78-2.40
818 Hotel/restaurant manageresses	38	1.21	0.85-1.65	1.07	0.76-1.47
819 Housekeeping workers NOS	55	0.86	0.65-1.12	0.85	0.64-1.11
82 Waiters	649	1.08	1.00-1.16	1.10	1.01-1.18 *
820 Waiters in restaurants	318	1.14	1.02-1.27	1.20	1.07-1.33 *
821 Waiters in cafés etc.	331	1.02	0.91-1.13	1.01	0.90-1.12
83 Caretakers and cleaners	2441	0.95	0.91-0.99	1.02	0.98-1.06 *
830 Caretakers	273	0.92	0.82-1.04	0.99	0.88-1.11
831 Cleaners	2150	0.95	0.91-0.99	1.02	0.98-1.06 *
839 Caretakers/cleaners NOS	18	1.53	0.91-2.43	1.41	0.83-2.23
84 Hygiene and beauty services	323	1.19	1.06-1.32	1.12	1.00-1.24 *
840 Hairdressers and barbers	262	1.22	1.07-1.37	1.12	0.99-1.26 *
841 Beauticians	12	0.86	0.45-1.51	0.81	0.42-1.41
842 Pedicurists	4	0.81	0.22-2.09	0.76	0.21-1.95
843 Sauna attendants etc.	45	1.21	0.88-1.62	1.27	0.92-1.70
85 Laundry and pressing	177	0.77	0.66-0.89	0.81	0.69-0.93 *
850 Launderers	138	0.72	0.61-0.85	0.75	0.63-0.88 *
851 Pressers	38	1.03	0.73-1.41	1.10	0.78-1.52
87 Photography	21	1.30	0.80-1.99	1.16	0.72-1.77
89 Services NOS	28	1.11	0.74-1.61	1.17	0.78-1.70
890 Hotel porters	3	0.54	0.11-1.58	0.58	0.12-1.70
891 Service workers NOS	25	1.27	0.82-1.88	1.34	0.87-1.98
9 Work not classified elsewhere	50	0.85	0.63-1.12	0.91	0.67-1.20
91 Occupation not specified	47	0.82	0.60-1.09	0.88	0.65-1.17
ECONOMICALLY INACTIVE PERSONS	18935	0.99	0.97-1.00	0.99	0.98-1.01